VITAMINS AND HORMONES

VOLUME 46

VITAMINS AND HORMONES
ADVANCES IN RESEARCH AND APPLICATIONS

Editor-in-Chief

G. D. AURBACH

Metabolic Diseases Branch
National Institute of Diabetes and Digestive and Kidney Diseases
National Institutes of Health
Bethesda, Maryland

Editor

DONALD B. MCCORMICK

Department of Biochemistry
Emory University School of Medicine
Atlanta, Georgia

Volume 46

ACADEMIC PRESS, INC. Harcourt Brace Jovanovich, Publishers

San Diego   New York   Boston
London   Sydney   Tokyo   Toronto

Academic Press, Inc.
San Diego, California 92101

United Kingdom Edition published by
ACADEMIC PRESS LIMITED
24-28 Oval Road, London NW1 7DX

QP
801
.V5
A9
1990

71455

Library of Congress Catalog Card Number: 43-10535

ISBN   0-12-709846-1   (alk. paper)

PRINTED IN THE UNITED STATES OF AMERICA
91 92 93 94   9 8 7 6 5 4 3 2 1

Contents

Structure and Regulation of G Protein-Coupled Receptors: The β_2-Adrenergic Receptor as a Model

SHEILA COLLINS, MARTIN J. LOHSE, BRIAN O'DOWD, MARC G. CARON, AND ROBERT J. LEFKOWITZ

Cellular and Molecular Mechanisms in the Regulation and Function of Osteoclasts

T. J. CHAMBERS AND T. J. HALL

Expression and Function of the Calcitonin Gene Products

MONE ZAIDI, BALJIT S. MOONGA, PETER J. R. BEVIS, A. S. M. TOWHIDUL ALAM, STEPHEN LEGON, SUNIL WIMALAWANSA, IAIN MACINTYRE, AND LARS H. BREIMER

Pantothenic Acid in Health and Disease

ARUN G. TAHILIANI AND CATHY J. BEINLICH

Biochemical and Physiological Functions of Pyrroloquinoline Quinone

MINORU AMEYAMA, KAZUNOBU MATSUSHITA, EMIKO SHINAGAWA, AND OSAO ADACHI

Preface

In this volume of *Vitamins and Hormones,* our readers are once again presented with the most timely and up-to-date reviews on topics of current interest.

Recent developments in the field of hormone receptors have centered around the study of adrenergic receptors as molecularly cloned proteins. S. Collins and her co-authors review this area and also provide a highly utilitarian comparison of amino acid sequences for many members of this protein family which is characterized by seven transmembrane-spanning hydrophobic regions.

T. J. Chambers and T. J. Hall present an important analysis of the fast-paced field of osteoclast maturation and function. Osteoclasts are the cells that control bone resorption, and their development and actions are regulated by a panoply of systemic hormones, locally acting cytokines, growth factors, and cell adhesion molecules. This presentation will be of value to investigators in the field as well as to the general reader.

M. Zaidi and his colleagues present a comprehensive description of the expression and function of calcitonin gene products. Expression of these genes is differentially regulated via alternative mRNA splicing between the endocrine and central nervous systems, with calcitonin produced in the thyroid, and CGRP (calcitonin-gene related peptide) type compounds produced in the CNS (CGRP) and pancreas (amylin).

Pantothenic acid is an important vitamin that is a key component of coenzyme A (the cofactor essential for a multitude of active ester reactions). The interwoven biochemistry and physiology of pantothenic acid is discussed by A. G. Tahiliani and C. J. Beinlich. They have developed an impressive treatise on the complex synthetic control and metabolism of this vitamin.

A rapidly changing field is the study of pyrroloquinoline quinones, a class of compounds important in enzymatic dissimilation of methanol, ethanol, and a number of other substrates. M. Ameyama and colleagues provide a new and extensive discourse on these cofactors,

analyzing the clinical and basic nutritional significance of these metabolically important quinones.

We express our gratitude to Academic Press and its staff for their
help in the preparation of this volume.

G. D. AURBACH
DONALD B. MCCORMICK

Structure and Regulation of G Protein-Coupled Receptors: The β₂-Adrenergic Receptor as a Model

SHEILA COLLINS,* MARTIN J. LOHSE,**
BRIAN O'DOWD,† MARC G. CARON,*
AND ROBERT J. LEFKOWITZ*

*The Howard Hughes Medical Institute
Departments of Medicine, Biochemistry, and Cell Biology
Duke University Medical Center
Durham, North Carolina 27710

**Laboratory of Molecular Biology-Gene Center
Max-Planck Institute of Biochemistry
D-8033 Martinsried, Germany

†Department of Pharmacology
University of Toronto
Toronto, Ontario M5S 1A8, Canada

I. Introduction

Over the past few years we have witnessed remarkable advances in our understanding of the molecular basis of transmembrane signaling. One of the major classes of cell surface receptors is coupled to specific intracellular effectors via guanine nucleotide-binding regulatory proteins (G proteins). Based upon the earlier pharmacological development of highly specific, high-affinity radioligands, all of the major catecholamine-related G protein-coupled receptors have now been purified, cloned, and sequenced. From this information, in turn, has come the cloning of discrete receptor "sub"-subtypes, several of which were not previously known to exist. Similarly, there has been a dramatic expansion of the family of G proteins (Birnbaumer, 1990). Multiple

1

forms of G_s have been shown to be generated by alternative splicing, while distinct genes for several unique forms of G_i, as well as novel G proteins coupled to ion channels, have been cloned. In this chapter we outline the major findings concerning the structure and coupling properties of G protein-coupled receptors, and describe what is currently known about the pathways and mechanisms regulating trans-membrane signaling at the receptor level. Much of our present knowledge derives from detailed studies in many laboratories on the structure and regulation of the β_2-adrenergic receptor (β_2AR) in particular.

II. PRIMARY SEQUENCE ANALYSIS OF G PROTEIN-COUPLED RECEPTORS

Since the cloning of the first G protein-coupled receptor (Dixon *et al.*, 1986), this gene family has grown considerably and includes such diverse members as the receptors which bind amine ligands (adrenergic, serotonergic, dopaminergic), muscarinic acetylcholine ligands, peptides (substance P, substance K, angiotensin), glycoprotein hormones [luteinizing hormone/chorionic gonadotropin (CG), follicle-stimulating hormone, thyroid-stimulating hormone] and the visual pigments. Structural similarities among these groups of G protein-coupled receptors are evident from an alignment of the primary sequences of 30 receptors (Fig. 1A and B). Each protein consists of a single polypeptide chain, and hydrophobicity plots suggest that these receptors span the plasma membrane seven times (Fig. 2). This topographical organization is analogous to that demonstrated for bacteriorhodopsin (Dunn *et al.*, 1981). It is also found in other, nonhomologous proteins such as β-hydroxy-β-methylglutaryl (HMG)-CoA reductase (Chin *et al.*, 1984), the mating factor receptors from *Saccharomyces* (Nakayama *et al.*, 1985), halo-opsin (Schobert *et al.*, 1988), and the cannabanoid receptor (Matsuda *et al.*, 1990). The significance of the seven transmembrane motif is not yet clear, but it must be uniquely suited for transmitting a signal from the external surface, via a ligand-induced conformational change in the receptors, to the internal surface of the plasma membrane.

The number of receptors included in this gene family is increasing rapidly. As has been found for the family of DNA-binding nuclear receptors (e.g., steroid receptors), a number of new putative G protein-coupled receptors have been cloned (Libert *et al.*, 1989) by low stringency screening methods. The identities of these "orphan" receptors and their ligands await further study.

A number of highly conserved amino acid residues are found within or near the seven transmembrane segments (TMS). If we limit the comparison to only those receptors that bind protonated amine ligands (i.e., adrenergic, muscarinic, serotonergic, and dopaminergic), we find even greater conservation of sequence. These conserved features are combined and highlighted in the model of the G protein-coupled receptors shown in Fig. 3. Many of these conserved residues are located on the side of the membrane closest to the cytoplasm, perhaps because these residues are for coupling to common cytoplasmic elements (e.g., G proteins). Thirty-two residues are conserved in these types of receptors; 29 of these are found in or near the seven TMS, and 25 of these are again located on the side of the TMS nearest the cytoplasm. Interestingly, only TMS III has a majority of conserved substitutions (including one identical aspartic acid residue, Asp-113 in β_2AR) on the side of the receptor facing the outside of the cell (Fig. 3). On the basis of site-specific mutagenesis experiments, Strader *et al.* (1987a) have proposed that Asp-113 in β_2AR acts as the counter ion for the cationic amine group on the ligand. Thus, while the TMS of these receptors generally show the least degree of similarity on the extracellular side of the receptor in TMS III, only conserved substitutions were permitted in residues surrounding the aspartic acid counter ion. Perhaps these conserved residues in TMS III also constitute part of the ligand binding domain.

The only structural features that vary appreciably among the receptors aligned in Fig. 1 are the sizes of the third cytoplasmic loops and carboxy termini. (In addition, the glycoprotein hormone receptors displayed in Fig. 1B show exceedingly long amino-terminal extensions.) Receptors with longer carboxyl tails tend to have shorter third cytoplasmic loops and vice versa. A possible explanation for this pattern suggests that certain common structural or functional components of these receptors may be found either in the third cytoplasmic loop or carboxy tails. These regions characteristically gain more acidic character with increased distance from the plasma membrane and generally share similar chemical composition. Evidence indicates that several of these receptors can be phosphorylated by various kinases (see Section III,A for more detailed discussion).

One other notable feature common to all of the receptors aligned in Fig. 1 is the presence of at least one proline residue in TMS IV. The adrenergic, dopaminergic, and serotonergic receptors also display a conserved proline residue in TMS II. Each of these prolines could induce an important structural twist in the TMS. From crystallographic studies of bacteriorhodopsin, Henderson and Unwin (1975) suggested that such a twist in the TMS could interlock amino acid side chains from adjacent TMS. For example, three of the TMS in bacteriorhodop-

A

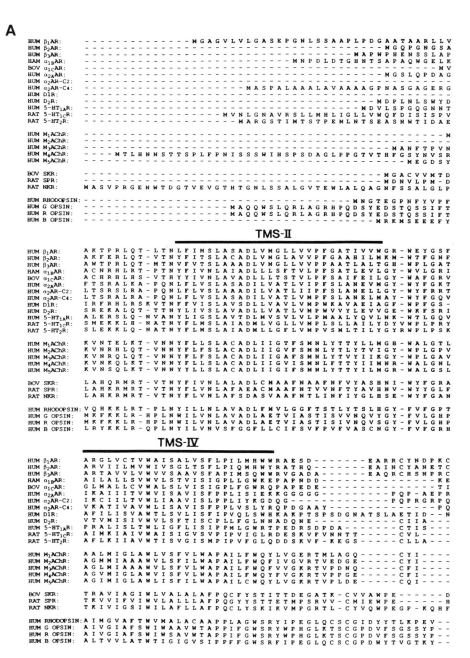

FIG. 1. Alignment of primary sequences for 30 of the G protein coupled-receptors using the single letter amino acid symbols. (A) Twenty-five receptors arranged by families. TMS-I–TMS-VII indicate putative membrane spanning domains. (B) Alignment of the glycoprotein hormone receptors as a separate group highlights their extraordinarily

```
                                              TMS-I
                                            ─────────
P A S P P A S L L P P A S E S P E P L S Q Q W T A G M G L L M A L I V L L I V A G N V L V I V A I   83
F L L A P N R S H A P D H D V T Q Q R D E V W V V G M G I V M S L I V L A I V F G N V L V I T A I   58
W P D L P T L A P N T A N T S G L P G V P W E A A L A G A L L A L A V L A T V G G N L L V I V A I   62
D A N F T G P N Q T S S N S T L P Q L D V T R A I S V G L V L G A F I L F A I V G N I L V I L S V   70
F L S G N A S D S S N C T H P P P P V N I S K A I L L G V I L G G L I L F G V L G N I L V I L S V   51
N A S W N G T E A P G G G A R A T P Y S L Q V T L T L V C L A G L L M L L T V F G N V L V I I A V   58
- - - - - - - - - - - - M D H Q D P Y S V Q A T A A I A A A I T F L I L F T I F G N A L V I L A V   37
S G G V A N A S G A S W G P P R G Q Y S A G A V A G L A A V V G F L I V F T V V G N V L V V I A V   76
- - M R T L N T S A M D G T G L V V E R T L C S Y P H C L F P S L L I L S T L L G N T L V C A A V   47
D D L E R Q N W S R P F N G S D G K A D R P H Y N Y Y A T L L T L L I A V I V F G N V L V C M A V   59
T S P P A P F E T G G N T T G I S D V T V S Y Q V I T S L L L G T L I F C A V L G N A C V V A A I   61
A G I V T D T F N S S D G G R L F Q F P D G V Q N W P A L S I V V I I I M T I G G N I L V I M A V   79
N R T N L S C E G Y L P P T C L S I L H L Q E K N W S A L L T T V V I I L T I A G N I L V I M A V   77

N T S A P P A V S P N I T V L A P G K G P W Q V A F I G I T T G L L S L A T V T G N L L V L I S F   50
- M N N S T N S S N N S L A L T S P Y K T F E V V F I V L V A G S L S L V T I I G N I L V M V S I   48
G S S G N Q S V R L V T S S S H N R Y E T V E M V F I V L V A G S L S L V T V V G N I L V M L S I   57
A A G N F S S P D G T T D D P L G G H T V W Q V V F I A F L T G I L A L V T I I G N I L V I V S F   93
H N A T T V N G T P V N H Q P L E R H R L W E V I T I A A V T A V V S L I T I V G N V L V M I S F   55

I N I S S G L D S N A T G I T A F S M P G W Q L A L W T A A Y L A L V L V A V M G N A T V I W I I   58
S D L F P N I S T N T S E S N Q F V Q P T W Q L L W A A A Y T V I V V T S V V Q G N L I V I W I I   57
A T T Q A P S Q V R A N L T N Q F V Q P S W R I A L W S L A Y G L V V A V A V F G N L I V I W I I   97

S N A T G V V R S P F E Y P Q Y Y L A E P W Q F S M L A A Y M F L L I V L G F P I N F L T L Y V T   62
Y T N S N S T R G P F E F P N Y H I A P R W V Y H L T S V W M I F V V I A S V F T N G L V L A A T   78
Y T N S N S T R G P F E G P N Y H I A P R W V Y H L T S V W M I F V V T A S V F T N G L V L A A T   78
L F K N I S S V G P W D G P Q Y H I A P V W A F Y L Q A A F M G T V F L I G F P L N A M V L V A T   59

                  TMS-III
                ──────────
F C E L W T S V D V L C V T A S I E T L C V I A L D R Y L A I T S P F R Y Q S L L T - R A R   174
W C E F W T S I D V L C V T A S I E T L C V I A V D R Y F A I T S P F K Y Q S L L T - K N K   149
G C E L W T S V D V L C V T A S I A L A V D R Y L A V T N P L R Y G A L V T - K R C   153
F C D I W A A V D V L C C T A S I L S L C A I S I D R Y I G V R Y S L Q Y P T L V T - R R K   161
F C N V W A A V D V L C C T A S I M G L C I I S I D R Y I G V S Y P L R Y P T I V T - Q K R   142
W C E I Y L A L D V L F C T S S I V H L C A I S L D R Y W S I T Q A I E Y N L K R T P - R R   149
W C E V Y L A L D V L F C T S S I V H L C A I S L D R Y W A V S R A L E Y N S K R T P - R R   128
W C G V Y L A L D V L F C T S S I V H L C A I S L D R Y W S V T Q A V E Y N L K R T P - R R   167
F C N I W V A F D I M C T A S I L N L C V I S V D R Y W A I S S P F R Y E R K M T P - K A   139
H C D I F V T L D V M M C T A S I L N L C A I S I D R Y T A V A M P M L Y N T R Y S S K R R   151
T C D L F I A L C C T S S I L H L C A I A L D R Y W A I T D P I D Y V N K R T P - - R   151
L C P V W I S L D V L F S T A S I M H L C A I S L D R Y V A I R N P I E - H S R F N S R T K   171
L C A I W I Y L D V L F S T A S I M H L C A I S L D R Y V A I Q N P I H - H S R F N S R T K   169

A C D L W L A L D Y V A S N A S V M N L L L I S F D R Y F S V T R P L S Y R A K R T P - R R   141
V C D L W L A L D Y V V S N A S V M N L L I I S F D R Y F C V T K P L T Y P V K R T T - K M   139
V C D L W L A L D Y V V S N A S V M N L L I I S F D R Y F C V T K P L T Y P A R R T T - K M   148
A C D L W L A L D Y V A S N A S V M N L L V I S F D R Y F S I T R P L T Y R A K R T T - K R   184
A C D L W L A L D Y V A S N A S V M N L L V I S F D R Y F S I T R P L T Y R A K R T P - K R   146

F C Y F Q N L F P I T A M F V S I Y S M T A I A A D R Y M A I V H P F - - Q P R L S A P - G   147
Y C K F H N F F P I A A L F A S I Y S M T A V A F D R Y M A I I H P L - - Q P R L S A T - A   146
Y C R F Q N F F P I T A V F A S I Y S M T A I A V D R Y M A I I D P L - - K P R L S A T - A   186

G C N L E G F F A T L G G E I A L W S L V V L A I E R Y V V V C K P M S - N F R F G E - N H   152
M C V L E G Y T V S L C G I T G L W S L A I I S W E R W M V V C K P F G - N V R F D A - K L   168
M C V L E G Y T V S L C G I T G L W S L A I I S W E R W L V V C K P F G - N V R F D A - K L   168
V C A L E G F L G T V A G L V T G V S L A F L A F E R Y I V I C K P F G - N F R F S S - K H   149

                  TMS-V
                ─────────
C D F V T N R A Y A I A S S V V S F Y V P L C I M A F V Y L R V F R E A Q K Q V K K I D S C E R R   264
C D F F T N Q A Y A I A S S I V S F Y V P L V I M V F V Y S R V F Q E A K R Q L Q K I D K S E G R   239
C A F A S N M P Y V L L S S V V S F Y L P L L V M L F V Y A R V F V V A T R Q L R L L R G E L G R   244
C G V T E E P F Y A L F S S L G S F Y I P L A V I L V M Y C R V Y I V A K R T T K N L E A G V M K   243
C Q I N E E P G Y V L F S A L G S F Y V P L T I L L V M Y C R V Y V V A K R E S R G L K S G L K T   224
C E I N D Q K W Y V I S S C I G S F F A P C L I M I L V Y V R I Y Q I A K R R T R V P P S R R G P   236
C K L N Q E A W Y I L A S S I G S F F A P C L I M I L V Y L R I Y L I A K R S N R R G P R A K G G   212
C G L N D E T W Y I L S S C I G S F F A P C L I M G L V Y A R I Y R V A K R R T R T L S E K R A P   250
C D S S L S R T Y A I S S S V I S F Y I P V A I M I V T Y T R I Y R I A Q K Q I R R I A A L E R A   234
- - - - - N P A F V V Y S S I V S F Y V P F I V T L L V Y I K I Y I V L R R R R K R V N T K R S S   229
- - - - K D H G Y T I Y S T F G A Y F I P L L L M L V Y G R I F R A A F R V R K T H V R E V K E K   234
- - - - N D P N F V L I G S F V A F F I P L T I M V I T Y F L T I Y V L R R Q T L M L L R G H T E   255
- - - - - D D N F V L I G S F V A F F I P L T I M V I T Y F L T I K S L Q K E A T L C V S D L S T   252

- Q F L S Q P I I T F G T A M A A F Y L P V T V M C T L Y W R I Y R E T E N R A R E L A A L Q G S   228
- Q F F S N A A V T F G T A I A A F Y L P V I I M T V L Y W H I S R A S K S R I K K D K K E P V A   226
- Q F L S N P A V T F G T A I A A F Y L P V I I M T V L Y I H I S L A S R S R I K K D K K E P V A   235
- Q F L S E P T I T F G T A I A A F Y M P V T I M T I L Y W R I Y K E T E K R T K E L A G L Q A S   271
- Q F L S E P T I T F G T A I A A F Y L P V S V M T I L Y C R I Y R E T E K R T K D L A D L Q G S   233

S G G K M L L L Y H L I V I A L I Y F L P L V V M F V A Y S V I G L T L W R R S V P G H Q A - - -   234
P N R T Y E K A Y H I C V T V L I Y F L P L L V I G Y A Y T V V G I T L W A S E I P G D S S - - -   233
T Y H I I V I I L V Y C F P L L M G Y V T I V G I T L W G G E I P G D T C D K Y H E Q L K A -   280

- - - - N N E S F V I Y M F V V H F T I P M I I I F F C Y G Q L V F T V K E A A A Q Q Q - - - - -   238
- - - - G V Q S Y M I V L M V T C C I T P L S I I V L C Y L Q V W L A I R A V A K Q Q K - - - - -   254
- - - - G V Q S Y M I V L M V T C C I T P L A I I M L C Y L Q V W L A I R A V A K Q Q K - - - - -   254
- - - - R S E S Y T W F L F I F C F I V P L S L I C F S Y T Q L L R A L K A V A A Q Q Q - - - - -   235
```

long amino-terminal extensions. TM-I–TM-VII indicate membrane spanning domains. LH, Luteinizing hormone; FSH, follicle-stimulating hormone; TSH, thyroid-stimulating hormone.

5

```
HUM β1AR:      F L G G P A R P P S P S P S P V P A P A P - - - - - - - - - - - - - - - - - - - - - -
HUM β2AR:      F H V Q N L S Q - - - - - - - - - - - - - - - - - - - - - - - - - - - - - - - - - -
HUM β3AR:      F P P E E S - P P A P S R S L A P A P V G - - - - - - - - - - - - - - - - - - - - -
HAM α1BAR:     E M S N S K E L T L R I H S K N - - - - - - - - - - - - - - - - - - - - - - - - - -
BOV α1CAR:     D K S D S E Q V T L R I H R K N - - - - - - - - - - - - - - - - - - - - - - - - - -
HUM α2AR:      D A V A A P P G G T E R R P N G L G P E R S A G P G G A A E A E P L P T Q L N G A P G E P A P A G
HUM α2AR-C2:   P G Q G E S K Q P R P D H G G A L A S A K L P A L A S V A S A R E V N G H S K S T G E K E E G E
HUM α2AR-C4:   V G P D G A S P T T E N G L G A A A G E A R T G T A R P R P P T W S R T R A A Q R P R G G A P G
HUM D1R:       A V H A K N C Q T T T G - - - - - - - - - - - - - - - - - - - - - - - - - - - - - - -
HUM D2R:       R A F R A H L R A P L K G N C T H P E D M K L C T V I M K S N G S F P V N R R R V E A A R R A Q
HUM 5-HT1AR:   T G A D T R H G A S P A P Q P K K S V N G E S G S R N W R L G V E S K A G G A L C A N G A V - -
RAT 5-HT1CR:   E E L A N M S L N F L N C C C K K N G G - - - - - - - - - - - - - - - - - - - - - - - -
RAT 5-HT2R:    R A K L A S F S F L P Q S S L - - - - - - - - - - - - - - - - - - - - - - - - - - - - -

HUM M1AChR:    E T P G K G G G S S S S S E R S Q P G A E G S P E T P P G R C C R C C R A P R L L Q A Y S W K E
HUM M2AChR:    N Q D P V S P S L V Q G R I V K P N N N N M P S S D D G L E H N K I Q N G K A P R D P V T E N C
HUM M3AChR:    E K K A K T L A F L K S P L M K Q S V K K P P P G E A A R E E L R N G K L E E A P P P A L P P P
HUM M4AChR:    G T E A E T E N F V H P T G S S R S C S S Y E L Q Q Q S M K R S N R R K Y G R C H F W F T T K S
HUM M5AChR:    D S V T K A E K R K P A H R A L F R S C L R C P R P T L A Q R E R N Q A S W S S S R R S T S T T

BOV SKR:       - - - - - - - - - - - - - - - - - - - - - - - - - - - - - - - - - - - - - - - - - - -
RAT SPR:       - - - - - - - - - - - - - - - - - - - - - - - - - - - - - - - - - - - - - - - - - - -
RAT NKR:       - - - - - - - - - - - - - - - - - - - - - - - - - - - - - - - - - - - - - - - - - - -

HUM RHODOPSIN: - - - - - - - - - - - - - - - - - - - - - - - - - - - - - - - - - - - - - - - - - - -
HUM G OPSIN:   - - - - - - - - - - - - - - - - - - - - - - - - - - - - - - - - - - - - - - - - - - -
HUM R OPSIN:   - - - - - - - - - - - - - - - - - - - - - - - - - - - - - - - - - - - - - - - - - - -
HUM B OPSIN:   - - - - - - - - - - - - - - - - - - - - - - - - - - - - - - - - - - - - - - - - - - -


HUM β1AR:      - - - - - - - - - - - - - - - - - - - - - - - - - - - - - - - - - - - - - - - - - - -
HUM β2AR:      - - - - - - - - - - - - - - - - - - - - - - - - - - - - - - - - - - - - - - - - - - -
HUM β3AR:      - - - - - - - - - - - - - - - - - - - - - - - - - - - - - - - - - - - - - - - - - - -
HAM α1BAR:     - - - - - - - - - - - - - - - - - - - - - - - - - - - - - - - - - - - - - - - - - - -
BOV α1CAR:     - - - - - - - - - - - - - - - - - - - - - - - - - - - - - - - - - - - - - - - - - - -
HUM α2AR:      - - - - - - - - - - - - - - - - - - - - - - - - - - - - - - - - - - - - - - - - - S S S
HUM α2AR-C2:   - - - - - - - - - - - - - - - - - - - - - - - - - - - - - - Q K E G V C G A S P E D E
HUM α2AR-C4:   - - - - - - - - - - - - - - - - - - - - - - - - - - - - - - - - - - - - - - - - - - -
HUM D1R:       - - - - - - - - - - - - - - - - - - - - - - - - - - - - - - - - - - - - - - - - - - -
HUM D2R:       - - - - - - - - - - - - - - - - - - - - - - - - - - - - - - - - - - - - T R Y S P I
HUM 5-HT1AR:   - - - - - - - - - - - - - - - - - - - - - - - - - - - - - - - - - - - - - - - - - - -
RAT 5-HT1CR:   - - - - - - - - - - - - - - - - - - - - - - - - - - - - - - - - - - - - - - - - - - -
RAT 5-HT2R:    - - - - - - - - - - - - - - - - - - - - - - - - - - - - - - - - - - - - - - - - - - -

HUM M1AChR:    - - - - - - - - - - - - - - - - - - - - - - - - - - - - - - - - - - - - - - - - L T S
HUM M2AChR:    - - - - - - - - - - - - - - - - - - - - - - - - - - - - - - D D E I T Q D E N T V S T S L
HUM M3AChR:    - - - - - - - - - - - - - - - - - - - - - - - - - - - - P A T E L S T T E A T T P A M P A
HUM M4AChR:    L K L P G H S T I L N S T K L P S S D N L Q V P E E E L G M V D L E R K A D K L Q A Q K S V D D
HUM M5AChR:    - - - - - - - - - G K E S P G E E F S A E E T E E T F V K R E T E K S D Y D T P N Y L L S P A A

BOV SKR:       - - - - - - - - - - - - - - - - - - - - - - - - - - - - - - - - - - - - - - - - - - -
RAT SPR:       - - - - - - - - - - - - - - - - - - - - - - - - - - - - - - - - - - - - - - - - - - -
RAT NKR:       - - - - - - - - - - - - - - - - - - - - - - - - - - - - - - - - - - - - - - - - - - -

HUM RHODOPSIN: - - - - - - - - - - - - - - - - - - - - - - - - - - - - - - - - - - - - - - - - - - -
HUM G OPSIN:   - - - - - - - - - - - - - - - - - - - - - - - - - - - - - - - - - - - - - - - - - - -
HUM R OPSIN:   - - - - - - - - - - - - - - - - - - - - - - - - - - - - - - - - - - - - - - - - - - -
HUM B OPSIN:   - - - - - - - - - - - - - - - - - - - - - - - - - - - - - - - - - - - - - - - - - - -
```

TMS-VI

```
HUM β1AR:      A P L A N G R A G K R R P S R L V A L R E Q K A L K T L G I I M G V F T L C W L P F F L A N V V
HUM β2AR:      V E Q D G R T G H G L R R S S K F C L K E H K A L K T L G I I M G T F T L C W L P F F I V N I V
HUM β3AR:      - - - - G V P A C G R R P A R L L P L R E H R A L C T L G L I M G T F T L C W L P F F L A N V L
HAM α1BAR:     K G K H N P R S S I A V K L F K F S R E K K A A K T L G I V V G M F I L C W L P F F I A L P L
BOV α1CAR:     K N K T H - - - - - F S V R L L K F S R E K K A A K T L G I V V G C F V L C W L P F F L V M P I
HUM α2AR:      R G R S A S G L P R R R A G A G G Q N R E K R F T F V L A V V I G V F V V C W F P F F F T Y T L
HUM α2AR-C2:   G R G V G A I G G Q W W R R R A Q L T R E K R F T F V L A V V I G V F V L C W F P F F F S Y S L
HUM α2AR-C4:   L S R R R R A R S S V C R R K V A Q A R E K R F T F V L A V V M G V F V L C W F P F F F I Y S L
HUM D1R:       N G K P V E C S Q P E S S F K M S F K R E T K V L K T L S V I M G V F V C C W L P F F I L N C I
HUM D2R:       N G K T R T S L K T M S R R K L S Q Q K E K K A T Q M L A I V L G V F I I C W L P F F I T H I L
HUM 5-HT1AR:   S F E R K N E R N A E A K R K M A L A R E R K T V K T L G I I M G T F I L C W L P F F I V A L V
RAT 5-HT1CR:   K P R R K K E K R P R G T M Q A I N N E K K A S K V L G I V F F V F L I M W C P F F I T N I
RAT 5-HT2R:    S I H R E P G S Y A G R R T M Q S I S N E Q K A C K V L G I V F F L F V V M W C P F F I T N I M

HUM M1AChR:    G Q K P R G K E Q L A K R K T F S L V K E K K A A R T L S A I L L A F I L T W T P Y N I M V L V
HUM M2AChR:    A R K I V K M T K Q P A K K P P P S R E K K V T R T I L A I L L A F I I T W A P Y N V M V L I
HUM M3AChR:    R K F A S I A R N Q V R K K R Q M A A R E R K V T R T I F A I L L A F I L T W T P Y N V M V L V
HUM M4AChR:    R F A L K T R S Q I T K R K R M S L V K E K K A A Q T L S A I L L A F I L T W T P Y N V M V L V
HUM M5AChR:    G L N P N P S H Q M T K R K R V V L V K E R K A A Q T L S A I L L A F I I T W T P Y N I M V L V

BOV SKR:       - - - - - - - - - - H G A N L R H L Q A K K K F V K T M V L V V V T F A I C W L P Y H L Y F I L
RAT SPR:       - - - - - - - - - - - D R Y H E Q V S A K R K V V K M M I V V V C T F A I C W L P F H V F F L L
RAT NKR:       - - - - - - - - - - K R K V V K M M I I V V V T F A I C W L P Y H V Y F L L

HUM RHODOPSIN: - - - - - - - - - - - E S A T T Q K A E K E V T R M V I I M V I A F L I C W V P Y A S V A F Y
HUM G OPSIN:   - - - - - - - - - - - E S E S T Q K A E K E V T R M V V V M V L A F C F C W G P Y A F F A C F
HUM R OPSIN:   - - - - - - - - - - - E S E S T Q K A E K E V T R M V V V M I F A Y C V C W G P Y T F F A V F
HUM B OPSIN:   - - - - - - - - - - - E S A T T Q K A E R E V S R M V V V M V G S F C V C Y V P Y A A F A M Y
```

FIG. 1A (*Continued*).

```
- - - - - - - - - - - - - - - - - - - - - - - - - - - - - - - - - - - - - - - - - - - - - - -    285
- - - - - - - - - - - - - - - - - - - - - - - - - - - - - - - - - - - - - - - - - - - - - - -    246
- - - - - - - - - - - - - - - - - - - - - - - - - - - - - - - - - - - - - - - - - - - - - - -    264
- - - - - - - - - - - - - - - - - - - - - - - - - - - - - - - - - - - - - - - - - - - - - - -    259
- - - - - - - - - - - - - - - - - - - - - - - - - - - - - - - - - - - - - - - - - - - - - - -    240
P R D T D A L D L E E S - - - - - - - - - - - - - - - - - - - - - - - - - - - - - - - - - - -    296
T P E D T G T R A L P P S W A A L P N S G Q G - - - - - - - - - - - - - - - - - - - - - - - -    283
P L R R G G R R - - - - - - - - - - - - - - - - - - - - - - - - - - - - - - - - - - - - - - -    306
E L E M E M L S S T S P P E R - - - - - - - - - - - - - - - - - - - - - - - - - - - - - - - -    246
                                                                                                292
                                                                                                280
                                                                                                267
                                                                                                267

E E E E D E G S M E S - - - - - - - - - - - - - - - - - - - - - - - - - - - - - - - - - - - -    287
V Q G E E K E S S N D S T S V S A V A S N M R - - - - - - - - - - - - - - - - - - - - - - - -    297
P R P V A D K D T S N E S S S G S A T Q N T K E R - - - - - - - - - - - - - - - - - - - - - -    308
W K P S S E Q M D Q D H S S S D S W N N N D A A A S L E N S A S S D E E D I G S E T R A I Y S I V    368
G K P S Q A T G P S A N W A K A E Q L T T C S S Y P S S E D E D K P A T D P V L Q V V Y K S Q - -    328

- - - - - - - - - - - - - - - - - - - - - - - - - - - - - - - - - - - - - - - - - - - - - - -    234
- - - - - - - - - - - - - - - - - - - - - - - - - - - - - - - - - - - - - - - - - - - - - - -    233
- - - - - - - - - - - - - - - - - - - - - - - - - - - - - - - - - - - - - - - - - - - - - - -    280

- - - - - - - - - - - - - - - - - - - - - - - - - - - - - - - - - - - - - - - - - - - - - - -    238
- - - - - - - - - - - - - - - - - - - - - - - - - - - - - - - - - - - - - - - - - - - - - - -    254
- - - - - - - - - - - - - - - - - - - - - - - - - - - - - - - - - - - - - - - - - - - - - - -    254
- - - - - - - - - - - - - - - - - - - - - - - - - - - - - - - - - - - - - - - - - - - - - - -    235


- - - - - - - - - - - - - - - - - - - - - - - - - - - - - - P P G P P R P A A A A A T    298
- - - - - - - - - - - - - - - - - - - - - - - - - - - - - - - - - - - - - - - - - - - - -    246
- - - - - - - - - - - - - - - - - - - - - - - - - - - - - - - T C A P P E - - - - - - -    270
- - - - - - - - - - - - - - - - - - - - - - - - - - - - - - - - F H E D T L S S T    268
- - - - - - - - - - - - - - - - - - - - - - - - - - - - - - - - A Q V G G S G V T S A    251
D H A E R P P G P R R P E R G P R G K G K A R A S Q V K P G D S L R G A G R G R R G S G R R L Q G    348
A E E E E E E E E E E C E P Q A V P V S P A S A C S P P L Q Q P Q G S R V L A T L R G Q V L L    345
R A G A E G G A G G A D G Q G A G P G A A Q S G A L T A S R S P G P G G R L S R A S S R S V E F F    355
- - - - - - - - - - - - - - - - - - - - - - - - - - - - - - - - - - - - - - - - - - - - -    246
P P S H H Q L T L P D P S H H G L H S T P D S P A K P E K N G H A K D H P L I A K I F E I Q T M P    347
- - - - - - - - R Q G D D G A A L E V I E V H R V G N S K E H L P L P S E A G P T P C A P A    318
- - - - - - - - - - - - - - - - - - - - - - - - - - - - - E E E N A P N P N P D Q    358
- - - - - - - - - - - - - - - - - - - - - - - - - - - - - - - - S S E K L F Q R    275

S E G E E P G S E V V I K M P M V D P E A Q A P T K Q P P R S S P N T V K R P T K K G R D R A G K    339
G H S K D E N S K Q T C I R I G T K T P K S D S C T P T N T T V E V V G S S G Q N G D E K Q N I V    261
P P L Q P R A L N P A S R W S K I Q I V T K Q T G N E C V T A I E I V P A T P A G M R P A A N V A    374
G G S F P K S F S K L P I Q L E S A V D T A K T S D V N S S V G K S T A T L P L S F K E A T L A K    465
A H R P K S Q K C V A Y K F R L V V K A D G N Q E T N N G C H K V K I M P C P F P V A K E P S T K    416

- - - - - - - - - - - - - - - - - - - - - - - - - - - - - - - - - - - - - - - - - - - - - - -    234
- - - - - - - - - - - - - - - - - - - - - - - - - - - - - - - - - - - - - - - - - - - - - - -    233
- - - - - - - - - - - - - - - - - - - - - - - - - - - - - - - - - - - - - - - - - - - - - - -    280

- - - - - - - - - - - - - - - - - - - - - - - - - - - - - - - - - - - - - - - - - - - - - - -    238
- - - - - - - - - - - - - - - - - - - - - - - - - - - - - - - - - - - - - - - - - - - - - - -    254
- - - - - - - - - - - - - - - - - - - - - - - - - - - - - - - - - - - - - - - - - - - - - - -    254
- - - - - - - - - - - - - - - - - - - - - - - - - - - - - - - - - - - - - - - - - - - - - - -    235
```

TMS-VII

```
K A F H R E L - - - - - - - - - - - V P D R L F V F F N W L G Y A N S A F N P I I Y C R S - P D F R    384
H V I Q D N L - - - - - - - - - - - I R K E V Y I L L N W I G Y V N S G F N P L I Y C R S - P D F R    332
R A L G G P S L - - - - - - - - - - K P P D A V F K V V F W L G Y F N S C L N P I I Y P C S S K E F K    352
G S L F S T L - - - - - - - - - - - R P S E T V F K I A F W L G Y L N S C I N P I I Y P C S S Q E F K    356
G S F F P D F - - - - - - - - C S - - V P R T L F K F F F W F G Y C N S S L N P V I Y T I F N Q D F R    334
T A V G - - - - - - - - - - - C S - - V P R T L F K F F F W F G Y C N S S L N P V I Y T I F N Q D F R    434
G A I C P K H - - - - - - - - C K - - V P H G L F Q F F F W I G Y C N S S L N P V I Y T V F N Q D F R    434
Y G I C R E A - - - - - - - - C Q - - V P G P L F K F F F W I G Y C N S S L N P V I Y T V F N Q D F R    444
L P F C G S G E T Q P F - C I - - - D S N T F D V F V W F G W A N S S L N P I I Y A F N - A D F R    338
N I H C D - - - - - - - - C N - - I P P V L Y S A F T W L G Y V N S A V N P I I Y T T F N I E F R    434
L P F C E S S - - - - - - - C H - - M P T L L G A I I N W L G Y S N S L L N P V I Y A Y F N K D F Q    407
S V L C G K A - - - - - - - C N Q K L M E K L L N V F V W I G Y V C S G I N P L V Y T L F N K I Y R    378
A V I C K E S - - - - - - - C N E N V I G A L L N V F V W I G Y L S A V N P L V Y T L F N K T Y R    369

S T F C K D C - - - - - - - - - - V P E T L W E L G Y W L C Y V N S T I N P M C Y A L C N K A F R    426
N T F C A P C - - - - - - - - - - I P N T V W T I G Y W L C Y I N S T I N P A C Y A L C N A T F K    448
N T F C Q S C - - - - - - - - - - I P D T V W S I G Y W L C Y V N S T I N P A C Y A L C N A T F K    461
N T F C D S C - - - - - - - - - - I P K T F W N L G Y V L C Y I N S T V N P V C Y A L C N K T F R    552
S T F C D K C - - - - - - - - - - V P V T L W H L G Y W L C Y V N S T V N P I C Y A L C N R T F R    503

G T F Q E D I Y C H - - - - - - K F I Q Q V Y L A L F W L A M S S T M Y N P I I Y C C L N H R F R    315
P Y I N P D L Y L K - - - - - - K F I Q Q V Y L A S M W L A M S S T M Y N P I I Y C C L N D R F R    313
T A I Y Q Q L N R W - - - - - - K Y I Q Q V Y L A S F W L A M S S T M Y N P I I Y C C L N K R F R    351

I F T H Q G S - - - - - - - - - N F G P I F M T I P A F F A K S A A I Y N P V I Y I M M N K Q F R    314
A A A N P G Y - - - - - - - - - P F H P L M A A L P A F F A K S A T I Y N P V I Y V F M N R Q F R    330
A A A N P G Y - - - - - - - - - A F H P L M A A L P A Y F A K S A T I Y N P V I Y V F M N R Q F R    330
M V N N R N H - - - - - - - - - G L D L R L V T I P S F F S K S A C I Y N P I I Y C F M N K Q F Q    311
```

```
HUM β1AR:    KAFQGLLCCARRAARRRHATHGDRPRASGCLARPGPPPSPGAASDDDDD
HUM β2AR:    IAFQELL-CLRRSSLKAYGNGYSSNGNTGEQSGYHVEQEKENKLLCEDLP
HUM β3AR:    SAFRRLL-CRCGRRLPPEPCAAARPALFPSGVPAARSSPAQPR-LCQRLD
HAM α1BAR:   RAFMRILGCQCRSGRRRRRRRRLGACAYTYRPWTRGGSLERSQSRKDSLD
BOV α1CAR:   RAFQNVLRIQCLRRKQSSKHTLGYTLHAPSHVLEGQHKDLVRIPVGSAET
HUM α2AR:    RAFKKIL-CRGDRKRRIV:-------------------------------
HUM α2AR-C2: RAFRRIL-CRPWTQTAW:--------------------------------
HUM α2AR-C4: PSFKHIL-FRRRRRGFRQ:-------------------------------
HUM D1R:     KAFSTLLGCYRLCPATNNAIETVSINNNGAAMFSSHHEPRGSISKECNLV
HUM D2R:     KAFLKILHC:--------------------------------------
HUM 5-HT1AR: NAFKKIIKCNFCRQ:----------------------------------
RAT 5-HT1cR: RAFSKYLRCDYKPDKKPPVRQIPRVAATALSGRELNVNIYRHTNERVARK
RAT 5-HT2R:  SAFSRYIQCQYKENRKPLQLILVNTIPALAYKSSQLQVGQKKNSQEDAEQ

HUM M1AChR:  DTFRLLLLCRWDKRRWRKIPKRPGSVHRTPSRQC:----------------
HUM M2AChR:  KTFKHLLMCHYKNIGATR:-------------------------------
HUM M3AChR:  KTFRHLLLCQYRNIGTAR:-------------------------------
HUM M4AChR:  TTFKMLLLCQCDKKKRRKQQYQQRQSVIFHKRAPEQAL:-----------
HUM M5AChR:  KTFKMLLLCRWKKKKVEEKLYWQGNSKLP:--------------------

BOV SKR:     SGFRLAFRCCPWVTPTEEDKMELTYTPSLSTRVNRCHTKEIFFMSGDVAP
RAT SPR:     LGFKHAFRCCPFISAGDYEGLEMKSTRYLQTQSSVYKVSRLETTISTVVG
RAT NKR:     AGFKRAFRWCPFIQVSSYDELELKTTRFHPTRQSSLYTVSRMESVTVLFD

HUM RHODOPSIN: NCMLTTICCGKNPLGDDEASATVSKTETSQVAPA:--------------
HUM G OPSIN:   NCILQLFGKKVDDGSELSSASKTEVSSVSSVSPA:--------------
HUM R OPSIN:   NCILQLFGKKVDDGSELSSASKTEVSSVSSVSPA:--------------
HUM B OPSIN:   ACIMKMV-CGKAMTDESDTCSSQKTEVSTVSSTQVGPN:----------


HUM β1AR:    --------------------------------------------------
HUM β2AR:    --------------------------------------------------
HUM β3AR:    --------------------------------------------------
HAM α1BAR:   RRGRLDSGPLFTFKLLGEPESPGTEGDASNGGCDATTDLANGQPGFKSNM
BOV α1CAR:   GPSTPSMGENHQIPTIKIHTISLSENGEEV:-------------------
HUM α2AR:    --------------------------------------------------
HUM α2AR-C2: --------------------------------------------------
HUM α2AR-C4: --------------------------------------------------
HUM D1R:     TVSTQPELADESCHTCSSQKLEEIALGLAIKKLRYGETLRCQESPLLLSN
HUM D2R:     --------------------------------------------------
HUM 5-HT1AR: --------------------------------------------------
RAT 5-HT1cR: --------------------------------------------------
RAT 5-HT2R:  --------------------------------------------------

HUM M1AChR:  --------------------------------------------------
HUM M2AChR:  --------------------------------------------------
HUM M3AChR:  --------------------------------------------------
HUM M4AChR:  --------------------------------------------------
HUM M5AChR:  --------------------------------------------------

BOV SKR:     --------------------------------------------------
RAT SPR:     --------------------------------------------------
RAT NKR:     --------------------------------------------------

HUM RHODOPSIN: ------------------------------------------------
HUM G OPSIN:   ------------------------------------------------
HUM R OPSIN:   ------------------------------------------------
HUM B OPSIN:   ------------------------------------------------
```

FIG. 1A (*Continued*).

sin are more strongly tilted away from the perpendicular axis than the others, lending a left-handed supercoil conformation to that protein (Henderson and Unwin, 1975).

A. Posttranslational Modification of Receptors

1. *Glycosylation*

Covalently attached carbohydrate, particularly at the amino-terminal region, is a characteristic of many of these receptors. Each of the adrenergic receptors contains N-linked complex oligosaccharides (O'Dowd *et al.*, 1989). The hamster β_2AR also contains high mannose-type

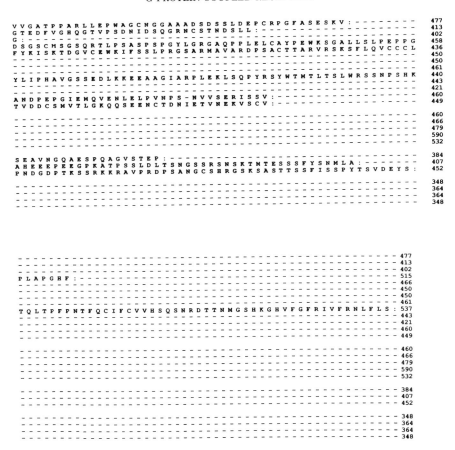

oligosaccharides. For the canine and porcine brain D_2-dopaminergic receptors, complex oligosaccharides have been found (Jarvie and Niznik, 1989), while the D_2-dopaminergic receptor isolated from the anterior pituitary contains hybrid oligosaccharides (Jarvie *et al.*, 1988). Some of the "orphan" receptors recently cloned by polymerase chain reaction (PCR) and referred to earlier display very short NH$_2$-terminal domains devoid of the N-X Ser-Thr glycosylation motif (Libert *et al.*, 1989), suggesting that these receptors are members of a new subclass of nonglycosylated G protein-coupled receptors. An α_2AR isolated from rat cerebral cortex may also represent a nonglycosylated G protein-coupled receptor (Lanier *et al.*, 1988). To date, only the oligosaccharides

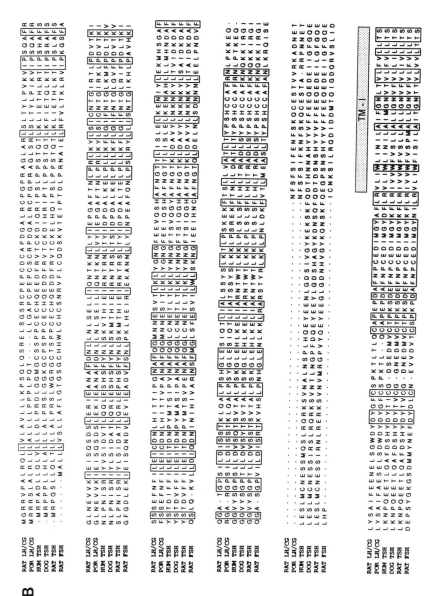

Fig. 1B.

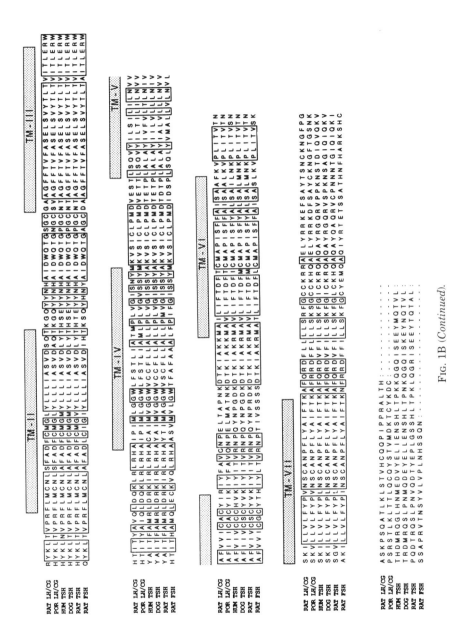

Fig. 1B (Continued).

11

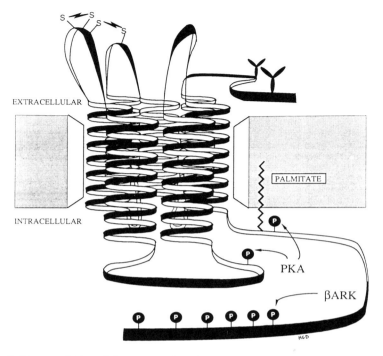

Fig. 2. Representation of the topography of β_2AR in the plasma membrane and post-translational modifications. Extracellular cysteine residues which may be involved in disulphide bond formation, as well as amino-terminal sites of glycosylation and putative sites of phosphorylation by PKA/PKC and βARK. Fatty acylation of a cysteine residue in the carboxyl tail (zigzag line) may anchor the amino-terminal segment of the tail to the plasma membrane.

attached to bovine rhodopsin have been studied by nuclear magnetic resonance (NMR) techniques (Applebury and Hargrave, 1986). The function of N-linked glycosylation in the β_2AR has been studied by site-specific mutagenesis (Dixon *et al.*, 1987). It appears that glycosylation is not required for either ligand binding or functional coupling to G proteins. Glycosylation may, however, play a role in receptor trafficking through the cell as well as regulation (Terman and Insel, 1988).

2. *Palmitoylation*

Earlier reports by O'Brien and colleagues (O'Brien and Zatz, 1984) indicated that rhodopsin was modified by covalent attachment of the fatty acid, palmitic acid. More recently, the two adjacent cysteine residues (Cys-322 and Cys-323) in the carboxyl tail of bovine rhodopsin

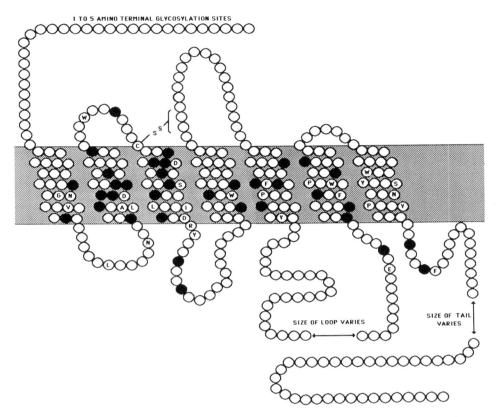

Fig. 3. Distribution of conserved amino acids among the adrenergic, serotonergic, dopaminergic, and muscarinic receptors. Amino acids identical in all receptors are indicated by letters, whereas conserved substitutions are indicated by black circles.

were found to be palmitoylated (Ovchinnikov *et al.*, 1988). In the alignment of amino acid sequences shown in Fig. 1., many of the receptors also contain at least one cysteine in approximately the same position. We reported that the human β_2AR is also palmitoylated, and that mutation of Cys-341 to a Gly results in a nonpalmitoylated form of the receptor (O'Dowd *et al.*, 1989). In a model identical to that proposed for rhodopsin (Ovchinnikov *et al.*, 1988), this posttranslational modification by palmitoylation would promote the association of the amino-terminal portion of the carboxy tail with the plasma membrane, thus forming a fourth intracellular loop (Fig. 2). In this model an agonist- or light-induced conformational change in the receptor might be mediated by release of the fatty acid group, thereby causing detachment of the amino-terminal region of the tail from the membrane. In each of the receptors shown in Fig. 1, the conserved cysteine residue is close to a region of positively charged amino acids. Bach *et al.* (1988) have suggested that such a cluster of positively charged amino acids may define a type of consensus acylation site. Moreover, these positively charged residues would likely promote association of the carboxyl tail with the membrane via electrostatic interactions with the negatively charged phospholipid head groups in the membrane.

A role for palmitoylation of the human β_2AR in receptor–G_s coupling (O'Dowd *et al.*, 1989) has been established. Mutant, nonpalmitoylated β_2AR (Cys-341→Gly) showed a markedly reduced ability to form a guanyl nucleotide-sensitive, high-affinity agonist-binding state characteristic of wild-type receptors, and was also impaired in its ability to activate adenylyl cyclase (O'Dowd *et al.*, 1989). Together with the highly conserved nature of this cysteine residue, from this data one might speculate that palmitoylation represents a general (but not necessarily universal) feature in members of the G protein-coupled receptor family. For other receptors lacking a cysteine residue at the equivalent position in the carboxyl tail, it will be interesting to determine whether they are palmitoylated at cysteine residues located elsewhere in the molecule.

3. *Disulphide Bond Formation in* β_2AR

The presence of several other conserved cysteine residues in the G protein-coupled receptors may indicate the importance of intracellular disulfide bridges. Based on altered ligand binding characteristics of β_2AR mutants lacking either Cys-106 or Cys-184, Dixon *et al.* (1987) suggested the existence of a disulphide bond between the two residues in the native protein (Fig. 2). Residue Cys-106 in β_2AR is conserved in every receptor. It has been estimated (Dohlman *et al.*, 1990) that altogether there are seven pairs of disulphide bonded cysteines in the β_2AR, with at least two of these pairs being essential for normal agonist binding. In a series of β_2AR mutants containing valine (Dohlman *et al.*, 1990) or serine residues (Fraser, 1989) substituted for cysteines, agonist binding was most impaired with loss of the vicinal cysteines 190 and 191. Dohlman *et al.* (1990) found that Cys-106 and Cys-184 were also necessary for proper ligand binding and functional activity.

4. *Phosphorylation*

As rhodopsin is phosphorylated on a series of serines and threonines in the cytoplasmic C-terminus of the protein by a specific retinal enzyme termed rhodopsin kinase, so by analogy is the β_2AR phosphorylated. Serine or threonine residues in the vicinity of acidic amino acids are thought to be susceptible to phosphorylation by an enzyme called β-adrenergic receptor kinase (βARK) (Benovic et al., 1986a). In addition to the β_2AR, the α_2AR (Benovic et al., 1987a), and muscarinic (Kwatra et al., 1989) receptors, as well as rhodopsin itself (Benovic et al., 1986b) can be phosphorylated by βARK in a completely agonist- or light-dependent fashion. Such putative βARK sites, however, appear to be confined to either the middle portion of intracellular loop 3 or the carboxyl tails in any given receptor, but not both (Fig. 2).

Other kinases capable of phosphorylating the β_2AR both in vitro and in vivo include the cAMP-dependent protein kinase (PKA) (see Fig. 2) and protein kinase C (PKC) (Benovic et al., 1988). Phosphorylation of the receptor by PKA and βARK appear to have important functional consequences, as discussed in Section III,B.

B. RECEPTOR COUPLING TO G PROTEINS

Establishing which regions of the receptor determine G protein recognition and coupling specificity has been a major goal of investigations into the structure and function of this receptor family. From a collection of chimeric α_2–β_2-adrenergic receptors, one construct, wherein β_2AR sequences encoding the entire third loop and contiguous sequence from the fifth and sixth TMS were replaced with the analogous region of the platelet α_2AR (Kobilka et al., 1988), was capable of coupling to Gs (albeit at levels below the native β_2AR). Similar functional analyses of chimeric muscarinic receptors have also indicated that regions of the cytoplasmic third loop are involved in the coupling of mAChR I and mAChR II with different G proteins (Kubo et al., 1988). Substitution of β_2AR amino acid residues in the carboxyl-most portion of the third cytoplasmic loop (263–274, 267–274, and 271–274) with sequence from platelet α_2AR produced three mutant β-adrenergic receptors with profound impairment in ability to couple to Gs (O'Dowd et al., 1988) (Fig. 4). Thus, it appears that some of the amino acids that confer G protein specificity reside in this region. Paradoxically, a deletion mutant of the β_2AR lacking simply 11 amino acids, 263–274, showed only a modest reduction in coupling to Gs, whereas a smaller deletion in this region (267–273) showed greater impairment in coupling ability. To understand these results we hypothesized that a realignment of Arg-259–Arg-260 in the 11-amino acid deletion mutant reconstructed an important charge distribution (Fig. 4) which approximated that of the wild type, thereby allowing G_s coupling. An additional series of mutant β_2ARs bearing substitutions of platelet α_2AR sequence, but now in the amino-terminal region of the third cytoplasmic loop, were still capable of efficient coupling to G_s (O'Dowd

β_2AR SPECIES	COUPLING IMPAIRMENT	C-TERMINUS OF INTRACELULAR LOOP III	TMS-VI
		252 267	
WILD TYPE	0%	- - G R T G H G L R R S S K F C L K E [H K] A L K	T - -
D263-273 + S259-260	-100%	- - - - - - - - - - - - - - G R T G H G L G A S S	T - -
D263-273	-15%	- - - - - - - - - - - - - G R T G H G L [R R] S S	T - -
D267-273	-50%	- - - - - - - - - - G R T G H G L [R R] S S K F C L	T - -
S267-274	-75%	- - G R T G H G L R R S S K F C L R E [K R] F T F	V - -
S271-274	-65%	- - G R T G H G L R R S S K F C L K E [H K] F T F	V - -

FIG. 4. Amino acid residues at the carboxy terminus of intracellular loop 3 of β_2AR following various deletion (D) and substitution (S) mutations. Percent coupling impairment refers to the decrease in the maximal level of agonist-induced adenylyl cyclase activity.

et al., 1988). Substitution of two basic residues, 226–228 (A-K-R), in β_2AR (conserved in other receptors aligned in Fig. 1) with the unrelated and uncharged sequence (G-A-G) caused virtually complete abolition of coupling. Thus, it appears that the function of this region of the receptor is to bind common elements in the different G proteins, but not to determine specificity. Further modification of this working hypothesis would seem to be required by the observations of Wong *et al.* (1990). In their study, substitution of a 12-amino acid segment from the amino-terminal portion of the third cytoplasmic loop of the turkey βAR into the mAChR I (coupled to inositol phospholipid metabolism) confers upon this chimera the full ability to stimulate adenylyl cyclase in addition to inositol *tris*-phosphate (IP_3) generation. Evidence for the participation of cytoplasmic loop 2 in G protein selectivity was also discussed in this study. From the sum of these studies, it seems likely that multiple cytoplasmic regions of the receptor will participate in the formation of a three-dimensional surface for G protein interaction. Additional work with several different receptor subtypes will refine these models.

III. Regulation of Receptor-Mediated Transmembrane Signaling

Stimulation of β-adrenergic receptors leads to the generation of an intracellular messenger, cAMP. This simple transmembrane signaling process, however, is subject to a complex set of regulatory phenomena. These regulatory mechanisms can be categorized as follows:

1. *Level of regulation.* Three main levels of regulation have been identified: receptor functionality; localization of receptors within the cells; and regulation of receptor number by variations of synthesis and degradation.

2. *Time frame.* It has become customary to differentiate between rapid effects, complete within a few minutes, and slow effects, that take place over hours.

3. *Inducing agents.* Feedback mechanisms that affect only the response to the inducing agent are generally termed homologous mechanisms. Changes in responsiveness that are caused by other, unrelated agents are termed heterologous.

All but a few regulatory mechanisms cause loss of receptor responsiveness, generally referred to as "densensitization." The only mechanism reported so far that actually increases responsiveness of the system, i.e., leads to sensitization, is an increase in receptor synthesis, which can be brought about by a variety of agents (see Section III,C,2). Desensitization of β-adrenergic receptors as it is observed experimentally, as well as clinically, is characterized by loss of receptor responsiveness to a stimulus of constant intensity. The phenomenon is most readily observed after exposure to β agonists (i.e., the homologous stimulus), but may also be caused by other agents that cause an elevation of intracellular cAMP. It involves a complex set of events that take place at different levels of regulation and over greatly varying periods of time. In the following section the mechanisms regulating receptor responsiveness will be discussed according to the level at which regulation occurs.

A. REGULATION OF RECEPTOR FUNCTIONALITY

The functionality of β-adrenergic receptors corresponds to their capacity to activate the stimulatory guanine nucleotide-binding protein, G_s. This signaling function is subject to strict regulation. During the most rapid (seconds to minutes) phase of homologous and heterologous desensitization, the loss of G_s activation by the receptors has often been referred to as "uncoupling" of receptors, and G_s.

The first suggestion that such uncoupling is due to alterations in the receptors rather than other components of the signaling cascade came from the observation that after desensitization, stimulation of adenylyl cyclase by receptor agonists was more profoundly affected than stimulation of G_s (by treatment with NaF) or adenylyl cyclase itself (by treatment with forskolin). Experimental verification of this hypothesis initially involved the fusion of desensitized membranes with untreated donor membranes that served to report receptor function. In the first of such experiments, Green and Clark (1981) investigated the β-receptor-stimulated adenylyl cyclase activity of membranes from isoproterenol-desensitized S49 *cyc−* cells, a mutant cell line lacking G_s (the α_s subunit is not expressed). After fusion with wild-type S49 cell membranes, which served to supply the G_s necessary for receptor stimulation of adenylyl cyclase activity, they observed a loss of "desensitization" of β-receptor-stimulated adenylyl cyclase. This finding indicated that the β-receptor, rather than G_s, played a crucial role in the desensitization process. More direct evidence for an alteration of the receptor itself was obtained by fusing either desensitized plasma membranes (Kassis and Fishman 1984; Kassis *et al.*, 1986) or partially purified receptors from desensitized membranes (Strulovici *et al.*, 1984) with donor membranes devoid of β-receptors. These studies showed that the β_2-receptors from desensitized cells were reduced in ability to stimulate adenylyl cyclase.

Biochemical evidence for a modification of β-adrenergic receptors during desensitization was first provided by Stadel *et al.* (1982). Desensitized β-receptors (from turkey erythrocytes) visualized by photoaffinity labeling showed an altered electrophoretic mobility as compared with native receptors; this was suggested to be due to a covalent modification. The nature of this modification was elucidated by prelabeling cells with radioactive phosphate before desensitization, and subsequent analysis of the purified receptors from native or desensitized cells. These experiments showed that β-receptor agonist-induced desensitization is paralleled by receptor phosphorylation with 2–3 phosphate groups incorporated per receptor (Stadel *et al.*, 1983a; Sibley *et al.*, 1984, 1985). The kinetics of receptor phosphorylation and functional uncoupling of the receptor were later found similar, suggesting that the two events are closely linked (Sibley *et al.*, 1984, 1985).

Two protein kinases appear to be capable of, and are thought to be responsible for, agonist-induced phosphorylation: cAMP-dependent protein kinase A (PKA), and a novel, receptor-specific kinase, (βARK), (Benovic *et al.*, 1986a, 1987b). PKA phosphorylates purified β_2AR and impairs its signaling function as assessed by reconstitution with purified G_s (Benovic *et al.*, 1985). Inhibition of β-receptor function after phosphorylation by PKA has also been shown using plasma membranes and the catalytic (active) subunit of PKA (Nambi *et al.*, 1985; Kunkel *et al.*, 1989). β_2ARs display two consensus sequences for PKA

(Arg-Arg-Ser-Ser), located in the carboxy-terminus of the third intracellular loop and in the amino-terminus of the cytoplasmic tail. The
site in the third loop appears to be the preferred substrate (Bouvier *et
al.*, 1989; Clark *et al.*, 1989). How phosphorylation of these sites results
in impaired coupling to G_s is presently unknown. Since, however, both
regions carrying phosphorylation sites may be involved in coupling to
G_s (Strader *et al.*, 1987b; O'Dowd *et al.*, 1988), it is conceivable that the
attachment of a phosphate group at these sites directly impairs the
coupling process.

The involvement of PKA in agonist-induced desensitization of β-
receptors is suggested by a variety of experimental data. First, as
previously noted, PKA-mediated phosphorylation impairs β-receptor
function both in membranes and in reconstituted systems with purified components (Nambi *et al.*, 1985; Benovic *et al.*, 1985). Second,
agonist-induced desensitization in whole cells can be partially mimicked by membrane-permeable analogs of cAMP (Sibley *et al.*, 1985).
Third, desensitization by low concentrations of agonist was found to be
deficient in the *kin–* mutant S49 cells which lack PKA activity (Clark
et al., 1988). Fourth, agonist-induced desensitization is deficient in
cells carrying mutated $β_2$-receptors which lack the concensus sites for
PKA-mediated phosphorylation (Hausdorff *et al.*, 1989). And finally, in
permeabilized cells, a peptide inhibitor of PKA (PKI) partially inhibits
agonist-induced desensitization (Lohse *et al.*, 1990a). It is important to
note that most of the studies showing involvement of PKA in the
process of agonist-induced desensitization suggested that this phenomenon is only partially mediated by PKA.

The existence of another kinase that may participate in desensitization was implicated in experiments with the *kin–* variant of S49,
wherein high concentrations of agonists induced not only desensitization of β-adrenergic receptors, but also receptor phosphorylation
(Strasser *et al.*, 1986). This finding led to the discovery, purification,
and eventual cloning of the β-adrenergic receptor kinase (Benovic *et
al.*, 1986a, 1987b, 1989). This novel kinase phosphorylates almost exclusively the agonist-occupied form of receptors, making it an attractive candidate for the highly receptor-specific process of "homologous
desensitization." In addition to $β_2$AR, receptors, the kinase also phosphorylates the agonist-occupied $α_2$-adrenergic and muscarinic receptors as well as light-activated rhodopsin (Benovic *et al.*, 1986b, 1987a;
Kwatra *et al.*, 1989), emphasizing further the similarities in these
receptor systems. The discovery of a βARK-related cDNA clone suggests the possibility of a family of receptor kinases, the specificities of
which remain to be unraveled (Benovic *et al.*, 1989). β-adrenergic re-

ceptor kinase catalyzes phosphorylation of multiple serines and threonines of the β_2AR, with most sites apparently localized in the carboxy-terminal cytoplasmic tail of the receptor (Dohlman et al., 1987). Serine and threonine residues adjacent to acidic residues appear to be favored substrates (Onorato, 1991), but the exact location of these phosphorylation sites is still to be determined.

Several lines of experimental data support the contention that βARK mediates the agonist-specific or homologous pattern of desensitization. First, in a system reconstituted with purified components, βARK-mediated phosphorylation of β_2-receptors reduces receptor function as assessed by ability to activate G_s (Benovic et al., 1987c). Second, agonist-induced desensitization and receptor phosphorylation in cell lines expressing mutant β_2-receptors which lack the putative βARK phosphorylation sites is reduced and delayed. And finally, in permeabilized A431 cells, heparin, a potent inhibitor of βARK, markedly reduces agonist-induced phosphorylation of β_2-receptors and virtually abolishes homologous desensitization (Lohse et al., 1989). Phosphorylation of β_2-receptors by βARK seems, however, insufficient by itself to significantly inhibit receptor function. This became evident when upon purification to homogeneity, βARK showed reduced inhibitory activity in a reconstituted system as compared to results with cruder preparations (Benovic et al., 1987c). This observation is very reminiscent of the situation in the rhodopsin system. Light-dependent phosphorylation of rhodopsin by rhodopsin kinase only modestly inhibits rhodopsin activation of its G protein, transducin. Full inhibition requires an additional retinal protein, called arrestin, which binds to and thereby inactivates phosphorylated rhodopsin (Wilden et al., 1986). The significant parallels between the two systems raised the possibility that a protein analogous to arrestin might serve to inhibit the function of βARK-phosphorylated β-receptors. Indeed, retinal arrestin can markedly enhance the inhibitory effects of βARK-mediated phosphorylation in a reconstituted system (Benovic et al., 1987b). However, the high concentrations of arrestin required, along with the lack of expression of arrestin in most nonretinal tissues, indicate that the observed inhibition cannot be exerted by arrestin itself.

The cDNA for such an arrestin-like protein has indeed been cloned, and the protein has been called β-arrestin (Lohse et al., 1990b). When transiently expressed in COS-7 cells and purified from the cytosol, β-arrestin inhibits the function of β_2ARs, as assessed by receptor stimulation of G_s in a reconstituted system of purified proteins. β-Arrestin shows a clear preference both for βARK-phosphorylated β_2AR over nonphosphorylated receptors, and for β_2AR over rhodopsin. Thus, the current view is that first, βARK phosphorylates agonist-occupied receptors; this modification then promotes the binding of β-arrestin thereby blocking activation of G_s by the receptor.

Studies have been undertaken to define the role of PKA and βARK in different types of desensitization (Hausdorff et al., 1989; Liggett et al., 1989; Lohse et al., 1989, 1990a; Lohse, 1990). From these experiments the following picture emerges: the PKA pathway can be activated by low concentrations of β-receptor agonists as well as a wide variety of other agents that raise intracellular cAMP content. Because of the amplification in most cases between receptor activation and activation of PKA, low concentrations of agonists (e.g., 10 nM isoproterenol) are sufficient for this pathway. Since agonist occupancy only slightly alters PKA-mediated receptor phosphorylation, activated PKA will phosphorylate a wide variety of receptors. Thus, the PKA pathway can be triggered by many types of receptors and will inhibit many types of receptors. This appears to be the basis for at least one heterologous form of desensitization. On the other hand, βARK-mediated phosphorylation requires agonist occupancy of receptors. Since agonist occupancy is complete only at much higher concentrations of agonist than are required for activation of PKA, the βARK pathway requires about 100 times greater concentrations of agonist. Remember, too, that βARK will only phosphorylate those receptors that are agonist occupied, while leaving all other receptors unaffected. This specific pattern appears to be responsible for the homologous, receptor-specific form of desensitization. This need for high agonist concentrations suggests that this mechanism may be operative mainly at synapses, where such high concentrations prevail.

Because stimulation of β_2AR leads to activation of PKA, under physiological circumstances the βARK pathway will never be activated without concomitant activation of the PKA pathway. In other words, a purely homologous pattern of desensitization does not exist in normal cells. An exact assessment of the quantitative role of PKA in desensitization to high concentrations of β-receptor agonists is complicated by the fact that it is very dependent on the assay conditions used to measure desensitization, in particular the Mg^{2+} concentration in the adenylyl cyclase assay (Clark et al., 1987). Overall, it appears that the contribution of βARK to desensitization induced by high agonist concentrations will be at least as large, if not significantly larger, than that of PKA (Hausdorff et al., 1989; Liggett et al., 1989; Lohse et al., 1990a).

B. REGULATION OF RECEPTOR LOCALIZATION

In order to be active, β-receptors must be localized in the plasma membrane, where they are capable of binding extracellular ligands and of activating G_s. Upon exposure to agonists, β-receptors are redistributed to an as yet ill-defined membrane compartment not accessible to agonists and spatially removed from G_s. This membrane compartment is characterized as follows: it is accessible to hydrophobic, but not to hydrophilic ligands such as isoproterenol or the antagonist CGP12177 (Hertel *et al.*, 1983; Toews and Perkins, 1984); agents that permeabilize membranes restore accessibility to hydrophilic ligands (Hertel *et al.*, 1983; Lohse *et al.*, 1990a); it appears lighter on sucrose gradient fractionation of plasma membranes, leading to the designation *light vesicle fraction* (Harden *et al.*, 1980); and receptors in this compartment do not exhibit high-affinity form of agonist binding (Harden *et al.*, 1980). The latter is most likely due to lack of G_s in this membrane compartment (Waldo *et al.*, 1983; Stadel *et al.*, 1983b).

Receptor agonists are the only agents identified so far causing this translocation process, often referred to as *sequestration*. Since sequestration appears to require agonist occupancy of receptors, the concentration–response relationship for these two processes is identical (Toews and Perkins, 1984; Lohse *et al.*, 1990a). The extent and kinetics of β-receptor sequestration vary from cell type to cell type, but usually 30–50% of the total pool of β-receptors are sequestered after 10–20 minute exposure to high agonist concentrations, whereas less than 10% are sequestered under control conditions. Sequestration of β-receptors is somewhat slower than receptor uncoupling or phosphorylation (Waldo *et al.*, 1983). While this indicates a temporal sequence in agonist-induced alterations of β-receptors, there appears to be no causal link. In fact, studies with mutant receptors lacking the phosphorylation sites for βARK and PKA (Strader *et al.*, 1987b; Bouvier *et al.*, 1988; Hausdorff *et al.*, 1989) as well as experiments using inhibitors of these two kinases (Lohse *et al.*, 1990a) show that sequestration proceeds normally even without agonist-induced phosphorylation. Thus, aside from the requirement for agonist occupancy, the signal responsible for triggering sequestration of β-receptors is not clear.

While early studies involving mutant β_2-receptors suggested that regions of the receptor involved in coupling to G_s may be required for sequestration (Strader *et al.*, 1987b), this hypothesis has been questioned by several lines of evidence. First, several mutant receptors have been identified that are impaired in coupling to G_s and yet show a normal pattern of sequestration (Hausdorff *et al.*, 1990; Campbell *et al.*, 1991). Second, early studies by Mahan *et al.*, (1985) showed that G_s is not required for agonist-induced sequestration of β-receptors.

The functional significance of sequestration is also far from clear. Whereas initial studies suggested that it may play a major role in rapid homologous desensitization, this, it is now clear, is not the case. In fact, one can predict that due to a large receptor reserve, in most cells sequestration of 30% of the β-receptors will not markedly affect response (Lohse, 1990). In addition, since agonist-induced phosphorylation of β-receptors precedes sequestration (see previous paragraph) the sequestered receptors will already be functionally uncoupled from G_s. Consequently, experiments examining the effects of manipulations that prevent sequestration have failed to show a contribution of sequestration to desensitization. Only in experimental situations where agonist-induced phosphorylation is prevented will sequestration reduce the signaling capacity of the β-receptor system (Lohse *et al.*, 1990a). An alternative functional role of sequestration was proposed by Sibley *et al.* (1986). They observed that internalized β-receptors show less phosphorylation than those remaining in the plasma membrane. This suggests the possibility that the receptors might be specifically dephosphorylated in the sequestered vesicles, and then be recycled back to the cell surface to regenerate fully functional receptors. The recycling of receptors back to the cell surface occurs relatively rapidly, with a half-life of about 5 minutes (Hertel and Staehelin, 1983).

In summary, although agonist-induced sequestration of β-adrenergic receptors had been observed a decade ago, very little is known about the triggering events, the mechanism and the functional significance of this process.

C. REGULATION OF RECEPTOR NUMBER

1. *Down-Regulation*

Down-regulation is defined as the loss of receptor binding sites in the cell with an accompanying loss in effector stimulation. Whereas uncoupling and sequestration are very rapid processes which take place within seconds to minutes after agonist exposure, down-regulation occurs following more prolonged stimulation (> 1 hour). Despite intense research efforts, the molecular mechanisms underlying down-regulation are poorly understood. Phosphorylation-dependent proteolysis of the receptor is one possibility. In the photoreceptor system, phosphorylation of rhodopsin may facilitate the action of several proteases (Bouvier *et al.*, 1989). Recovery from down-regulation has been shown, in some cases, to require new protein synthesis; in others cases it has not (see reviews in Benovic *et al.*, 1988; O'Dowd *et al.*, 1991). There is evidence (Mahan *et al.*, 1985; Shear *et al.*, 1976; Su *et al.*, 1980) that receptor–G_s coupling alone, in the absence of cAMP generation and the activation of PKA, can promote β_2AR down-regulation. The PKA pathway also appears to contribute to the process of down-regulation (Bouvier *et al.*, 1989; Collins *et al.*, 1989b; Hadcock and Malbon, 1988; Hadcock *et al.*, 1989a). This overlap of pathways is reminiscent of the situation for rapid desensitization, wherein the participation of multiple mechanisms ensures prompt termination of signal transmission. New insight into the process of adrenergic receptor down-regulation has been obtained through the construction and expression of mutant receptors, and the use of the cloned receptor genes as probes for studying receptor gene expression during the course of down-regulation. In this manner, the contributions of receptor–G_s coupling and the role of the PKA pathway are being evaluated at the molecular level.

a. *Agonist-Dependent Pathway.* Several groups (Mahan *et al.*, 1985; Shear *et al.*, 1976; Su *et al.*, 1980) showed that variants of the mouse S49 lymphoma cell series that either lack PKA activity (*kin−*) or display perturbed G_s–effector coupling (H21a) are nevertheless capable of β_2AR down-regulation. However, mutants with abnormal receptor-G_s coupling (*cyc−, unc*) show a blunted (but not blocked) down-regulation of β_2AR. These studies raised the possibility that *physical* (protein–protein) interactions between β_2AR and G_s were more important than the actual *functional* coupling and activation of adenylyl cyclase for triggering receptor down-regulation. While these studies were descriptive in nature, they provided an important foundation for subsequent molecular approaches. Campbell *et al.* (1991) addressed the issue of physical receptor–G_s coupling in down-regulation using a collection of human β_2AR mutants generated by site-directed mutagenesis techniques. These mutant receptors displayed varying degrees of impairment in coupling to G_s. Their ability to undergo agonist-induced down-regulation appeared to reflect their capacities to physically couple to G_s. Since such receptors are consequently incapable of stimulating adenylyl cyclase, it was reasoned that provision of exogenous cAMP (dibutyryl cAMP) and phosphodiesterase inhibitors might correct abnormal down-regulation patterns. No significant increase in the rate or extent of down-regulation was obtained, however, implying that the primary defect was not a lack of PKA activation. Therefore, while the evidence to date supports the notion of a cAMP-independent pathway in βAR down-regulation, the mechanism for this is unknown. Moreover, it is important to note that although mutant receptors in these studies were fully impaired for coupling to G_s, down-regulation response was not completely blocked.

b. Role of Second Messenger Pathways. The study of receptor gene expression during down-regulation has demonstrated that second messengers do, in fact, contribute to the process of down-regulation. Using the hamster smooth muscle cell line DDT_1MF-2, Hadcock and Malbon (1988) and Collins *et al.* (1989b) found that prolonged exposure to either β-adrenergic agonists or cAMP analogs (or agents such as forskolin which directly stimulate adenylyl cyclase) produced a loss of receptor binding sites, accompanied by substantial decreases in $β_2AR$ mRNA levels. These groups, therefore, showed that the second messenger cAMP, in the absence of any contribution from agonist occupancy, was able to promote $β_2AR$ down-regulation. Hadcock and Malbon (1988) observed that while agonist-promoted down-regulation of receptors was quite rapid and actually preceded the decline in mRNA levels, cAMP treatment resulted in a more modest decrease in $β_2AR$ mRNA. Generally in agreement, the studies of Collins *et al.* (1989b) indicated that decreases in $β_2AR$ mRNA, either in response to prolonged agonist or cAMP treatment, tended to precede the loss of receptor number. In addition, treatment with dibutyryl cAMP or forskolin produced an equally effective reduction in $β_2AR$ mRNA levels, although the effect on receptor density was clearly less dramatic. Since the role of agonist activation of the receptor is the stimulation of adenylyl cyclase and the generation of cAMP, the ability of cAMP to mimic the decrease in both receptor mRNA levels and (in part) receptor number, suggests that the PKA pathway is intimately involved in these processes. Yet, in both studies, the observation that agonists produce more rapid, or more effective, receptor down-regulation has been interpreted as further evidence for the apparent role of an agonist-promoted, *cAMP-independent* mechanism in receptor down-regulation, as noted earlier.

A good correlation between activation of the PKA pathway and decreases in $β_2AR$ mRNA levels has been observed for the S49 mouse lymphoma mutants (Hadock *et al.*, 1989a). Agonist or forskolin treatment of wild-type S49 cells reduced $β_2AR$ mRNA levels by 50%, while $β_2AR$ mRNA and receptor down-regulation were both unaffected in *kin−* cells, which lack PKA activity. Receptor mRNA levels in the $β_2AR–G_s$ coupling mutants, *cyc-* and *unc,* were lowered only upon activation of PKA by forskolin. Unexpectedly, the novel mutant *H21a,* (normal receptor–G_s coupling but defective G_s–cyclase coupling), nevertheless generated a more modest (~25%) but significant decrease of β_2AR mRNA, leading the authors to propose that receptor-G_s activation of a PKA-independent pathway, such as calcium and potassium channels (Brown and Birnbaumer, 1990) may also serve to regulate β_2AR mRNA levels. Unfortunately, ligand binding data for *H21a* or other mutants was not presented in this study, in order to correlate receptor density with mRNA levels during down-regulation. Since the study of agonist-induced down-regulation by Campbell also did not measure β_2AR mRNA levels, it is not possible to relate the effects of these coupling mutants to the partial decrease of β_2AR mRNA observed by Malbon and colleagues (Hadcock *et al.*, 1989a) for the *H21a* mutant of S49.

Evidence that posttranscriptional mechanisms regulate adrenergic receptor gene expression has recently appeared (Bouvier *et al.*, 1989; Hadcock *et al.*, 1989b; Oron *et al.*, 1987). Examining the role of cAMP alone in promoting β_2AR down-regulation in greater detail, Bouvier *et al.* (1989) compared wild-type β_2AR with mutated receptors in which one or both consensus sites for PKA phosphorylation were substituted with irrelevant amino acids. Since previous studies of the β_2AR have clearly established the participation of PKA phosphorylation in the process of rapid desensitization it was of interest to know what role, if any, these same phosphorylation sites play in the cAMP-dependent down-regulation of β_2AR.

The functional consequences of these mutations were evaluated in cell lines expressing the receptor under the control of a viral promoter. After exposure to dibutyryl cAMP or forskolin, cAMP-induced phosphorylation of the mutant β_2ARs was completely abolished, but cAMP-induced down-regulation of the receptor was only moderately slowed relative to the wild-type cells. Thus, the initial delay in the rate of down-regulation of the mutant receptor induced by cAMP is most likely due to an alteration in phosphorylation. However, it is clear from these results that although phosphorylation contributes to, it is not the major factor, governing the process of down-regulation. The more significant finding in this study was the dramatic decrease in β_2AR mRNA levels in both wild-type and mutant cells, which preceded the decline in receptor number. Therefore, since down-regulation of β_2AR mRNA in the transfected cells can occur in the *absence* of a promoter, we proposed (Bouvier *et al.*, 1989) that posttranscriptional events must play a role in the regulation of β_2AR expression. Effects on mRNA stability have been demonstrated for a number of cAMP-regulated genes (Hod and Hanson, 1988; Jungmann *et al.*, 1983; Smith and Liu, 1988). For G protein-coupled receptors in particular, down-regulation of the thyrotropin-releasing hormone receptor was accompanied by a rapid decrease in the level of translatable receptor mRNA (Oron *et al.*, 1987), and it was speculated that some form of post-transcriptional control was involved.

Evidence in support of this idea has been presented by Malbon and colleagues (Hadcock *et al.*, 1989b). They detected a decrease in the half-life of the β_2AR mRNA following prolonged agonist exposure of DDT$_1$MF-2 cells. Further studies will reveal whether this is a general mechanism for regulating β_2AR and other G protein-coupled receptors, or occurs only in select cells and physiological conditions. It is tempting to speculate that the 3'-untranslated region (UTR) of the mRNA for the β_2AR, as well as other G_s-coupled receptors, may be the focus of such regulation. Among the receptors cloned to date that are known to couple to stimulation of adenylyl cyclase, several [β_2AR (Kobilka *et al.*, 1987), D_1R (Dearry *et al.*, 1990), LH/CG-R (McFarland *et al.*, 1989), FSH-R (Sprengel *et al.*, 1990), and TSH-R (Akamizu *et al.*, 1990)] contain 3'-UTRs that are rich in AU sequence and other features correlated with highly regulated, short-lived mRNAs (Ross 1988; Shaw and Kamen 1986). In this context it is noteworthy that in their report of the cloning of the rat TSH-R, Akamizu *et al.* (1990) also demonstrated that TSH-R down-regulation was accompanied by a greater than 50% decrease in TSH-R mRNA. This down-regulation of TSH-R mRNA could be mimicked by cAMP analogues or forskolin; essentially identical to what has been previously described for the β_2AR.

A posttranscriptional pattern of regulation may not be confined to the β_2AR or G_s-coupled receptors. In a study of the α1AR (α_{1B} subtype), which is coupled to phosphoinositide turnover and calcium mobilization via PKC, down-regulation of α1ARs in rabbit vascular smooth muscle cells (RSMC) was accompanied by a rapid, but transient, down-regulation of α_{1B} mRNA (Izzo *et al.*, 1990). Up to 80% of the receptor message was lost by 4 hours of treatment with the adrenergic agonist norepinephrine, followed by a gradual return to control levels by 24 hours. Regulation was specific to the α1AR since the decrease in α_{1B} mRNA was blocked by prazosin, an α_1-antagonist, but not by the β-antagonist propranolol. Since exposure of RSMC to phorbol esters or norepinephrine causes rapid uncoupling of the receptor from phosphatidylinositol turnover and CA^{2+} mobilization (Colucci and Alexander, 1986; Cotecchia *et al.*, 1985), it is reasonable to speculate that the second messenger pathways associated with α_1AR activation may participate in the regulation of α_{1B} mRNA. Thus, the transient nature of the effect of norepinephrine on α_{1B} mRNA may be a consequence of this uncoupling event.

2. Up-Regulation and Endocrine Modulation

a. Steroid Hormones. Some of the first studies to address transcriptional control of adrenergic receptors focused upon regulation by steroid hormones, whose major mode of action is the direct modulation of target gene transcription. Early studies demonstrated that glucocorticoids increase β-agonist-stimulated adenylyl cyclase activity and β_2AR number (reviewed in Davies and Lefkowitz, 1984; Collins *et al.*, 1989a). The cloning of the β_2AR made it possible to extend these original observations and directly address the role of regulation of β_2AR gene expression. Increases in β_2AR density and adrenergic responsiveness in DDT_1MF-2 smooth muscle cells treated with glucocorticoid agonists were preceded by a rapid elevation of β_2AR mRNA (Collins *et al.*, 1988). Direct increases in the rate of β_2AR gene transcription were shown to be the mechanistic basis for this increase (Collins *et al.*, 1988). Sequence elements within the 5'-flanking region of the β_2AR gene with > 85% homology to a 15-base-pair (bp) glucocorticoid response element (GRE) consensus sequence (Evans, 1988) may be responsible for this regulation.

In another report, treatment of cells with a combination of β-agonist and dexamethasone demonstrates the dynamic regulation and adaptation of β_2AR gene expression to multiple hormonal signals. In this study (Hadcock *et al.*, 1989b), Malbon and colleagues found that the agonist-induced down-regulation of β_2AR and mRNA levels in DDT_1MF-2 cells described previously (Collins *et al.*, 1989b; Hadock and Malbon, 1988) could be reversed by treatment with dexamethasone. The enhanced rate of β_2AR gene transcription in response to the steroid was sufficient to increase receptor RNA levels and overcome the down-regulation. Conversely, receptor up-regulation, resulting from initial treatment with steroid, was gradually lowered by the subsequent addition of agonist and the development of down-regulation. This study was also interesting from a clinical perspective because treatment of asthmatics with β-agonists over time may result in refractoriness to this form of therapy, while glucocorticoids, which are frequently employed in the treatment of acute asthma, are potentially able to overcome this refractoriness (Nelson, 1986).

The effects of sex steroids on adrenergic activity and receptor number have also been described. Catecholamines appear to be integral signaling components in the ventral prostate and other reproductive tissues for maintaining their steroid sensitivity. Studies *in vivo* have shown that expression of the β_2AR gene in the ventral prostate is regulated by androgens in a manner similar to that observed for glucocorticoids (Collins *et al.*, 1989a).

b. *Cyclic AMP.* Another aspect of adrenergic receptor up-regulation that has recently been described is "autoregulation": the ability of the receptor/effector complex to directly regulate the transcription of its own genes. The β_2AR is the first G protein-coupled receptor for which such a feedback loop has been demonstrated (Collins *et al.*, 1990). Preliminary evidence indicates that such a process may exist for other G protein-coupled receptors as well (see the following discussion). We (Collins *et al.*, 1989b) have observed that short-term (minutes) exposure to β-agonists or cAMP analogues produced a 3- to 5-fold elevation in β_2AR mRNA. This increase was due to direct transcriptional stimulation of the β_2AR gene, with no effect on β_2AR mRNA stability at these early times. These newly synthesized transcripts are efficiently translated as indicated by their localization to heavy polysomes (S. Collins, unpublished observations). The enhancement in mRNA levels is transient and followed, upon more prolonged exposure, by a typical pattern of down-regulation, characterized by the reduction in receptor number and a shortening of β_2AR mRNA half-life as described earlier. For several other cAMP-regulated genes which display early and transient accumulation of mRNA, dynamic changes in both the transcription rate and mRNA stability occur (Hod and Hanson, 1988; Jungmann *et al.*, 1983). Thus, the β_2AR gene conforms to this regulatory paradigm.

The transcriptional response of several genes to cAMP has been localized to a distinct DNA sequence, termed the cAMP response element (CRE) (Roesler *et al.*, 1988), in their 5'-flanking promoter regions. Most CREs contain a variation of the palindromic sequence motif TGACGTCA which is recognized by a 43-kDa phosphoprotein (cAMP response element binding protein, CREB) present in many cells. This protein has been purified (Yamamoto *et al.*, 1988), cloned (Gonzalez *et al.*, 1989; Hoeffler *et al.*, 1988), and its ability to stimulate the transcription of target genes shown to be modified by phosphorylation (Gonzalez and Montminy, 1989), thus linking ligand–receptor interactions at the cell surface with the regulation of gene expression.

More recent studies indicate that in addition to the cAMP pathway, CREB can be activated by changes in intracellular Ca^{2+}, thus affording the possibility for cross-talk between signaling systems. This example also highlights how the same transcription factor and recognition element can be economically deployed by the cell to respond to diverse second messenger pathways. Promoter-reporter gene fusions constructed between the 5'-flanking region of the human β_2AR gene and the coding region of the bacterial chloramphenicol acetyltransferase (CAT) gene conferred cAMP-inducible CAT activity (Collins *et al.*, 1989b), establishing that the promoter region of the β_2AR contains elements responsible for the transcriptional enhancing activity of cAMP. This element has now been more precisely defined (Collins *et al.*, 1990) by site-directed mutagenesis, gel-shift analysis, and DNA footprinting (Fig. 5). The sequence GTACGTCA located at -57 to -50 bp in the β_2AR promoter is a CRE which is recognized and stimulated by the CREB transcription factor. This sequence thus serves as an enhancer of β_2AR gene transcription. The presence of comparable CRE sequences in the 5'-flanking regions of the three mammalian β_2AR genes cloned to date (Allen *et al.*, 1988; Kobilka *et al.*, 1987; Nakada *et al.*, 1989) suggests that this may be a fundamental regulatory mechanism for this gene. It will be important to establish the role of this sequence in both basal and tissue-specific expression of the β_2AR, as the CREs from several genes are obligatory for their expression (Roesler *et al.*, 1988). Evidence that other members of the G protein-coupled receptor family may be similarly modulated by cAMP (Sakaue and Hoffman, 1990) or other second-messenger pathways (Fukamouchi *et al.*, 1990) has recently emerged. Hershey *et al.* (1991) have located a putative Ca^{2+}/CRE in the promoter of the substance P receptor gene in a position equivalent to the β_2AR CRE. These findings suggest the existence of common autoregulatory mechanisms involving the same second messenger cascades that these receptors activate.

IV. CONCLUSIONS

In summary, the recent cloning of the β-adrenergic receptor and other members of the adrenergic receptor family and related molecules has led to a virtual explosion of information and understanding about the structure of this ubiquitous and diverse class of receptor molecules, and of the ways in which their unique structures determine their function. Seven transmembrane regions, likely α-helical in structure, cluster together within the membrane to form a ligand binding pocket. Agonists interact with this receptor binding pocket and somehow trigger conformational changes in the cytosolic portions of the receptor molecule. The conformational changes occurring in regions of the third cytoplasmic loop and carboxy-terminal domain in

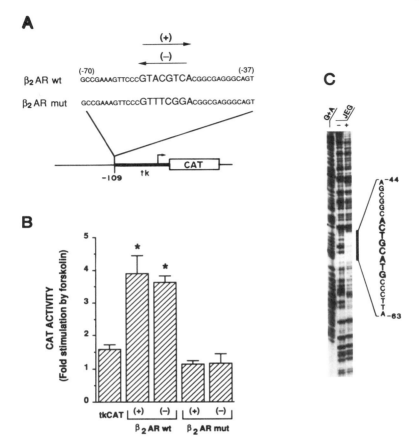

FIG. 5. Identification of a cAMP response element (CRE) in the promoter of the β_2AR gene. (A) A single copy of a 34-bp oligonucleotide encompassing the wild-type (wt) β_2AR CRE (large letters) or a mutant version thereof (mut) plus flanking sequences (smaller letters) was inserted upstream of the thymidine kinase (tk) promoter in either the forward (+) or reverse (−) orientation relative to the direction of transcription (raised arrow) to generate the CAT reporter constructs β_2(+)CAT and β_2(−)CAT. (B) Stimulation of CAT activity by forskolin following transfection of the β_2AR wt and β_2AR mut constructs into JEG-3 cells. The results shown are the average of 4–6 experiments (*, $p < .001$). (C) DNase I footprinting analysis of the human β_2AR CRE with CRE binding protein (CREB)-containing JEG-3 nuclear extract. In the presence (+) but not the absence (−) of JEG-3 extract a protected region, centered on the sequence GTACGTCA at -57 bp to -50 bp, is visualized. A Maxam–Gilbert G+A sequencing reaction is included for orientation. (From Collins et al., 1990.)

closest opposition to the plasma membrane are then transmitted to the
α subunit of G proteins. Phosphorylation of the receptor by several
protein kinases, on distinct cytosolic domains, appears to be a major
factor controlling receptor function. Evidence suggests that an additional protein, β-arrestin, is required to effect the "homologous" form
of desensitization triggered by agonist occupancy and βARK phosphorylation of the receptor. Thus, β-arrestin appears to play a major
and very specific role in regulating the sensitivity of the β_2AR and
possibly other G protein-coupled receptors. Finally, changes in receptor gene expression regulating receptor number and contributing to
overall responsiveness of these receptor systems, can be effected
through either heterologous hormones or agonist-dependent, second-
messenger-mediated autoregulation. Evidence for posttranscriptional
regulation of G protein-coupled receptor mRNA levels underscores the
variety and complexity of heretofore unanticipated molecular pathways controlling receptor expression. Clearly, we are just at the beginning of our efforts to understand how receptor structure determines
receptor function and how, in molecular terms, receptor function is
regulated.

ACKNOWLEDGMENTS

We thank Mark Hnatowich for help with the alignment of the receptors in Fig. 1,
Henrik Dohlman for the preparation of Fig. 2, and Donna Addison for secretarial
support.

REFERENCES

Akamizu, T., Ikuyama, S., Saji, M., Kosugi, S., Kozak, C., McBridge, O. W., and Kohn, L.
    D. (1990). Cloning, chromosomal assignment, and regulation of the rat thyrotropin
    receptor: expression of the gene is regulated by thyrotropin, agents that increase
    cAMP levels, and thyroid autoantibodies. *Proc. Natl. Acad. Sci. U.S.A.* **87,** 5677–
    5681.
Allen, J. M., Baetge, E. E., Abrass, I. B., and Palmiter, R. D. (1988). Isoproterenol
    response following transfection of the mouse β_2-adrenergic receptor gene into Y1
    cells. *EMBO J.* **7,** 133–138.
Applebury, M. L., and Hargrave, P. A. (1986). Molecular biology of the visual pigments.
    Vision Res. **26,** 1881–1895.
Bach, R., Konigsberg, W. H., and Nemerson, Y. (1988). Human tissue factor contains
    thioester-linked palmitate and stearate on the cytoplamic half-cystine. *Biochem-
    istry* **27,** 4227–4231.
Benovic, J. L., Pike, L. J., Cerione, R. A., Staniszewski, C., Yoshimasa, T., Codina, J.,
    Birnbaumer, L., Caron, M. G., and Lefkowitz, R. J. (1985). Phosphorylation of the
    mammalian β-adrenergic receptor by cyclic AMP-dependent protein kinase: Regula-
    tion of the rate of receptor phosphorylation and dephosphorylation by agonist occu-
    pancy and effects on coupling of the receptor to the stimulatory guanine nucleotide
    regulatory protein. *J. Biol. Chem.* **260,** 7094–7101.
Benovic, J. L., Strasser, R. H., Caron, M. G., and Lefkowitz, R. J. (1986a). β-Adrenergic

receptor kinase: Identification of a novel protein kinase which phosphorylates the agonist-occupied form of the receptor. *Proc. Natl. Acad. Sci. U.S.A.* **83**, 2797—2801.

Benovic, J. L., Mayor, F., Jr., Somers, R. L., Caron, M. G., and Lefkowitz, R. J. (1986b). Light dependent phosphorylation of rhodopsin by the β-adrenergic receptor kinase. *Nature (London)* **322**, 869–872.

Benovic, J. L., Regan, J. W., Matsui, H., Mayor, F., Jr., Cotecchia, S., Leeb-Lundberg, L. M. F., Caron, M. G., and Lefkowitz, R. J. (1987a). Agonist-dependent phosphorylation of the α₂-adrenergic receptor by the β-adrenergic receptor kinase. *J. Biol. Chem.* **262**, 17251–17253.

Benovic, J. L., Mayor, F., Jr., Staniszewski, C., Lefkowitz, R. J., and Caron, M. G. (1987b). Purification and characterization of the β-adrenergic receptor kinase. *J. Biol. Chem.* **262**, 9026–9032.

Benovic, J. L., Kuhn, H., Weyland, I., Codina, J., Caron, M. G., and Lefkowitz, R. J. (1987c). Functional desensitization of the isolated β-adrenergic receptor by the β-adrenergic receptor kinase: Potential role of an analog of the retinal protein arrestin (48kDa protein). *Proc. Natl. Acad. Sci. U.S.A.* **84**, 8879–8882.

Benovic, J. L., Bouvier, M., Caron, M. G., and Lefkowitz, R. J. (1988). Regulation of adenylyl cyclase-coupled β-adrenergic receptors. *Annu. Rev. Cell Biol.* **4**, 405–428.

Benovic, J. L., DeBlasi, A., Stone, W. C., Caron, M. G., and Lefkowitz, R. J. (1989). β-adrenergic receptor kinase: primary structure delineates a multigene family. *Science* **426**, 235–240.

Birnbaumer, L. (1990). G proteins in signal transduction. *Annu. Rev. Pharmacol. Toxicol.* **30**, 675–705.

Bouvier, M., Hausdorff, W., DeBlasi, A., O'Dowd, B. F., Kobilka, B. K., Caron, M. G., and Lefkowitz, R. J. (1988). Mutations of the β₂-adrenergic receptor which remove phosphorylation sites delay the onset of agonist promoted desensitization. *Nature (London)* **333**, 370–373.

Bouvier, M., Collins, S., O'Dowd, B. F., Campbell, P. T., DeBlasi, A., Kobilka, B. K., MacGregor, C., Irons, G. P., Caron, M. G., and Lefkowitz, R. J. (1989). Two distinct pathways for cAMP-mediated down regulation of the β₂-adrenergic receptor. *J. Biol. Chem.* **264**, 16786–16792.

Brown, A., and Birnbaumer, L. (1990). Ionic channels and their regulation by G protein subunits. *Annu. Rev. Physiol.* **52**, 197–213.

Campbell, P. T., Hnatowich, M., O'Dowd, B. F., Caron, M. G., Lefkowitz, R. J. L., and Hausdorff, W. P. (1991). Mutations of the human β₂-adrenergic receptor that impair coupling to G_s interfere with receptor down-regulation but not sequestration. *Mol. Pharmacol.* **39**, 192–198.

Chin, D. J., Gil, G., Russell, D. W., Liscum, L., Luskey, K. L., Basu, S. K., Okayama, H., Berg, P., Goldstein, J. L., and Brown, M. S. (1984). Nucleotide sequence of 3-hydroxy-3-methylglutaryl coenzyme A reductase, a glycoprotein of endoplasmic reticulum. *Nature, (London)* **30**, 613–617.

Clark, R. B., Friedman, J., Johnson, J. A., and Kunkel, M. W. (1987). β-Adrenergic receptor desensitization of wild-type but not cyc⁻ lymphoma cells unmasked by submillimolar Mg^{2+}. *FASEB J.* **1**, 289–297.

Clark, R. B., Kunkel, M. W., Friedman, J., Goka, T. J., and Johnson, J. A. (1988). Activation of cAMP-dependent protein kinase is required for heterologous desensitization of adenylyl cyclase in S49 wild-type lymphoma cells. *Proc. Natl. Acad. Sci. U.S.A.* **85**, 1442–1446.

Clark, R. B., Friedman, J., Dixon, R. A. F., and Strader, C. D. (1989). Identification of a specific site required for rapid heterologous desensitization of the β-adrenergic receptor by cAMP-dependent protein kinase. *Mol. Pharmacol.* **36**, 343–348.

Collins, S., Caron, M. G., and Lefkowitz, R. J. (1988). β-Adrenergic receptors in hamster smooth muscle cells are transcriptionally regulated by glucocorticoids. *J. Biol. Chem.* **263**, 9067–9070.

Collins, S., Bolanowski, M. A., Caron, M. G., and Lefkowitz, R. J. (1989a). Genetic regulation of β-adrenergic receptors. *Annu. Rev. Physiol.* **51**, 203–215.

Collins, S., Bouvier, M., Bolanowski, M. A., Caron, M. G., and Lefkowitz, R. J. (1989b). Cyclic AMP stimulates transcription of the β_2-adrenergic receptor gene in response to short term agonist exposure. *Proc. Natl. Acad. Sci. U.S.A.* **86**, 4853–4857.

Collins, S., Altschmied, J., Herbsman, O., Caron, M. G., Mellon, P. L., and Lefkowitz, R. J. (1990). A cAMP response element in the β_2AR gene confers transcriptional autoregulation by cAMP. *J. Biol. Chem.* **265**, 19330–19335.

Colucci, W. S., and Alexander, R. W. (1986). Norepinephrine-induced alterations in the coupling of alpha$_1$-adrenergic receptor occupancy to calcium efflux in rabbit aortic smooth muscle cells. *Proc. Natl. Acad. Sci. U.S.A.* **83**, 1743–1746.

Cotecchia, S., Leeb-Lundberg, L. M. F., Hagen, P.-O., Lefkowitz, R. J., and Caron, M. J. (1985). Phorbol ester effects on α_1 adrenoceptor binding and phosphatidylinositol metabolism in cultured vascular smooth muscle cells. *Life Sci.* **37**, 2389–2398.

Davies, A. O., and Lefkowitz, R. J. (1984). Regulation of β-adrenergic receptors by steroid hormones. *Annu. Rev. Physiol.* **46**, 119–1130.

Dearry, A., Gingrich, J. A., Falardeau, P., Fremeau, R. G., Bates, M. D., and Caron, M. G. (1990). Molecular cloning and expression of the gene for a human D$_1$ dopamine receptor. *Nature (London)* **347**, 72–76.

Dixon, R. A. F., Kobilka, B. K., Strader, D. J., Benovic, J. L., Dohlman, H. G., Frielle, T., Bolanowski, M. A., Bennett, C. D., Rands, E., Diehl, R. F., Mumford, R. A., Slater, E. E., Sigal, I. S., Caron, M. G., Lefkowitz, R. J., and Strader, C. D. (1986). Cloning of the gene and cDNA for mammalian β-adrenergic receptor and homology with rhodopsin. *Nature (London)* **321**, 75–79.

Dixon, R. A. F., Sigal, I. S., Candelore, M. R., Register, R. B., Scattergood, W., Rands, E., and Strader, C. D. (1987). Structural features required for ligand binding to the β-adrenergic receptor. *EMBO J.* **6**, 3269–3275.

Dohlman, H. G., Bouvier, M., Benovic, J. L., Caron, M. G., and Lefkowitz, R. J. (1987). The multiple membrane spanning topography of the β_2-adrenergic receptor. Localization of the sites of binding, glycosylation and regulatory phosphorylation by limited proteolysis. *J. Biol. Chem.* **262**, 14282–14288.

Dohlman, H. G., Caron, M. G., DeBlasi, A., Frielle, T., and Lefkowitz, R. J. (1990). Role of extracellular disulfide-bonded cysteines in the ligand binding function of the β_2-adrenergic receptor. *Biochemistry* **29**, 2335–2342.

Dunn, R., McCoy, J., Simsek, M., Majumdar, A., Chang, S. H., Rajbhandary, U. L., and Khorana, H. G. (1981). The bacteriorhodopsin gene. *Proc. Natl. Acad. Sci. U.S.A.* **78**, 6744–6748.

Evans, R. M. (1988). The steroid and thyroid hormone receptor superfamily. *Science* **240**, 889–895.

Feldman, R. D., McArdle, W., and Lai, C. (1986). Phenylarsine oxide inhibits agonist-induced changes in photoaffinity labeling but not agonist-induced desensitization of the β-adrenergic receptor. *Mol. Pharmacol.* **30**, 459–462.

Fraser, C. M. (1989) Site-directed mutagenesis of β-adrenergic receptors. Identification of conserved cysteine residues that independently affect ligand binding and receptor activation. *J. Biol. Chem.* **264**, 9266–9270.

Fukamouchi, F., Hough, C., and Chuang, D.-M. (1990). Regulation of m_2- and m_3-muscarinic receptor mRNA in cultured cerebellar granule cells. *FASEB J.* **4,** A460. (Abstr.)

Gonzalez, G. A., and Montminy, M. R. (1989). Cyclic AMP stimulates somatostatin gene transcription by phosphorylation of CREB at serine 133. *Cell* **59,** 675–680.

Gonzalez, G. A., Yamamoto, K. K., Fischer, W. H., Karr, D., Menzel, P., Biggs, W. H., III, Vale, W. W., and Montminy, M. R. (1989). A cluster of phosphorylation sites on the cAMP-regulated factor CREB predicted by its sequence. *Nature (London)* **337,** 749–752.

Green, D. A., and Clark, R. B. (1981). Adenylate cyclase coupling proteins are not essential for agonist-specific desensitization of lymphoma cells. *J. Biol. Chem.* **256,** 2105–2108.

Hadcock, J. R., and Malbon, C. C. (1988). Down-regulation of β-adrenergic receptors: agonist-induced reduction in receptor mRNA levels. *Proc. Natl. Acad. Sci. U.S.A.* **85,** 5021–5025.

Hadcock, J. R., Ros, M., and Malbon, C. C. (1989a). Agonist regulation of β-adrenergic receptor mRNA. Analysis in S49 mouse lymphoma mutants. *J. Biol. Chem.* **264,** 13956–13961.

Hadcock, J. R., Wang, H., and Malbon, C. C. (1989b). Agonist-induced destabilization of β-adrenergic receptor mRNA. Attenuation of glucocorticoid induced up-regulation of β-adrenergic receptors. *J. Biol. Chem.* **264,** 19928–19933.

Harden, T. K., Cotton, C. V., Waldo, G. L., Lutton, J. K., and Perkins, J. P. (1980). Catecholamine-induced alteration in sedimentation behavior of membrane bound β-adrenergic receptors. *Science* **210,** 441–443.

Hausdorff, W. P., Bouvier, M., O'Dowd, B. F., Irons, G. P., Caron, M. G., and Lefkowitz, R. J. (1989). Phosphorylation sites on two domains of the β_2-adrenergic receptor are involved in distinct pathways of receptor desensitization. *J. Biol. Chem.* **264,** 12657–12665.

Hausdorff, W. P., Hnatowich, M., O'Dowd, B. F., Caron, M. G., and Lefkowitz, R. J. (1990). A mutation of the β_2-adrenergic receptor impairs agonist activation of adenylyl cyclase without affecting high affinity agonist binding. *J. Biol. Chem.* **265,** 1388–1393.

Henderson, R., and Unwin, P. N. (1975). Three dimensional model of purple membranes obtained by electron microscopy. *Nature (London)* **257,** 28–32.

Hertel, C., and Staehelin, M. (1983). Reappearance of β-adrenergic receptors after isoproterenol treatment in intact C6-cells. *J. Cell Biol.* **97,** 1538–1543.

Hertel, C., Staehelin, M., and Perkins, J. P. (1983). Evidence for intravesicular β-adrenergic receptors in membrane fractions from desensitized cells: Binding of the hydrophilic ligand CGP12177 only in the presence of alamethicin. *J. Cyclic Nucleotide Protein Phosphorylation Res.* **9,** 119–128.

Hod, Y., and Hanson, R. W. (1988). Cyclic AMP stabilizes the mRNA for phosphoenol pyruvate carboxykinase (GTP) against degradation. *J. Biol. Chem.* **263,** 7747–7752.

Hoeffler, J. P., Meyer, T. E., Yun, Y., Jameson, J. L., and Habener, J. F. (1988). Cyclic AMP-responsive DNA-binding protein-structure based on a cloned placental cDNA. *Science* **242,** 1430–1433.

Hoffman, Y. M., Peegel, H., Sprock, M. J. E., Zhang, O.-Y., and Menon, K. J. J. (1991). Evidence that human chorionic gonadotropin/luteinizing hormone receptor down-regulation involves decreased levels of receptor messenger ribonucleic acid. *Endocrinology* **128,** 388–393.

Izzo, N. J., Seidman, C. E., Collins, S., and Colucci, W. S. (1990). α_1-Adrenergic receptor mRNA level is regulated by norepinephrine in rabbit aortic smooth muscle cells. *Proc. Nat'l. Acad. Sci. U.S.A.* **87**, 6268–6271.

Jarvie, K. R., and Niznik, H. B. (1989). Deglycosylation and proteolysis of photolabeled D_2 dopamine receptors of the porcine anterior pituitary. *J. Biochem. (Tokyo)* **106**, 17–22.

Jarvie, K. R., Niznik, H. B., and Seeman, P. (1988). Dopamine D_2 receptor binding subunits of $M_r \simeq$ 140,000 and 94,000 in brain: Deglycosylation yields a common unit of $M_r \simeq$ 44,000. *Mol. Pharmacol.* **34**, 91–97.

Jungmann, R. A., Kelley, D. C., Miles, M. F., and Milkowski, D. M. (1983). Cyclic AMP regulation of lactate dehydrogenase. *J. Biol. Chem.* **258**, 5312–5318.

Kassis, S., and Fishman, P. H. (1984). Functional alteration of the β-adrenergic receptor during desensitization of mammalian adenylate cyclase cy β-agonists. *Proc. Natl. Acad. Sci. U.S.A.* **81**, 6686–6690.

Kassis, S., Olasmaa, M., Sullivan, M., and Fishman, P. H. (1986). Desensitization of the β-adrenergic receptor-coupled adenylate cyclase in cultured mammalian cells: Receptor sequestration versus receptor function. *J. Biol. Chem.* **261**, 12233–12237.

Kobilka, B. K., Frielle, T., Dohlman, H. G., Bolanowski, M. A., Dixon, R. A. F., Keller, P., Caron, M. G., and Lefkowitz, R. J. (1987). Delineation of the intronless nature of the genes for the human and hamster $β_2$-adrenergic receptor and their putative promoter regions. *J. Biol. Chem.* **262**, 7321–7327.

Kobilka, B. K., Kobilka, T. S., Daniel, K., Regan, J. W., Caron, M. G., and Lefkowitz, R. J. (1988). Chimeric $α_2$-,$β_2$-adrenergic receptors: Delineation of domains involved in effector coupling and ligand binding specificity. *Science* **240**, 1310–1316.

Kubo, T,. Bujo, H., Akiba, I., Nakai, J., Mishina, M., and Numa, S. (1988). Location of a region of the muscarinic acetylcholine receptor involved in selective effector coupling. *FEBS Lett.* **241**, 119–125.

Kunkel, M. W., Friedman, J., Shenolikar, S., and Clark, R. B. (1989). Cell-free heterologous desensitization of adenylyl cyclase in S49 lymphoma cell membranes mediated by cAMP-dependent protein kinase. *FASEB J.* **3**, 2067–2074.

Kwatra, M. M., Benovic, J. L., Caron, M. G., Lefkowitz, R. J., and Hosey, M. M. (1989). Phosphorylation of chick heart muscarinic cholinergic receptors by the β-adrenergic receptor kinase. *Biochemistry* **28**, 4543–4537.

Lanier, S. M., Homcy, C. J., Patenaude, C., and Graham, R. M. (1988). Identification of structurally distinct $α_2$-adrenergic receptors. *J. Biol. Chem.* **263**, 14491–14496.

Libert, F., Parmentier, M., Lefort, A., Dinsart, C., Van Sande, J. V., Maenhaut, C., Simons, M.-J., Dumont, J. E., and Vassart, G. (1989). Selective amplification and cloning of four new members of the G protein-coupled receptor family. *Science* **244**, 569–572.

Liggett, S. B., Bouvier, M., Hausdorff, W. P., O'Dowd, B. F., Caron, M. G., and Lefkowitz, R. J. (1989). Altered patterns of agonist-stimulated cAMP accumulation in cells expressing mutant $β_2$-adrenergic receptors lacking phosphorylation sites. *Mol. Pharmacol.* **36**, 641–646.

Lohse, M. J. (1990). Quantitation of receptor desensitization by an operational model of agonism. *J. Biol. Chem.* **265**, 3210–3211.

Lohse, M. J., Lefkowitz, R. J., Caron, M. G., and Benovic, J. L. (1989). Inhibition of β-adrenergic receptor kinase prevents rapid homologous desensitization of $β_2$-adrenergic receptors. *Proc. Natl. Acad. Sci. U.S.A.* **86**, 3011–3015.

Lohse, M. J., Benovic, J. L., Caron, M. G., and Lefkowitz, R. J. (1990a). Multiple pathways of rapid $β_2$-adrenergic receptor desensitization: delineation with specific inhibitors. *J. Biol. Chem.* **265**, 3202–3209.

Lohse, M. L., Benovic, J. L., Codina, J., Caron, M. G., and Lefkowitz, R. J. (1990b). β-Arrestin, a protein that regulates β-adrenergic receptor function. *Science* **248,** 1547–1550.

Mahan, L. C., Koachman, A. M., and Insel, P. A. (1985). Genetic analysis of β-adrenergic receptor internalization and down-regulation. *Proc. Natl. Acad. Sci. U.S.A.* **82,** 129–133.

Matsuda, L. A., Lolait, S. J., Brownstein, M. J., Young, A. C., and Bonner, T. I. (1990). Structure of a cannabinoid reeptor and functional expression of the cloned cDNA. *Nature (London)* **346,** 561–564.

McFarland, K. C., Sprengel, R., Phillips, H. S., Kohler, M., Rosemblit, N., Nikolics, K., Segaloff, D. L., and Seeburg, P. H. (1989). Lutropin-choriogonadotropin receptor: An unusual member of the G protein-coupled receptor family. *Science* **245,** 494–499.

Nakada, M. T., Haskell, K. M., Ecker, D. J., Stadel, J. M., and Crooke, S. T. (1989). Genetic regulation of β_2-adrenergic receptors in 3T3-L1 fibroblasts. *Biochem. J.* **260,** 53–59.

Nakayama, N., Miyajima, A., and Arai, K. (1985). Nucleotide sequences of STE2 and STE3, cell type-specific sterile genes from saccharomyces cerevisiae. *EMBO J.* **4,** 2643–2648.

Nambi, P., Peters, J. R., Sibley, D. R., and Lefkowitz, R. J. (1985). Desensitization of the turkey erythrocyte β-adrenergic receptor in a cell-free system. *J. Biol. Chem.* **260,** 2165–2171.

Nelson, H. S. (1986). Adrenergic therapy of bronchial asthma. *J. Allergy Clin. Immunol.* **77,** 771–785.

O'Brien, P. J., and Zatz, M. (1984). Acylation of bovine rhodopsin by [³H]palmitic acid. *J. Biol. Chem.* **259,** 5054–5057.

O'Dowd, B. F., Hnatowich, M., Regan, J. W., Leader, W. M., Caron, M. G., and Lefkowitz, R. J. (1988). Site-directed mutagenesis of the cytoplasmic domains of the human β_2-adrenergic receptor: Localization of regions involved in a G protein-receptor coupling. *J. Biol. Chem.* **263,** 15985–15992.

O'Dowd, B. F. Hnatowich, M., Caron, M. G., Lefkowitz, R. J., and Bouvier, M. (1989). Palmitoylation of the human β_2-adrenergic receptor. *J. Biol. Chem.* **264,** 7564–7569.

O'Dowd, B. F., Collins, S., Bouvier, M., Caron, M. G., and Lefkowitz, R. J. (1991). Structural, functional and genetic aspects of receptors coupled to G proteins. *In* "Molecular Biology of Receptors Which Couple to G-Proteins" (M. Brann, ed.). Birkhauser, Cambridge, Massachusetts (in press).

Onorato, J. J., Regan, J. W., Caron, M. G., Lefkowitz, R. J., and Benovic, J. L. (1991). The role of acidic amino acids in determining the substrate specificity of the β-adrenergic receptor kinase. *Biochemistry* **30,** 5118–5125.

Oron, Y., Straub, R. E., Traktman, P., and Gershengorn, M. D. (1987). Decreased TRH receptor mRNA activity precedes homologous down regulation: assay in oocytes. *Science* **238,** 1406–1408.

Ovchinnikov, Y. A., Abdulaev, N. G., and Bogachuk, A. S. (1988). Two adjacent cysteine residues in the C-terminal cytoplasmic fragment of bovine rhodopsin are palmitylated. *FEBS Lett.* **230,** 1–5.

Roesler, W. J., Vandenbark, G. R., and Hanson, R. W. (1988). Cyclic AMP and the induction of eukaryotic gene transcription. *J. Biol. Chem.* **263,** 9063–9066.

Ross, J. (1988). Messenger RNA turnover in eukaryotic cells. *Mol. Biol. Med.* **5,** 1–14.

Sakaue, M., and Hoffman, B. B. (1991). cAMP regulates transcription of the α_2A adrenergic receptor gene in HT-29 cells. *J. Biol. Chem.* **266,** 5743–5749.

Schobert, B., Lanyi, J. K., and Oesterheld, D. (1988). Structure and orientation of halorhodopsin in the membrane: a proteolytic fragmentation study. *EMBO J.* **4**, 905–911.

Segaloff, D. L., Wang, H., and Richards, J. S. (1990). Hormonal regulation of luteinizing hormone/chorionic gonadotropin receptor mRNA in rat ovarian cells during follicular development and luteinization. *Mol. Endocrinol.* **4**, 1856–1865.

Shaw, G., and Kamen, R. (1986). A conserved AU sequence from the 3' untranslated region of GM-CSF mRNA mediates selective mRNA degradation. *Cell* **46**, 659–667.

Shear, M., Insel, P. A., Melmon, K. L., and Coffino, P. (1976). Agonist specific refractoriness induced by isoproterenol. *J. Biol. Chem.* **251**, 7572–7576.

Sheng, M., and Greenberg, M. E. (1990). The regulation and function of c-fos and other immediate early genes in the nervous system. *Neuron* **4**, 477–485.

Sheng, M., McFadden, G., and Greenberg, M. E. (1990). Membrane depolarization and calcium induce c-fos transcription via phosphorylation of transcription factor CREB. *Neuron* **4**, 571–582.

Sibley, D. R., Peters, J. R., Nambi, P., Caron, M. G., and Lefkowitz, R. J. (1984). Desensitization of turkey erythrocyte adenyly cyclase: β-adrenergic receptor phosphorylation is correlated with attenuation of adenyly cyclase activity. *J. Biol. Chem.* **259**, 9742–9749.

Sibley, D. R., Strasser, R. H., Caron, M. G., and Lefkowitz, R. J. (1985). Homologous desensitization of adenylyl cyclase is associated with phosphorylation of the β-adrenergic receptor. *J. Biol. Chem.* **260**, 3883–3886.

Sibley, D. R., Strasser, R. H., Benovic, J. L., Daniel, K., and Lefkowitz, R. J. (1986). Phosphorylation/dephosphorylation of the β-adrenergic receptor regulates its functional coupling to adenylyl cyclase and subcellular distribution. *Proc. Natl. Acad. Sci. U.S.A.* **83**, 9408–9412.

Smith, J. D., and Liu, A. Y.-C. (1988). Increased turnover of the messenger RNA encoding tyrosine aminotransferase can account for the desensitization and de-induction of tyrosine aminotransferase by 8-bromo-cyclic AMP treatment and removal. *EMBO J.* **7**, 3711–3716.

Sprengel, R., Braun, T., Nikolics, K., Segaloff, D. L., and Seeburg, P. H. (1990). The testicular receptor for follicle stimulating hormone: Structure and functional expression of cloned cDNA *Mol. Endocrinol.* **4**, 525–530.

Stadel, J. M., Nambi, P., Lavin, T. N., Heald, S. L., Caron, M. G., and Lefkowitz, R. J. (1982). Catecholamine-induced desensitization of turkey erythrocyte adenylyl cyclase: Structural alterations in the β-adrenergic receptor revealed by photoaffinity labeling. *J. Biol. Chem.* **257**, 9242–9245.

Stadel, J. M., Nambi, P., Shorr, R. G. L., Sawyer, D. F., Caron, M. G., and Lefkowitz, R. J. (1983a). Catecholamine-induced desensitization of turkey erythrocyte adenylyl cyclase is associated with phosphorylation of the β-adrenergic receptor. *Proc. Natl. Acad. Sci. U.S.A.* **80**, 3173–3177.

Stadel, J. M., Strulovici, B., Nambi, P., Lavin, T. N., Briggs, M. M., Caron, M. G., and Lefkowitz, R. J. (1983b). Desensitization of the β-adrenergic receptor of frog erythrocytes: Recovery and characterization of the down regulated receptors in sequestered vesicles. *J. Biol. Chem.* **258**, 3032–3038.

Strader, C. D., Sigal, I. S., Register, R., Candelore, M. R., Rands, E., and Dixon, R. A. F. (1987a). Identification of residues required for ligand binding to the β-adrenergic receptor. *Proc. Natl. Acad. Sci. U.S.A.* **94**, 4384–4388.

Strader, C. D., Sigal, I. S., Blake, A. D., Cheung, A. H., Register, R. B., Rands, E., Zemcik, B. A., Candelore, M. R., and Dixon, R. A. F. (1987b). The carboxyl terminus of the hamster β-adrenergic receptor expressed in mouse L cells is not required for receptor sequestration. *Cell* **49,** 855–863.

Strasser, R. H., Sibley, D. R., and Lefkowitz, R. J. (1986). A novel catecholamine activated adenosine 3′, 5′-phosphate independent pathway for β-adrenergic receptor phosphorylation in wild-type and mutant S49 lymphoma cells. *Biochemistry* **25,** 1371–1377.

Strulovici, B., Cerione, R. A., Kilpatrick, B. F., Caron, M. G., and Lefkowitz, R. J. (1984). Direct demonstration of impaired functionality of a purified desensitized β-adrenergic receptor in a reconstituted system. *Science* **225,** 837–840.

Su, Y. F., Harden, T. K., and Perkins, J. P. (1980). Catecholamine specific desensitization of adenylyl cyclase: Evidence for a multiple step process. *J. Biol. Chem.* **255,** 7410–7419.

Terman, B. I., and Insel, P. A. (1988). Use of 1-deoxymannogirimycin to show that complex oligosaccharides regulate cellular distribution of the α_1-adrenergic receptor glycoprotein in BC_3H_1 muscle cells. *Mol. Pharmacol* **34,** 8–14.

Toews, M. L., and Perkins, J. P. (1984). Agonist-induced changes in β-adrenergic receptors in intact cells. *J. Biol. Chem.* **259,** 2227–2235.

Waldo, G. L., Northup, J. K., Perkins, J. P., and Harden, T. K. (1983). Characterization of an altered membrane form of the β-adrenergic receptor produced during agonist-induced desensitization. *J. Biol. Chem.* **258,** 13900–13908.

Wang, H., Segaloff, D. L., and Ascoli, M. (1991). Lutropin/Choriogonadotropin downregulates its receptor by both receptor-mediated endocytosis and acAMP-dependent reduction in receptor mRNA. *J. Biol. Chem.* **266,** 780–785.

Wilden, U., Hall, S. W., and Kuhn, H. (1986). Phosphodiesterase activation of photoexcited rhodopsin is quenched when rhodopsin is phosphorylated and binds the intrinsic 48 kDa protein of rod outer segments. *Proc. Natl. Acad. Sci. U.S.A.* **83,** 1174–1178.

Wong, S. K-F., Parker, E. M., and Ross, E. M. (1990). Chimeric muscarinic cholinergic β-adrenergic receptors that activate G_s in response to muscarinic agonists. *J. Biol. Chem.* **265,** 6219–6224.

Yamamoto, K. K., Gonzalez, G. A., Biggs, W. H., III, and Montminy, M. R. (1988). Phosphorylation-induced binding and transcriptional efficacy of nuclear factor CREB. *Nature (London)* **334,** 494–498.

Cellular and Molecular Mechanisms in the Regulation and Function of Osteoclasts

T. J. CHAMBERS AND T. J. HALL

Department of Histopathology
St. George's Hospital Medical School
London SW17 ORE, England

I. INTRODUCTION

The morphogenesis and restructuring of bone depends upon the integrated activity of the cells that form bone (osteoblasts) and the cells that resorb bone (osteoclasts). Cells of the osteoblastic lineage not only form bone but appear to be pivotal in regulating bone resorption. Current evidence suggests that osteoblastic cells may be involved in osteoclast formation, in the induction and localization of osteoclastic bone resorption, and in the regulation of activity of resorptive cells. The mechanisms involved in osteoclast attachment and subsequent resorption of mineralized bone have been the focus of considerable research effort over the last few years, and the results of such studies are reviewed in Section II, before we review evidence concerning osteoclast formation and lineage, and the induction and regulation of osteoclastic bone resorption (Section III). The reader is also referred to other reviews on this topic (Nijweide *et al.*, 1986; Marks and Popoff, 1988; Vaes, 1988; Baron, 1989).

II. Molecular Mechanisms of Osteoclastic Bone Resorption

A. Osteoclastic Adhesion to Bone Surfaces

In order to resorb bone, the osteoclast must be attached to the bone surface, and research into the attachment process has, over the last few years, yielded much information on the mechanisms involved. The site of the osteoclast that forms the intimate attachment to the bone surface is referred to as the sealing zone, which is a circumferential ringlike structure that separates the osteoclast membrane into two defined areas that have distinct roles during bone resorption. The basolateral surface of bone-attached osteoclast is in contact with the extracellular fluid, while the apical membrane within the sealing zone and in close apposition to the bone surface, forms into a highly convoluted surface referred to as the ruffled border. It is at the ruffled border membrane that protons and vacuolar proteinases are extruded into the hemivacuole or resorption lacuna.

Studies have revealed some of the mechanisms by which osteoclasts recognize and bind to bone surfaces (reviewed in Horton and Davies, 1989). The integrins are cellular adhesion molecules that comprise a large family of heterodimeric cell surface glycoproteins (Hynes, 1987), and recognize a variety of extracellular matrix-associated ligands, many of which contain the Arg-Gly-Asp (RGD) tripeptide recognition sequence (Ruoslahti and Pierschbacher, 1986). An adhesion receptor on human osteoclasts was characterized biochemically by Davies *et al.* (1989), using two mouse monoclonal antibodies (termed 13C2 and 23C6; Horton *et al.*, 1985). These monoclonal antibodies were used to immunoprecipitate from human osteoclastoma tissue, a molecule termed the osteoclast functional antigen (OFA) (Davies *et al.*, 1989), which was shown to comprise a 140-kDa α-chain and an 85-kDa β-chain. The α-chain was identified as being immunologically cross-reactive with the α-chain of the vitronectin receptor, and the β-chain was found to be related to the platelet gpIIIa molecule (β_3 integrin; Davies *et al.*, 1989; Horton and Davies, 1989). The observations showing that OFA expression on bone cells is restricted to osteoclasts and preosteoclasts (Horton and Davies, 1989; Simpson and Horton, 1989), and that the monoclonal antibody 13C2 inhibits osteoclastic bone resorption in the bone slice assay (Chambers *et al.*, 1986), strongly suggest that OFA plays an important role in osteoclast function.

Several reports indicate that osteoclast podosomes, short microfilament-containing protrusions that act as cellular adhesive feet, are localized at the sealing zone in both avian and human osteoclasts

(Marchisio *et al.*, 1984; Zambonin-Zallone *et al.*, 1988, 1989; Teti *et al.*, 1989a). Furthermore, Zambonin-Zallone *et al.* (1989) found a β_3 integrin on human osteoclast podosomes, thus implying that OFA, which also contains a β_3 integrin, is located at the osteoclast sealing zone. Although monoclonal antibody 13C2 was shown to inhibit human osteoclastic bone resorption, it did not cause detachment of osteoclasts from bone slices (Chambers *et al.*, 1986), but rather caused cytoplasmic retraction, in a manner similar to the effects of calcitonin (CT) on osteoclasts (Chambers *et al.*, 1985a). Taken together, these results suggest that OFA is not the only adhesion receptor involved in osteoclast attachment to bone surfaces, but that it may play a crucial role in (1) tight attachment of the osteoclast to mineralized bone surfaces at the level of podosomes that constitute the osteoclast–bone attachment at the sealing zone; and (2) that OFA is involved in cytoskeletal organization within the resorbing osteoclast.

Integrins such as the vitronectin receptor are known to be transmembrane proteins that act as linkers between extracellular ligands and cytoskeletal components such as vinculin, talin, α-actinin and F-actin (reviewed in Geiger, 1983; Hynes, 1987). Evidence that such transmembrane linker effects are mediated by OFA in osteoclasts comes from the immunofluorescence studies of Marchisio *et al.* (1984), who demonstrated that vinculin, F-actin, and α-actinin are localized as a ring of dotlike structures in chick osteoclasts, such that their intracellular organization parallels the circumferential structure of the sealing zone. Similar immunofluorescent studies by Zambonin-Zallone *et al.* (1989) and Teti *et al.* (1989a) have also demonstrated that F-actin and vinculin are associated with the extracellular location of the β_3 integrin molecule in the belt of podosomes that are present at the attachment site of human osteoclasts spread on glass coverslips. Interestingly, Teti *et al.* (1989a) also showed that the number of osteoclasts with podosomes increased under acidic culture conditions and decreased with increasing pH, suggesting that local acidic conditions may stimulate osteoclast adhesion to bone surfaces. Similarly, high extracellular calcium concentrations (4 mM) were shown by the same group to decrease chick osteoclast podosome expression by approximately 50% (Miyauchi *et al.*, (1990). The significance of these results in the regulation of osteoclastic bone resorption is discussed in Section II,E.

The nature of the extracellular ligand(s) in mineralized bone that OFA may bind to has also been addressed. Osteoclast functional antigen is a member of the vitronectin receptor family, suggesting that its ligand(s) in bone may well contain the RGD tripeptide recognition sequence, and need not therefore be vitronectin itself. Several candidate ligands of bone containing the RGD sequence include osteopontin, thrombospondin, and bone sialoprotein. Osteopontin (Oldberg *et al.,* 1986) is of particular interest since its production by osteoblasts is increased by calcitriol (Yoon *et al.,* 1987), which is also known to stimulate osteoclastic bone resorption via an effect on osteoblasts (Chambers, 1985) (although production is suppressed by parathyroid hormone (PTH); Noda and Rodan, 1989). Thus, Reinholt *et al.* (1990) used antibodies to rat osteopontin to immunolocalize the molecule in ultrathin sections of young rat maxillae. They found osteopontin in the bone surface, below the sealing/clear zone of *in situ* resorbing osteoclasts, sparse below the ruffled border, and also associated with osteoblasts. Alternatively, since in our experience isolated osteoclasts excavate bone slices in the absence of serum, osteoblasts may not deposit osteopontin at the time of resorption, specifically in sealing zones, but may rather incorporate osteopontin into bone during osteogenesis. If so, osteopontin may be reduced below the ruffled border due to partial digestion. In the same study, however, antibodies to the human vitronectin receptor were immunolocalized specifically to the sealing zone of osteoclasts, suggesting that a vitronectin-type adhesion receptor is also involved in the attachment of rat osteoclasts to bone surfaces and that osteopontin is likely to be an extracellular recognition ligand in the bone matrix.

Clearly, the nature of all the molecules involved in osteoclast recognition and binding to bone surfaces and the mechanisms involved in regulating the attachment process are not yet fully identified. However, the results of the findings previously reviewed indicate that this is an area of growing interest that may have important therapeutic implications in the treatment of bone disease.

B. Role of Carbonic Anhydrase in Osteoclastic Bone Resorption

The putative function of osteoclast carbonic anhydrase in the resorptive process derives from studies with sulfonamide inhibitors of carbonic anhydrase that were developed as diuretics in the 1950s (reviewed in Maren and Sanyal, 1983; Maren, 1984). Early *in vivo* studies examined the effects of acetazolamide on serum calcium levels in nephrectomized rats (Waite *et al.,* 1970; Waite, 1972). Acetazolamide was shown to cause hypocalcemia, and to inhibit the hypercalcemia induced in rats treated with PTH, suggesting an effect on bone resorption (Waite *et al.,* 1970). This conclusion was supported by later studies by Conaway *et al.* (1973) and Kenny (1985), showing that acetazolamide treatment of limb-immobilized rats could partially inhibit the disuse loss of bone mass, which is apparently due to increased osteoclastic activity.

Evidence that carbonic anhydrase affects bone resorption came directly from the work of Minkin and Jennings (1972), who showed that known specific sulfonamide inhibitors of carbonic anhydrase—ethoxzolamide, acetazolamide, and methazolamide (in order of potency)—inhibited the release of radiocalcium from PTH-stimulated calvarial cultures. The fact that microscopical observations revealed no evidence for alterations in bone forming cells or osteoid formation in acetazolamide-treated calvaria supported the conclusion that the sulfonamides inhibit the resorptive process through inhibition of carbonic anhydrase.

The first observation that osteoclasts contain carbonic anhydrase was reported by Gay and Mueller (1974), using labeled inhibitor autoradiography. Tritiated acetazolamide was injected into hens and autoradiography was performed on sections of medullary bone. Grain patterns and concentrations showed preferential localization of tritiated acetazolamide in osteoclasts, whereas osteoblasts and osteocytes showed only background levels of labeling. Subsequently, several groups have shown, primarily by immunohistochemical staining with carbonic anhydrase-specific antibodies, that osteoclasts from birds and mammals contain carbonic anhydrase (Vaananen and Parvinen, 1983; Gay et al., 1984; Vaananen, 1984; Cao and Gay, 1985; Sundquist et al., 1987). There are currently thought to be at least nine isozymes of carbonic anhydrase, although only four (carbonic anhydrase isozymes I, II, III, and IV) have been characterized in any detail (Tashjian, 1989). The purification and isolation of carbonic anhydrase isozymes I and II from hemolysates taken from several mammalian species has allowed the development of carbonic anhydrase isozyme-specific antisera, and immunohistochemical studies using such antibodies have demonstrated that carbonic anhydrase isozyme II is present in rat (Vaananen and Parvinen, 1983; Sundquist et al., 1987) and human (Vaananen, 1984) osteoclasts.

In both avian and rat osteoclasts, carbonic anhydrase was found partly in the cytosol and partly in association with the ruffled border membrane (Gay et al., 1984; Cao and Gay, 1985; Sundquist et al., 1987). Clearly, localization of carbonic anhydrase at the ruffled border membrane portends that local production of protons at the relevant site for extrusion by proton transport systems (see Section II,C) is important for function of resorbing osteoclasts.

Cao and Gay (1985) reported some interesting studies on the effects of CT on the localization of carbonic anhdrase in avian osteoclasts. Cultured chick embryo metatarsi showed high levels of immunocytochemically stained carbonic anhydrase associated with osteoclast ruffled border membranes, as determined by morphometric analysis of micrographs. Osteoclasts in CT-treated metatarsi, however, showed a significant decrease in carbonic anhydrase associated with the ruffled border membrane. Since there is evidence to suggest that carbonic anhydrase associated with membranes is more stable and active (Gay et al., 1984), this may be one of the mechanisms by which CT controls osteoclastic bone resorption. It has also been shown that the activity of carbonic anhydrase in cultures of chick osteoclasts is rapidly increased (approximately 2-fold) after treatment with PTH (Silverton et al., 1987), and that CT did not prevent the PTH stimulation of carbonic anhydrase activity. Similar results were also reported by Hunter et al. (1988) using cultured chick osteoclasts and fluorescence to assess osteoclast acidity, showing that acetazolamide produced a steady decline in osteoclast acidity, while PTH produced a transient increase in osteoclast acidity which was attributed to activation of carbonic anhydrase activity. Calcitonin was shown to produce a decrease in osteoclast acidity, although his was less pronounced than the effect of acetazolamide, these results being in accord with previous studies by this group (Gay et al., 1984; Cao and Gay, 1985), as previously discussed. Parathyroid hormone may enhance the carbonic anhydrase activity of bone by inducing an increase in the number of mature osteoclasts in the bone tissue (Hall and Kenny, 1986; Vaes, 1988). However, the results of Silverton et al. (1987) and Hunter et al. (1988) suggest that a PTH-stimulated increase in osteoclast carbonic anhydrase activity may also be involved.

The in vivo and in vitro results with sulfonamide inhibitors of carbonic anhydrase and their inhibitory effect on bone resorption can be taken to indicate that carbonic anhydrase plays an important role in osteoclast bone resorption. However, the results of studies with sulfonamides and their inhibitory effect on bone resorption in organ culture show some discrepancies. Thus, in a study using ^{45}Ca-labeled fetal rat long bones, Raisz et al. (1988) found that acetazolamide and ethoxzolamide were much less potent inhibitors of radiocalcium release in PTH-stimulated organ cultures (approximately 10 times less potent) than was found in the earlier study of Minkin and Jennings (1972), discussed at the beginning of this section. This difference in inhibitory potency was noted by Raisz et al. (1988), and a proposed explanation was that the use of a 5% CO_2 in air atmosphere in their cultures would clearly favor the catalytic production of protons by osteoclast carbonic anhydrase and thus facilitate resorption, whereas Minkin and Jennings (1972) used an oxygen–nitrogen atmosphere for their organ cultures, under which conditions carbonic anhydrase activity may be more easily inhibited by sulfonamides. Thus, while *in vivo* experiments examining the effects of sulfonamides on PTH-stimulated bone resorption are complicated by possible effects of these agents on other tissues, the organ culture system, which has proved to be a reliable *in vitro* model for examining the direct effects of agents on bone, also has its limitations. In particular, the interpretation of results may be complicated by effects of compounds on osteoblasts, which regulate osteoclast function, or effects on cells other than osteoclasts, e.g., macrophages, which may assist in solubilizing ^{45}Ca from bone particles released from bone by osteoclasts (Vaes, 1988). Furthermore, the effective concentrations of compounds may be underestimated since their penetration into cultured bone may be limited, and consequently their access to osteoclasts. We have therefore assessed the effects of several sulfonamides in the bone slice assay (Chambers *et al.*, 1984a, 1985a), where osteoclasts disaggregated from neonatal rat long bones and sedimented onto slices of bovine cortical bone make discrete resorption pits which can be counted and their plane surface area measured. This assay is generally more sensitive, and less prone to indirect effects than organ culture systems. Ethoxzolamide and acetozalomide were found to be potent inhibitors of osteoclastic bone resorption ($IC_{50} \sim 0.1$ μM and 1 μM, respectively) in the bone slice assay (Hall *et al.*, 1991). In the PTH-stimulated organ culture experiments of Minkin and Jennings (1972) and Raisz *et al.* (1988) the IC_{50} results for ethoxzolamide were approximately 4 μM and 30 μM, respectively. Results with several other sulfonamides of lesser inhibitory activity correlated well with the order of inhibitory activity on the catalytic activity of purified human erythrocyte carbonic anhydrase II determined by the Maren assay (Maren, 1960). Thus, our results clearly demonstrated a direct, noncytotoxic inhibition of osteoclastic bone resorption by inhibitors of carbonic anhydrase that was correlated with inhibition of purified carbonic anhydrase II, supporting the view that it is carbonic anhydrase isozyme II that exists in osteoclasts (Hall *et al.*, 1991).

The majority of this work has used avian or nonhuman mammalian osteoclasts. Evidence for the role of carbonic anhydrase II in human osteoclast activity comes from the elegant genetic studies on patients with autosomal recessive osteopetrosis reported by Sly *et al.* (1983), who showed that carbonic anhydrase II deficiency is the primary defect in this syndrome.

In summary, there is convincing evidence from both immunocytochemical and sulfonamide inhibition studies that avian and
mammalian osteoclasts contain carbonic anhydrase which, in mammalian osteoclasts, has been identified as carbonic anhydrase isozyme
II. Studies with avian osteoclasts indicate that carbonic anhydrase
exists in both cytoplasmic and at high levels, ruffled border membrane
bound forms; the latter is well placed for producing protons which are
extruded into the hemivacuole during bone resorption. Sulfonamide
inhibition studies have provided convincing evidence that osteoclastic
bone resorption is absolutely dependent on the enzymic activity of
carbonic anhydrase, needed for production of protons for hemivacuole
acidification leading to the solubilization of bone mineral and providing an acidic environment optimal for activity of osteoclast acid proteinases which degrade the organic components of bone. The role of
protons in bone resorption and the mechanisms by which osteoclasts
secrete them into the hemivacuole are discussed in detail in Section
II,C.

C. Role of Protons and Proton Transport Systems in Osteoclastic Bone Resorption

A number of previous studies have suggested the possibility that
osteoclasts may resorb bone by secreting acid into an extracellular
acidic compartment during bone resorption (Neuman *et al.*, 1960;
Vaes, 1968; Arnett and Dempster, 1990), but direct evidence for low
pH in the resorptive hemivacuole has only been recently presented.
Baron *et al.* (1985) developed an *in vitro* system where active osteoclasts could be observed *in situ* on the endosteal surface of cultured
chick long bones. Incubation with the weak base Acridine Orange,
which is sequestered in protonated form in sealed acidic compartments, revealed large fluorescent discs associated with osteoclasts that
were considered to be extracellular due to their disappearance when
osteoclasts were removed from bone surfaces. The addition of ammonium chloride caused dissipation of the large fluorescent discs associated with osteoclasts, which rapidly reappeared after removal of the
ammonium chloride, suggesting that osteoclasts actively acidify the
extracellular hemivacuole. Similar studies by Anderson *et al.* (1986)
using osteoclasts *in situ* on mouse calvarial bone surfaces and Acridine
Orange fluorescence, found that osteoclast acidification was predict-
ably modulated by hormones and drugs known to stimulate (PGE_2,
PTH) or inhibit (CT) osteoclastic bone resorption. As will be discussed,
this paper was also the first to show inhibitory effects of Cl^-/HCO_3^-

exchange, H^+,K^+-ATPase and Na^+/H^+ antiporter inhibitors on osteoclasts. However, the most direct evidence for osteoclastic acidification of the hemivacuole, by microelectrode studies, was reported by Silver *et al.* (1988). In these elegant studies, rat and chick osteoclasts were observed *in vitro* on glass surfaces. *In vivo* studies were also performed by implanting bone fragments into transparent chambers in rabbits' ears. pH recordings from cultured osteoclast hemivacuoles showed a rapid acidification to pH 3 or less. Osteoclasts not properly attached or not resealing around the microelectrode did not form or sustain a low pH in the hemivacuole. *In vivo* measurements revealed a less acidic pH (minimum of pH 4.7, mean for 18 readings of pH 6.0) in the hemivacuole of actively resorbing osteoclasts on bone fragments, and calcium concentrations were high (mean for 18 readings of ~ 27 mM) in the same hemivacuoles. This observation led the authors to propose that protons were being consumed by the solubilization of calcium from bone mineral. An alternative explanation could be that the buffering capacity and/or the pH of extracellular fluid *in vivo* is greater than that of the culture medium. In this regard, the demonstration that reducing the pH of the culture medium to just below neutral can dramatically increase bone resorption in both the bone slice assay (Arnett and Dempster, 1986), and in organ cultures (Goldhaber and Rabadjija, 1987), is noteworthy and is reviewed in detail by Arnett and Dempster (1990).

The mechanism(s) by which osteoclasts secrete protons produced by carbonic anhydrase has been an area of intense research interest. Baron *et al.* (1985) used an antiserum raised against lysosomal membranes that cross-reacted with a 100-kDa H^+,K^+-ATPase in pig gastric mucosa, and found by immunocytochemistry that this molecule was exclusively localized at the ruffled border membrane of chick osteoclasts, indicating that this proton pump may be involved in proton transport into the hemivacuole. Further support for the use of this proton pump by osteoclasts came from inhibition studies with omeprazole, a specific and potent inhibitor of the gastric H^+,K^+-ATPase, in organ cultures (Tuukkanen and Vaananen, 1986). However, the concentrations of omeprazole (100 μM) required to significantly inhibit PGE_2 or PTH-stimulated radiocalcium release were considerably higher than those which inhibit gastric gland H^+,K^+-ATPase ($IC_{50} \sim 50$ nM; (Lindberg *et al.*, 1987). In our own experiments with omeproazole in the bone slice assay, we also found that 100 μM omeprazole was required to produce a significant inhibition of osteoclastic bone resorption (Hall and Chambers, 1990). We concluded that at such high concentrations omeprazole may be inhibiting osteoclast activity by other undefined mechanism(s), and Vaananen *et al.* (1990) detected no H^+,K^+-ATPase in rat osteoclasts by immunocytochemical staining with a monoclonal antibody specific for this proton pump.

   Studies show that two other proton transport systems may be potentially involved in osteoclastic bone resorption. Blair *et al.* (1989a) reported on a vacuolar electrogenic H^+-ATPase in chick osteoclasts that was localized to the ruffled border membrane adjacent to bone surfaces. Direct evidence for the involvement of the vacuolar proton pump in osteoclastic bone resorption was reported by Sundquist *et al.* (1990) using bafilomycin A, a macrolide antibiotic which is a relatively specific and potent inhibitor of vacuolar H^+-ATPases (Bowman *et al.*, 1988). Bafilomycin A almost totally inhibited rat osteoclastic bone resorption at a concentration of 10 nM, in the bone slice assay. The same group have also reported that antibodies to the vacuolar H^+-ATPase localize to the ruffled border membrane of both rat and avian osteoclasts (Vaananen *et al.*, 1990). During the exocytosis of vacuolar enzymes at the osteoclast ruffled border, membrane fusion of the vacuolar and ruffled border membranes during exocytosis would also result in the insertion of the H^+-ATPase proton pump into the ruffled border membrane, such that it would be oriented to extrude protons into the hemivacuole.

   Our own studies followed up the observation of Anderson *et al.* (1986) showing that amiloride, an inhibitor of the Na^+/H^+ antiporter (Moolenaar, 1986), is an inhibitor of PTH-stimulated osteoclast acidification in calvarial organ culture as determined by Acridine Orange fluorescence. We therefore tested the effects of amiloride and the more potent analogue dimethylamiloride (Vigne *et al.*, 1984), on disaggregated rat osteoclasts in the bone slice assay (Hall and Chambers, 1990). Amiloride and dimethyl amiloride both inhibited osteoclastic bone resorption in concentration-dependent fashion with IC_{50} values of 9 μM and 0.7 μM, respectively. Neither compound significantly affected osteoclast morphology or survival on bone slices at concentrations as high as 100 μM which inhibited osteoclastic bone resorption by >80%. We have also confirmed that bafilomycin A at concentrations of 10–100 nM completely inhibits osteoclastic bone resorption in the bone slice assay, and we found no evidence of overt cytotoxicity as determined by morphological examination of osteoclasts on glass cover slips (A. Gallagher, T. J. Chambers, and T. J. Hall, unpublished observations).

   It is difficult to reconcile the fact that inhibition of either the vacuolar proton pump or the Na^+/H^+ antiporter alone with selective inhibitors can result in total or near total inhibition of osteoclast bone resorption. However, in the absence of appropriate antibodies for determining membrane localization of the antiporter in osteoclasts, it is possible that the antiporter is required for "housekeeper" pH regulation at the basolateral surface of metabolically active osteoclasts attaching to bone surfaces prior to commencing proton secretion (disturbance of which function would prevent the cell from initiating bone resorption). Antiporter-mediated exchange of protons into the hemivacuole for sodium ions into osteoclasts suggests that the resorbing osteoclast would require considerable Na^+, K^+-ATPase activity in order to maintain membrane electrogenic potential, which is achieved by the energy-dependent exchange of three intracellular sodium ions for one extracellular potassium ion. Thus, it is interesting that Baron et al. (1986) have demonstrated high levels of Na^+, K^+-ATPase activity in both the apical and basolateral membranes of chick osteoclasts.

Another important question that has only recently been addressed relates to the fate of bicarbonate ions which are produced along with protons by the carbonic anhydrase-catalysed hydration of carbon dioxide. As previously described, protons are secreted into the hemivacuole at the osteoclast's apical ruffled border membrane, thus leaving the osteoclast in a potential state of intracellular alkalosis due to the remaining basic bicarbonate ions. The first indication of how osteoclasts may deal with this potential problem was reported by Anderson et al. (1986). They demonstrated that PTH stimulation of mouse osteoclast acidification, as assessed by Acridine Orange fluorescence, was inhibited in concentration-dependent fashion by 4-acetamido-4'-isocyano-stilbene-2,2'-disulfonic acid (SITS), a disulfonic stilbene derivative known to selectively inhibit the $HCO_3^- Cl^-$ or anion exchanger which is present in many cell types, including erythrocytes (Cabantchik et al., 1978), kidney tubule cells (Zeidel et al., 1986), and osteoblasts (Redhead and Baker, 1988). Teti et al. (1989b) also detected the anion exchanger in avian osteoclasts using pH-sensitive fluorescent probes to measure cytoplasmic pH changes while varying the ionic composition of the medium, and using inhibitors of the anion exchanger. Evidence that the anion exchanger is involved in osteoclastic bone resorption was reported by Klein-Nulend and Raisz (1989). Using the organ culture system it has been shown that SITS and 4,4'-diisothiocyanostilbene-2,2'-disulfonic acid (DIDS), another disulfonic stilbene derivative that inhibits the anion exchanger, both inhibited the release of radiocalcium from control and PTH-stimulated [45]Calcium-labeled foetal rat long bones. It should be noted that rat calvarial osteoblasts possess a functional anion exchanger (Redhead and Baker, 1988), so that in organ cultures, where osteoclastic bone resorption is regulated by osteoblasts, it is possible that SITS and

DIDS may be influencing bone resorption via an effect on osteoblasts as well as by a direct effect on osteoclasts. Our own studies using the bone slice assay clearly showed that DIDS directly inhibited osteoclastic bone resorption in a concentration-dependent manner (Hall and Chambers, 1989). The inhibition of bone resorption in the bone slice assay was only partial (~50% inhibition with 100 μM DIDS), as was found in control organ culture experiments treated with 100 μM DIDS (Klein-Nulend and Raisz, 1989, Fig. 1). In PTH-stimulated organ cultures, however, 100 μM DIDS inhibited radiocalcium release by ~70% and 90% at days 2 and 5 of assay, respectively (Klein-Nulend and Raisz, 1989, Fig. 2). The increased potency of DIDS inhibition in organ cultures is likely to be due to an inhibitory effect on PTH-activated osteoblasts and their stimulatory effect(s) on osteoclasts, as well as a direct effect on osteoclasts per se.

As previously described, the osteoclast is polarized when attached to bone surfaces during resorption. There is strong evidence showing that both carbonic anhydrase and the vacuolar H^+-ATPase are localized to the apical ruffled border membrane, such that protons are produced at the appropriate site for extrusion into the resorbing hemivacuole. The location of the Na^+/H^+ antiporter in osteoclasts awaits the availability of appropriate antibodies for immunolocalization studies. Kellokumpu et al. (1988) have found the anion exchanger in rat osteoclasts and, although the membrane localization was not described, it would seem likely that the anion exchanger will be found to be localized in the basolateral membrane such that the basic bicarbonate ions would be transported into the extracellular fluid (Marks and Popoff, 1988; Baron, 1989). Indeed, Blair et al. (1989b) have proposed that the basolateral exchange of bicarbonate for chloride ions is essential for proton secretion by the electrogenic vacuolar H^+-ATPase, the result being the ionically balanced, charge-coupled cosecretion of HCl into the hemivacuole.

D. ROLE OF OSTEOCLAST PROTEINASES IN BONE RESORPTION

The close correlation between bone resorption and the release of acid hydrolases in PTH-stimulated organ cultures led Vaes (1965, 1968) to propose that osteoclast-derived proteinases are involved in the resorption of the organic matrix of bone. There is now considerable evidence to support this view, and several other acid-dependent osteoclast vacuolar (lysosomal) enzymes including cathepsins and cysteine-proteinases, are also important in osteoclastic bone resorption (reviewed in Eeckhout et al., 1988; Vaes, 1988; see Section III,B). Considerable evidence exists to suggest that these proteinases are released specifically at the osteoclast apical ruffled border membrane. Ultrastructural studies show vacuolar fusion to and exocytosis into the resorbing hemivacuole at the ruffled border membrane. Vaes (1980) and Chambers *et al.* (1987) found that CT inhibits bone resorption and the release of a vacuolar acid phosphatase from osteoclasts. Baron *et al.* (1988) have used immunocytochemistry to show that osteoclast proteinases are vectorially transported from the golgi complex to the osteoclast ruffled border, where they may be released directly into the hemivacuole during bone resorption. Thus, the resorbing hemivacuole can be considered as an extracellular secondary lysosome, which carries out degradation of both the mineral and organic components of bone.

The organic matrix of bone consists primarily of type I collagen, but there is little evidence to suggest that osteoclasts produce a true collagenase that cleaves collagen into $\frac{1}{4}$ and $\frac{3}{4}$ fragments under neutral pH conditions (Blair *et al.*, 1986; Eeckhout *et al.*, 1988; Vaes, 1988). However, there are two possible mechanisms that may allow osteoclasts to degrade bone collagen. First, the low pH and high calcium concentration in the resorbing hemivacuole are conditions under which insoluble bone collagen becomes sensitive to "non-collagen-specific" proteolytic degradation (reviewed in Eeckhout *et al.*, 1988; Vaes, 1988). Second, there is evidence to suggest that a latent form of procollagenase is produced by osteoblasts during bone formation and/or during the resorptive phase of bone remodeling (Eeckhout *et al.*, 1986). This procollagenase may be activated by osteoclast proteinases in the resorbing hemivacuole, thus providing the initial cleavage of bone collagen and rendering it susceptible to further proteolysis by osteoclast acid proteinases (Eeckhout *et al.*, 1988; Vaes, 1988). Alternatively, as discussed in Section III,B (see also Vaes, 1988), it may be that osteoblast-derived collagenase is essential for the degradation of the unmineralized material that lines bone surfaces, thus allowing osteoclasts access to the mineralized bone surface in the initial stages of the bone resorption process.

The importance of osteoclast-derived proteinases in the degradation of the bone organic matrix is illustrated by the inhibitory effect of cysteine-proteinase inhibitors on osteoclastic bone resorption. In PTH-stimulated organ cultures, a carboxyalkyl peptide analogue of the collagen α-chain caused dose-dependent, reversible inhibition of bone resorption, without inhibiting the release of osteoclast vacuolar enzymes (Delaisse *et al.*, 1985). Furthermore, it was shown that cysteine-proteinase inhibitors reduced the bone resorptive activity of isolated osteoclasts cultured on dentine slices (Delaisse *et al.*, 1987).

Chambers *et al.* (1984a) and Blair *et al.* (1986) showed that osteoclasts can resorb the organic and inorganic components of bone. The biochemical and molecular mechanisms involved in osteoclastic bone resorption previously reviewed are now relatively well understood. However, the extracellular mechanism(s) involved in modulating osteoclasts during bone resorption have only recently been posed, as discussed in Section III,C.

E. ROLE OF CALCIUM IN OSTEOCLASTIC BONE RESORPTION

The extrusion of protons produced by osteoclast carbonic anhydrase into the resorptive hemivacuole by proton transport systems in the ruffled border membrane is clearly of primary importance in bone resorption, both in (1) providing an acidic environment in the hemivacuole, to enable acid hydrolases to degrade the organic components of bone, and (2) solubilizing the hydroxyapatite of bone mineral. The fate of the calcium solubilized from bone mineral and its role in regulating osteoclastic bone resorption has been the focus of considerable research interest. The effect of acid on the solubility of hydroxyapatite has been studied extensively (reviewed in Eeckhout *et al.*, 1988; Vaes, 1988; Arnett and Dempster, 1990). Direct determination of pH and calcium in resorbing hemivacuoles has been reported by Silver *et al.* (1988), as discussed in Section II,C; they found calcium concentrations between 17 and 40 mM Ca^{2+}. Functional evidence for the involvement of a Na^+/Ca^+ exchanger in osteoclastic bone resorption has been reported by Krieger and Tashjian (1980), and as discussed by Baron *et al.* (1986), the existence of the Na^+/Ca^+ exchanger in the basolateral membrane of osteoclasts could be responsible for the extrusion of calcium ions passively entering osteoclasts at the apical ruffled border membrane. Further, Akisaka *et al.* (1988) have reported on a Ca^{2+}-ATPase in chick osteoclast basolateral membranes, which may also be involved in the transcellular movement and extrusion of calcium ions from osteoclasts. There is now considerable evidence, however, to suggest that high extracellular calcium concentrations (2–20 mM), comparable to those found in resorbing hemivacuoles by Silver *et al.* (1988), can inhibit bone resorption by avian or rat osteoclasts (Malgaroli *et al.*, 1989; Zaidi *et al.*, 1989; Miyauchi *et al.*, 1990). The mechanisms involved are not entirely clear, but evidence from Miyauchi *et al.* (1990) showing that expression of the osteoclast adhesion structure, the podosome (see Section II,A), is significantly decreased in avian osteoclasts cultured on glass surfaces when exposed to 4 mM extracellular calcium, is particularly interesting. Zaidi *et al.* (1989) also showed that the inhibition of rat osteoclast bone resorption in the bone slice assay by 20 mM calcium was correlated with a decrease in enzyme release from the cells.

In the bone slice assay, disaggregated rat osteoclasts, without detectable osteoblastic influence, produce discrete resorption pits as viewed under the scanning electron microscope (Chambers *et al.*, 1984a; Chambers, 1989). However, it has been shown that osteoclasts, both *in vivo* and *in vitro* in bone cultures, where they are under the influence of osteoblasts, are motile cells that move across the surface of mineralized bone leaving tracks of resorption pits and/or trails of resorbed bone behind them (reviewed in Jones *et al.*, 1986). Thus, under physiological conditions, osteoclasts are likely to migrate during bone resorption. This infers a degree of polarization such that the high concentrations of vacuolar calcium may cause loosening of sealing zone attachment preferentially at one pole, perhaps the posterior pole of the translocating cell, so that as the osteoclast migrates across the bone surface, resorption is accompanied by the continuous or discontinuous release of calcium ions through a zone of relatively weaker attachment of the sealing zone at its posterior pole.

III. Cellular and Hormonal Regulation of Bone Resorption

A. Regulation of Osteoclast Formation

The life span of osteoclasts *in vivo* appears to be up to 2 weeks, with a half-life of around 6–10 days (Jaworski *et al.*, 1981; Loutit and Townsend, 1982; Marks and Schneider, 1982). Osteoclasts thus need to be continuously replenished for bone resorption to continue. Moreover, the rate of bone resorption *in vivo* correlates with the number of multinuclear cells: increased numbers of osteoclasts are seen in response to PTH, whereas CT administration causes a fall in osteoclast numbers (Baron and Vignery, 1981). The relationship between number and activity and the short half-life imply that regulation of osteoclast formation represents an important mechanism whereby osteoclastic function is regulated.

It has been established for 15 years through parabiosis experiments, quail-chick chimaeras, and bone marrow transplantation experiments that osteoclasts can be supplied to bone via the circulatory system, from a precursor derived ultimately from hemopoietic tissue (for reviews see Nijweide *et al.*, 1986; Marks and Popoff, 1988; Chambers, 1989). In view of the evidence that not only hemopoietic cells but elements of the stroma of hemopoietic tissue can be transplanted and can reach bone through the blood stream, the osteoclasts may have derived from hemopoietic cells, cells of the bone marrow stroma, or from some other unidentified precursor of hemopoietic tissue (Loutit and Nisbet, 1982; Chambers, 1989). Experiments in which limb rudiments were cocultured with hemopoietic cells showed that the cells that led to osteoclast formation in the rudiment exist in greatest number in the fraction that also contains the greatest number of hemopoietic stem cells (Scheven *et al.,* 1986). The hemopoietic stem cell indeed appeared responsible for osteoclast formation in the rudiment upon induction of osteoclast formation by coculture of rudiments with a single hemopoietic stem cell (Hagenaars *et al.,* 1989). The same conclusion was reached in experiments wherein a hemopoietic cell line was induced to form osteoclasts when incubated on bone marrow stromal cells (Hattersley and Chambers, 1989c). Since osteoclast formation was induced in the hemopoietic cell line even when nonvital stromal cells were used, these experiments additionally demonstrated that stromal cells induce osteoclasts in hemopoietic cells, rather than the converse.

Circumstantial evidence and phenotypic similarities, still being identified, quickly established the mononuclear phagocyte lineage as the favored candidate for osteoclast precursor (Loutit and Nisbet, 1979). Comparison of osteoclasts properties, however, with those of mononuclear phagocytes, also reveals significant distinctions between the two cell types. Osteoclasts lack many characteristics shared by all mononuclear phagocytes, yet possess properties lacking in mononuclear phagocytes, most notably CT receptors and the ability to excavate bone. The lineage of the osteoclast remains a highly controversial topic. The main possibilities are: that osteoclasts derive from induction of osteoclastic characteristics in relatively mature mononuclear phagocytes (monocytes or macrophages); that the osteoclast lineage represents a branch from the mononuclear phagocyte lineage at some earlier stage; or that the osteoclast is analogous to lineages such as erythroid or eosinophil in its lineage, and quite distinct from the mononuclear phagocyte lineage. Our conclusion in a review (Chambers, 1989), wherein the then available evidence was discussed in greater detail favored an origin for osteoclasts distinct from the mononuclear phagocyte series, because the phenotypic differences were so extensive as to make it unlikely for osteoclasts to develop from a cell already differentiated significantly toward the mononuclear phagocyte lineage. Moreover, attempts to induce osteoclastic differentiation from macrophages had failed. In this chapter we will discuss only more recent work.

Experimental systems have been developed wherein osteoclast-like cells are induced to differentiate *in vitro* from the hemopoietic tissue of several species. Work predominantly in human systems initially used multinuclearity as the criterion for osteoclasts, but other parameters more distinctive for osteoclasts *in vivo* are now utilized, including tartrate-resistant acid phosphatase (TRAP), CT-induced cytoplasmic retraction, osteoclast-specific monoclonal antibodies, bone resorption (MacDonald *et al.*, 1986, 1987; Chenu *et al.*, 1988; Hughes *et al.*, 1989; Kukita *et al.*, 1989; Kukita and Roodman, 1989; Takahashi *et al.*, 1989; Chenu *et al.*, 1990; Kukita *et al.*, 1990a,b; Kurihara *et al.*, 1990a,b; Thavarajah *et al.*, 1990), and most recently, CT receptor autoradiography (Kurihara *et al.*, 1990c).

In sections of normal bone, osteoclasts are distinguished from other cells by multinuclearity and TRAP-positivity (Burstone, 1958; Kaye, 1984). It seemed reasonable to use these characteristics as markers for osteoclasts *in vitro*. There is, however, no doubt that macrophages too can become multinuclear and TRAP-positive *in vivo* and *in vitro*, in circumstances that seem to have little to do with osteoclast formation (Yan *et al.*, 1972; Ketcham *et al.*, 1985; Snipes *et al.*, 1986; Bianco *et al.*, 1987; Hattersley and Chambers, 1989b). The question thus arises, whether the TRAP-positive multinuclear cells that develop in human bone marrow cultures are macrophage giant cells or osteoclasts. The scanty bone resorption seen in such cultures suggests the former. Bone slices *in vitro* are resolved at the rate of 10^{-3}–10^{-4} μm^2 per cell per day by freshly isolated human or murine osteoclasts, and per CT-receptor-positive cell in murine hemopoietic cultures (McSheehy and Chambers, 1986a, 1987; Hattersley and Chambers, 1989a). If the multinuclear TRAP-positive cells were mature in osteoclastic function, we should expect to see extensive resorption of the surface of the bone slices in the cultures. Yet the published photographs (Takahashi *et al.*, 1989; Kukita *et al.*, 1990b; Kurihara *et al.*, 1990b) suggest that resorption in such cultures is very slight. Consistent with this, we found that, despite the presence of many multinuclear cells, in only 9 out of 64 experiments was bone resorption seen, and then only in small amounts on a minority of bone slices (Flanagan *et al.*, 1991). This scanty resorption could be interpreted to mean that the multinuclear cells were: (1) immature osteoclasts; (2) in an environment suboptimal for resorption; or (3) represented the activity of a distinct, very rare subpopulation of mono- or multinuclear cells in these cultures.

The multinuclear cells in human bone marrow cultures show minor changes in shape in response to high concentrations of CT, but macrophages respond to high concentrations of CT and CGRP (Nong *et al.*, 1989), and the response of the bone marrow multinuclear cells was not characteristic of the osteoclastic response to CT seen in the rat (Flanagan *et al.*, 1991). There are no reports of CT-responses in human bone marrow multinuclear cells resembling that of rat osteoclasts. We also found, like others, that putatively osteoclast-specific monoclonal antibodies bind to multinuclear cells. The binding was, however, considerably weaker than that of freshly isolated osteoclasts, and as in published photographs, was of perinuclear distribution, in contrast to the peripheral, membrane distribution we found previously (Horton *et al.*, 1985). We found that the antigenic phenotype of the multinuclear cells was characteristic of macrophage polykaryons, and unlike that of osteoclasts. We believe that the osteoclast-like cells in human bone marrow cultures are yet to be proven osteoclastic in nature by the characteristics of CT responsiveness, bone resorption, and antigenic phenotype. Like osteoclasts, however, these cells are multinuclear and TRAP-positive. Opinion about the nature of these cells remains a matter of perspective. Were osteoclasts to derive from the mononuclear phagocyte lineage, development in macrophages of certain osteoclast characteristics such as multinuclearity and TRAP, even though found in some extraskeletal systems, could be taken to represent differentiation toward osteoclasts. On the other hand, the multinuclear cells continue to express typical macrophage characteristics foreign to osteoclasts, do not evidence convincing resorptive function, CT receptor expression, CT responsiveness, or reactivity with osteoclast-specific antibodies. These observations are more consistent with distinct lineages. That the multinuclear cells are macrophagic rather than osteoclastic is supported further by the observation that granulocyte macrophage-colony stimulating factor (GM-CSF) and macrophage CSF, both of which stimulate macrophage formation and function, also stimulate multinucleate giant cell formation in human bone marrow cultures (MacDonald *et al.*, 1986), but inhibit osteoclast formation in cultures of murine bone marrow cells (Hattersley and Chambers, 1990a; Shinar *et al.*, 1990). Analogously, prostaglandins (PGs) inhibit multinuclear cell formation in the human system (Chenu *et al.*, 1990), but stimulate murine osteoclast formation (Akatsu *et al.*, 1989; Collins and Chambers, 1991).

It is possible that these differences may be due to species, to differences in culture conditions, or (less likely) to differences in responsiveness. Certainly species differences do exist, but these favor the thesis that the multinuclear cells are likely to be macrophagic; in human bone marrow cultures, progress toward macrophages is the dominant outcome (Moore et al., 1980). Long-term maintenance of pro-liferation and differentiation of hemopoietic stem cells into neu-trophils and other hemopoietic cells is not maintained in the manner observed in murine bone marrow under the same conditions of culture. This species difference seems to extend to osteoclast formation: os-teoclast formation (bone resorption) is rare in human, intermediate in rabbit (Fuller and Chambers, 1987), and extensive in the murine sys-tem (Hattersley and Chambers, 1989a).

Induction of osteoclastic differentiation from hemopoietic precur-sors depends upon a stromal cell type found in bone marrow but not in the spleen (Takahashi et al., 1988; Udagawa et al., 1989; Hattersley and Chambers, 1990b). Differentiation is not induced in hemopoietic cells physically separated from stroma, but proceeds in cells in contact with stroma (Takahashi et al., 1988), even if the stromal cells are devitalized (Hattersley and Chambers, 1989c). This suggests that os-teoclast induction is mediated by a contact-dependent interaction. A similar mechanism is evident in other hemopoietic cells in liquid culture (Roberts et al., 1987; Kodama et al., 1991a). For other lineages, investigators have identified CSFs that are necessary for the survival, proliferation, and differentiation of hemopoietic cells (Metcalf, 1988). Such factors have been difficult to identify in the fluid phase of liquid bone marrow cultures, despite hemopoiesis in such cultures, but can be eluted from the bone marrow stromal cells (Gordon et al., 1987; Roberts et al., 1988). It is possible that hemopoiesis proceeds despite a general deficiency in CSFs putatively necessary for the process by virtue of cytokines bound to the matrix/surface of stromal cells that support hemopoiesis through contact interactions. We have attempted to extract potentially osteoclast-inductive cytokines from bone marrow stromal cells and stromal cell lines by elution or heparitinase treat-ment. Although CSFs for other lineages (including macrophages) are found in the eluates, such fractions do not induce osteoclast formation in hemopoietic spleen cell cultures (G. Hattersly and T. J. Chambers, unpublished observations).

We do not know the nature of the osteoclast-inducing stromal cell found in bone marrow but not in spleen. An osteoblastic origin is possible (Takahashi et al., 1988), but cell lines of known osteoblastic phenotype do not induce osteoclasts (Udagawa et al., 1989; Hattersley and Chambers, 1990b). Moreover, the stromal cell lines we have devel-oped that do induce osteoclast formation do not stimulate bone resorp-tion when cocultured with mature osteoclasts plus PTH (A. Gallagher, G. Hattersly, and T. J. Chambers, unpublished observations). This sug-gests that osteoclast induction and osteoclast stimulation may be effected via distinct processes. The differentiation potential of at least one of the stromal cell lines that induces osteoclasts (ST2 cells) (Udagawa *et al.,* 1989) is known to include that of osteoblasts, but such cells can differentiate into other phenotypes, including cartilage, fat and muscle (Ashton *et al.,* 1980; Owen, 1985; Grigoriadis *et al.,* 1988), and the phenotype of the ST2 cells during osteoclast induction is uncertain.

Osteoclast-inductive cell lines have been used to identify osteoclast precursors (Udagawa *et al.,* 1990). Alveolar macrophages, peritoneal macrophages, and monocytes formed macrophage colonies, 80% of which were reported to contain CT receptors when incubated on ST2-cell monolayers. Excavation of bone was also found. Moreover, unpublished data was cited in which macrophage colonies, induced in semisolid medium in M-CSF, similarly showed osteoclastic differentiation when incubated on ST2 cells. If this can be confirmed, it represents convincing evidence that osteoclasts derive from the mononuclear phagocyte series, and not merely from immature precursors but from mature cells.

We have performed similar experiments (J. Kerby and T. J. Chambers, unpublished results, 1991), using ST2 cells, and also a bone marrow stromal cell line we developed expressly for its capacity to induce osteoclasts. We were unable to induce osteoclastic differentiation in alveolar or peritoneal macrophages, or in macrophage colonies formed in semisolid medium in the presence of M-CSF and transferred to stromal cell monolayers. We have also incubated single colony-forming cells (derived from blast-cell colonies) on the stromal monolayers and found that CT receptors were not a feature of macrophage colonies, nor of granulocyte-macrophage colonies, but were found in multilineage colonies. This discrepancy is difficult to explain. Our results are consistent with those of Scheven *et al.* (1986) who found that osteoclast-forming cells copurified with hemopoietic stem cells; and with transplantation experiments wherein macrophages and macrophage colony-forming cells did not correct the osteoclast deficiency of one type of osteopetrosis, a type that is cured by bone marrow transplantation (Schneider and Byrnes, 1983; Schneider and Relfson, 1988). The results of Udagawa *et al.* (1990) are, however, consistent with work on the *op/op* mouse.

Osteopetrosis in the *op/op* mouse reflects an osteoclast deficiency (Marks and Lane, 1976) that cannot be cured by transplantation of normal bone marrow cells (Wiktor-Jedrzejczak *et al.,* 1982; Marks *et al.,* 1984). It has been known for some time that macrophage numbers are also low, probably due to deficient M-CSF production (Wiktor-Jedrzejczak *et al.,* 1982). M-CSF has been shown absent (Wiktor-

Jedrzejczak *et al.*, 1990; Felix *et al.*, 1990b) due to a mutation in the M-CSF gene, wherein a stop codon has been inserted early in the coding region (Yoshida *et al.*, 1990). Cure of the osteoclast defect has been achieved by M-CSF administration *in vivo* (Felix *et al.*, 1990a; Kodama *et al.*, 1991b). Cure of the bone disease required large amounts of M-CSF (Felix *et al.*, 1990a), but this may be due to the very short half-life (10 min) of M-CSF *in vivo* (Bartocci *et al.*, 1987).

The mononuclear phagocyte series is the only previously described target for M-CSF (except macrophage-like placental cells; Pollard *et al.*, 1987; Regenstreif and Rossant, 1989). The findings in the *op/op* mouse thus closely relate the ontogeny of the osteoclast to that of mononuclear phagocytes. A plausible model would be that osteoclasts derive from mononuclear phagocytes, presumably in response to some osteoclast-specific inductive signal, and that M-CSF is necessary to provide the precursors for this process. Our experience with osteoclast induction from mononuclear phagocytic precursors *in vitro* suggests that if such exists, osteoclasts must branch from the mononuclear phagocyte series at a very early stage, before commitment to macrophage colony formation. This is consistent with the expression of M-CSF receptors on primitive hemopoietic cells before commitment to the mononuclear phagocyte series (Metcalf, 1988).

Another possibility is that mononuclear phagocytes may be required as accessory cells for osteoclast formation. Although it has been suggested that bone marrow macrophages may play an essential role in hemopoiesis (Crocker and Gordon, 1985), hemopoiesis for cells other than the osteoclast is essentially normal in the *op/op* mouse (Wiktor-Jedrzejczak *et al.*, 1982), so that if there were such a requirement for macrophages as accessory cells in hemopoiesis, it is unique to osteoclastopoiesis. It is difficult to see a biological advantage to such a role for macrophages in osteoclast formation.

It is not likely that a single cytokine by itself accounts for the differentiation of two such phenotypically different cells. M-CSF promotes macrophage formation in semisolid medium. Osteoclasts are not formed under these circumstances as previously discussed. Presumably, a second signal is needed for osteoclast formation. The contact-dependent nature of osteoclast formation suggests that hemopoietic cells bearing M-CSF receptors require M-CSF together with a second factor that is provided by contact with bone marrow stromal cells, for differentiation into osteoclasts. This is supported by the observation that in liquid marrow cultures from normal mice, in which endogenous M-CSF is sufficient for osteoclast and macrophage formation, exogenous M-CSF increases macrophage but inhibits osteoclast formation (Hattersley and Chambers, 1990a; Shinar *et al.*, 1990). This result is consistent with the existence of a shared precursor, in which M-CSF, in competition with the osteoclast-inductive microenvironment, induces macrophage differentiation. Although both lineages commence with an M-CSF-dependent differentiation step, M-CSF appears to be essentially a macrophage-inductive cytokine.

B. INDUCTION OF BONE RESORPTION

Osteoclast progenitors are seeded into bone from the circulation during development. When these progenitors first arrive in the periosteum they are still proliferative and highly radiosensitive. They are at this stage CT-receptor- and TRAP-negative, but differentiate into postmitotic TRAP-negative cells, which then become TRAP-positive and, simultaneously or soon thereafter, CT-receptor-positive (see Nijweide et al., 1986; Marks and Popoff, 1988, for reviews; see also Taylor et al., 1989). It is known that osteoclasts can also be supplied from hematogenous precursors in later life, if osteoclasts are abnormally deficient, as found in osteopetrosis or after irradiation. It is not known, however, whether hematogenous supply represents normal physiology. It may be that hemopoietic tissue supplies a radiosensitive osteoclast stem cell to bone surfaces during development, that becomes dedicated to osteoclast production and sustains osteoclast number independent of either hemopoiesis or continued vascular supply. Alternatively, there may be continued recruitment of osteoclastic precursors through the vascular system, an embryonic characteristic, throughout life. In either case, these considerations suggest that a population of osteoclast precursors exists on bone surfaces that is capable of proliferation, but occult, since it consists of TRAP-negative, CT-receptor-negative mononuclear cells: the earliest precursor recognizable by morphological criteria is already TRAP-positive (Scott, 1967).

As discussed more fully elsewhere (Chambers, 1980), for the osteoclast, essentially a wandering cell derived form hematogenous precursors, to achieve the complex and dynamic patterns of localization that enable skeletal morphogenesis and restructuring, suggests that its localization is assisted by resident bone cells (osteocytes, bone-lining cells, and other cells of the osteoblastic lineage). Thus, osteoclastic precursors, whether already resident on bone surfaces or emigrating from the blood stream, are likely to be guided to resorptive sites and induced to mature by osteoblastic cells. Constituents of bone matrix, such as osteocalcin or type I collagen peptides are chemotactic for monocytes (Mundy et al., 1978; Malone et al., 1982; Mundy and Poser, 1983), but it is not known whether they are also chemotactic for preosteoclasts. Osteocalcin-deficient bone particles implanted sub-cutaneously are also less efficient than normal bone particles as re-cruiters of multinuclear cells, that resorb these particles (Lian *et al.*, 1984). Whether these multinucleate giant cells that surround the par-ticles are bonafide osteoclasts, however, is controversial. Although these cells apparently display several osteoclastic characteristics (Glowacki and Cox, 1986; Glowacki *et al.*, 1986; Goldring *et al.*, 1988; Peignoux-Deville *et al.*, 1989), such observations are not uniformly reproducible (Popoff and Marks, 1986; Walters and Schneider, 1987, 1988; Bagi and Miller, 1989; Peignoux-Deville *et al.*, 1989). Moreover, such cells lack at least some osteoclast-specific antigens and their mode of bone resorption seems to differ from that of osteoclasts (Popoff and Marks, 1986; Marks and Chambers, 1991).

Because factors that activate cells are often chemotactic if presented as a gradient, and because induction of osteoclastic differentiation and activation appears to be contact-dependent (see above and later), it is tempting to imagine that activation signals are emitted by bone-lining cells at a site deemed appropriate for resorption, and that these bind as a gradient to the surface of adjacent bone-lining cells/ECM, to produce a relatively stable solid-phase chemotactic gradient that could serve to guide precursors to the site and induce activation on arrival. It also seems likely, by analogy with interactions between cells in similar systems (e.g., endothelial cells and inflammatory cells) that bone-lin-ing cells modulate expression of osteoclastic adhesion molecules in a manner appropriate for osteoclast localization. Adhesion systems may exist that enable osteoclast migration, and the close adhesion needed in hemivacuole formation. Like other migratory cells, the osteoclast expresses tissue plasminogen activator (Grills *et al.*, 1990), which may facilitate migration through endothelium and over bone surfaces.

Once induced to a site appropriate for resorption, osteoblastic cells (most likely bone-lining cells) may initiate resorptive behavior in os-teoclasts via exposure of the mineral phase. Implantation of inorganic materials such as hydroxyapatite crystals into tissues evokes a mac-rophage foreign body response, leading to sequestration or dissolution of the implanted material (see Chambers, 1978). Presumably, there-fore, bone has evolved some means of protecting bone mineral from phagocytic attack. This protective mechanism is probably extra-cellular because upon death of bone-lining cells (as in osteonecrosis), bone does not evoke a foreign body response (Glimcher and Kenzora, 1979; Ham and Harris, 1972). The factor may well be the un-mineralized layer of organic material that is observed lining bone surfaces (Raina, 1972; Fornasier, 1980; Vanderwiel, 1980). Then, when bone resorption is required, bone-lining cells may remove the organic protective material, and induce exposure of mineral to contact with the specialized digestive cells of bone, the osteoclasts (Chambers, 1980).

We tested this hypothesis by using devitalized slices of cortical bone. Because these slices are sections of bone, mineral is exposed on the cut surface. Such slices, lacking the unmineralized organic covering resident on native surfaces, are spontaneously resorbed by osteoclasts *in vitro*. If, however, bone mineral is removed, resorption does not proceed (Chambers *et al.*, 1984b).

The hypothesis was also tested using native bone surfaces. Preexisting cells were removed from calvariae of adult rats, and osteoclasts were incubated on the endocranial surface. We found that osteoclasts did not excavate this (unmineralized surface), but did so if the unmineralized organic surface was first removed by collagenase (Chambers *et al.*, 1985b; Chambers and Fuller, 1985). Since osteoclasts are clearly capable of destruction of both inorganic and organic components of bone (Chambers *et al.*, 1984b) this indicates that contact with bone mineral induces osteoclasts to resorptive activity, while unmineralized organic material does not. We also found, consistent with the hypothesis, that osteoblasts are able to remove the surface layer of unmineralized organic material *in vitro*, in response to PTH, and expose underlying bone mineral. Bone so modified displays increased susceptibility to osteoclastic resorption, and this susceptibility is abrogated by demineralization (Chambers and Fuller, 1985).

Do these experimental results reflect physiological processes? Removal of organic material by osteoblasts took the unphysiological time of several days. For practical reasons we used a bone surface on which the unmineralized layer was approximately 10 μm deep (osteoid). It is likely that bone resorption *in vivo* is generally initiated on bone surfaces upon which bone formation has long since ceased. On such (resting) surfaces, the unmineralized organic layer is only a few hundred nanometers thick, and if bone-lining cells remove this at a similar rate to that we observed *in vitro*, mineral exposure could be effected in a relatively short time. The results are consistent with the events observed preceding resorption *in vivo*, where previously covered mineral becomes exposed onto the bone surface just before osteoclasts appear at the same site (Van Tran *et al.*, 1982). However, in the latter experiments, no assessment was made of the relative contributions to mineral exposure of surface digestion and continued mineralization.

The model [that mineral is protected from contact with osteoclasts (and mononuclear phagocytes) by unmineralized organic material, and that bone-lining cells initiate and localize osteoclastic resorption by localized neutral protease activity, which exposes mineral onto the bone surface and activates resorptive behavior in osteoclasts] enables a new interpretation of the significance of neutral protease release by osteoblastic cells. Osteoblastic cells produce collagenase and tissue plasminogen activator *in vitro,* and secrete increased amounts of these neutral proteases, and decreased amounts of protease inhibitor in the presence of PTH and other bone resorbing hormones (Hamilton *et al.,* 1984; Heath *et al.,* 1984; Sakamoto and Sakamoto, 1984; Thomson *et al.,* 1987a; Shen *et al.,* 1988; Pfeilschifter *et al.,* 1990). Collagenase production has not been detected in human bone cells *in vitro* (Rifas *et al.,* 1989). However, human bone cell systems do not reproduce *in vivo* behavior *in vitro,* as judged by bone formation, and osteoclast formation, as convincingly as rodent systems. Nevertheless, the cells do produce the neutral proteases gelatinase and tissue plasminogen activator *in vitro.* Collagenase has been identified in bone-lining cells *in situ* in circumstances of increased bone resorption, and synthesis in bone is increased by exposure to a resorptive stimulus (Sakamoto and Sakamoto, 1985; Eeckhout *et al.,* 1986; Delaisse *et al.,* 1988). This may suggest a role for collagenase-secreting cells as accessory cells in bone resorption (accessory cells remove collagen, osteoclasts digest mineral; Sakamoto and Sakamoto, 1985). However, even if, as is likely, collagenase is absent from osteoclasts (Blair *et al.,* 1986; Sakamoto and Sakamoto, 1986), it is not required by them for collagen digestion, since osteoclasts resorb both organic and inorganic components of bone (Chambers *et al.,* 1984a). Acid protease (cathepsin) release correlates with ^{45}Ca release in organ culture, and cysteine protease (including cathepsin) inhibitors inhibit bone resorption (Delaisse *et al.,* 1984): osteoclasts are likely to digest organic matrix through acid hydrolase secretion (see Section II,D).

A second possible explanation for osteoblastic neutral protease secretion is that these cells act as alternative bone resorptive cells. However, we found osteoblasts removed only the organic surface layer, and exposed but did not detectably resorb the underlying mineral. Also, there is neither ^{45}Ca release nor bone resorption in response to PTH in osteopetrotic mice with defective osteoclasts (Jilka and Hamilton, 1985).

Several observations support a role for osteoblastic neutral protease as the mechanism by which osteoclasts are induced to resorptive activity. According to this model, there are two distinct processes: osteoblastic neutral protease digestion of the organic layer, preceding and enabling acid hydrolytic resorption of bone. Inhibition or incompetence of the latter process, due to acetazolamide, CT, bisphosphonate, or in osteopetrosis, does not affect collagenase release and uncalcified collagen digestion in response to PTH (Jilka and Cohn, 1983; Jilka and Hamilton, 1985; Eeckhout *et al.*, 1986; Delaisse *et al.*, 1988), but there is failure to degrade mineralized tissue. On the other hand, digestion of unmineralized collagen in bone organ cultures is inhibited by a synthetic collagenase inhibitor (Delaisse *et al.*, 1985, 1988). Thus, neutral protease secretion when osteoclasts are inactive indeed accounts for digestion of unmineralized collagen, but cannot by itself account for bone resorption. Osteoclastic resorption seems dependent on this neutral protease secretion: collagenase and products of collagen digestion are detected before [45]Ca release (Sakamoto and Sakamoto, 1985); inhibition of collagenase by anticollagenase antibody (Sakamoto and Sakamoto, 1984), cartilage derived anticollagenase factor (Horton *et al.*, 1978), or a synthetic collagenase inhibitor (Delaisse *et al.*, 1985) inhibits PTH-stimulation of [45]Ca release in organ culture. Inhibition is not complete, but increases with time (Horton *et al.*, 1978); the explanation may be that osteoclasts already in contact with mineral continue to resorb, but there is inhibition of induction of osteoclasts to new resorptive sites in response to the hormone.

The model is consistent with the well-recognized preference of osteoclasts for the resorption of mineralized bone rather than osteoid *in vivo,* which is especially striking in osteomalacia. Although the surface of osteoid does not induce resorption, resorption has been reported to be induced by cut sections of osteoid (Jones *et al.*, 1985), presumably due to the nodules of early mineralization that exist between the bone surface and the mineral front. Osteoclasts do not resorb bone from which mineral has been completely removed (Chambers *et al.*, 1984b).

The model is based on the assumption that bone surfaces are lined by a layer of unmineralized material. This is indisputedly present, as osteoid, on bone-formative surfaces; the general consensus is that unmineralized material persists, after bone formation and mineralization has been completed, on resting surfaces (Raina, 1972; Fornasier, 1977; Vanderwiel, 1980). This view has been challenged, on the basis that resting bone surfaces appear similar whether or not they had been treated to remove organic material (Boyde and Hobdell, 1969; Boyde, 1972). If this be so, neutral proteases will not be required in the adult, where the majority of bone surfaces are resting, to enable osteoclastic access to bone mineral. Thus, much of the data cited previously concerning neutral protease secretion may reflect a requirement for collagenase that is special to the rapidly growing, incompletely mineralized bone used in those experiments. The observations may not reflect bone physiology in the adult organism, in which resorption generally occurs on resting surfaces.

Chow and Chambers (1991), therefore, undertook a formal scanning electron microscopical (SEM) study to assess the prevalence of unmineralized organic material on the endosteal surface of adult human rib, in which 85% of the bone surface was resting as assessed by light microscopy. Cells were removed from the bone surface; a total of 1200 SEM photographs were then taken. Organic material was then removed from the specimen by NaOCl, and the same surfaces were inspected again. When the appearances were compared with those of the photographs taken previously, in only three photographs could areas be identified in which the bone surface was not altered by removal of organic material from the specimen, a proportion entirely consistent with the model discussed earlier in this section, in which we would anticipate that such areas would occasionally exist. However, it is known that, superficial to the surface collagen fibers that are easily recognizable after dehydration for SEM, is a layer of glycosaminoglycans (GAGs) (Fornasier, 1977; Vanderwiel, 1980; Miller et al., 1989), constituting the most superficial component of the endosteal membrane, immediately subjacent to the bone-lining cells (Miller et al., 1980; Miller and Jee, 1987). Such molecules decrease dramatically in size with dehydration, and have not been noted in SEM observations of the bone surface. Collagen fibers are clearly seen on the surface despite submersion in these GAGs; thus, the GAGs, at least, on the bone surface are not mineralized. It is also noteworthy that resting bone surfaces show a special, electron-dense layer of organic material, the lamina limitans, a structure associated with cessation of mineralization (Scherft, 1972; Luk et al., 1974). This structure is absent from surfaces where mineral is extending (Luk et al., 1974), and may represent deposition of material that terminates calcification. Alternatively, material of resting bone surfaces may be of a special constitution less prone to mineralization than is osteoid, and may be laid down by osteoblasts at the termination of bone formation. Such an alternative is consistent with the existence of the endosteal membrane, between the lamina limitans and cells on the bone surface, which differs ultrastructurally from osteoid (Miller et al., 1980; Parfitt, 1984; Miller and Jee, 1987). Both of these possibilities suggest that the nature of the material secreted by osteoblasts may change immediately before cessation of bone formation. It would clearly be of interest to identify the cell products associated with this change of behavior, both for an understanding of the mechanism by which calcification is inhibited, and also as markers for the environmental stimuli that determine cessation of bone formation by osteoblastic cells.

Because the composition of bone-forming surfaces differs from that of resting surfaces, the conclusion that osteoclasts do not resorb osteoid cannot necessarily be extended to resting surfaces. For example, it is conceivable that such surfaces may, either in general or in the particular areas appropriate for resorption, possess adhesion or other molecules that are not found in osteoid that induce bone resorptive (acid hydrolytic) or neutral protease (tissue plasminogen activator) activity in osteoclasts, either of which may be sufficient to enable osteoclastic access to underlying mineral. Nevertheless, the hypothesis that neutral protease release by osteoblastic cells in response to bone resorbing hormones is a mechanism whereby osteoblasts localize and induce osteoclastic resorption, remains consistent with the available data.

C. MODULATION OF RESORPTIVE ACTIVITY

The same reasoning applicable to regulation of bone resorption by the osteoblastic lineage makes it likely that osteoblastic cells can modulate the activity of osteoclasts already actively engaged in bone resorption. Much of our current information on the regulation of bone resorption derives from studies using organ culture. While this is an effective means to identify the direct effect of a systemic hormone on bone, the many cellular interactions possible in organ culture make resolution of the mechanism difficult. We therefore developed methods whereby osteoclasts could be disaggregated from other bone cells, and dispersed at sufficiently low density that indirect actions were minimized. The hormonal responsiveness of such populations could then be compared with or without influence by other bone cells.

Osteoclasts appear to respond directly to CT. In time-lapse video recordings, osteoclasts, widely dispersed from other cells, respond to CT with complete cessation of cytoplasmic motility within 1 minute, thereafter showing gradual retraction of pseudopods (Chambers and Magnus, 1982). This effect is highly sensitive, prolonged, and appears at concentrations of CT as low as $3 \times 10^{-12} M$ (Chambers and Moore, 1983). This response is specific with no effect on macrophages or macrophage polykaryons. Calcitonin also inhibits bone resorption by isolated mammalian osteoclasts (Chambers et al., 1985a; Arnett and Dempster, 1987). A direct effect on osteoclasts is consistent with the detection of CT receptors on osteoclasts (Warshawsky et al., 1980; Rao et al., 1981; Nicholson et al., 1986a). These CT effects on osteoclasts, as in other target cells, are probably mediated by cyclic AMP (cAMP), since CT causes a dose-dependent rise in cAMP in osteoclasts (Nicholson et al., 1986b; Rifkin et al., 1988). Moreover, either dibutryl cAMP or forskolin, which increases cAMP by stimulating adenyl cyclase, induce changes in motility, shape, TRAP secretion, and bone resorption of isolated osteoclasts identical to those induced by CT (Chambers *et al.*, 1987; Nicholson *et al.*, 1988; Ransjö *et al.*, 1988; Murrills and Dempster, 1990). Increased intracellular calcium by CT may also be involved in signal transduction (see Section II). Calcitonin gene-related peptide and amylin display similar actions on osteoclasts at 1000 and 30 × higher concentrations, respectively (Zaidi *et al.*, 1987, 1990), probably as partial agonists of the CT receptor.

Isolated chicken osteoclasts seem to differ from mammalian osteoclasts, with bone resorption not being affected by CT (Arnett and Dempster, 1987; Murrills and Dempster, 1990), and no CT receptors demonstrable (Nicholson *et al.*, 1987). If, however, chickens are fed a low-calcium diet for 2 weeks before osteoclast isolation, CT receptors and responsiveness, including inhibition of bone resorption, can be detected, albeit at high CT concentrations (de Vernejoule *et al.*, 1988; Eliam *et al.*, 1988; Hunter *et al.*, 1988).

Parathyroid hormone stimulates bone resorption *in vivo* and in organ culture, but does not affect isolated osteoclasts in any of the assays wherein osteoclasts display the characteristically dramatic responses to CT. Parathyroid hormone does not affect osteoclastic motility or cell spreading (Chambers *et al.*, 1984c), TRAP release (Chambers *et al.*, 1987), cAMP production (Nicholson *et al.*, 1986b), or bone resorption (Chambers *et al.*, 1985a; de Vernejoul *et al.*, 1988; Nicholson *et al.*, 1989). This suggests that the preparations of osteoclasts are deficient in some cell type that mediates the PTH-responsiveness of bone. This deficiency can be restored by incubation of osteoclasts with osteoblastic cell lines, or primary cultures of osteoblastic cells (McSheehy and Chambers, 1986a; Nicholson *et al.*, 1989). Such cocultures respond to concentrations as low as 10^{-4} IU/ml of PTH, close to the physiological range, with increases in bone resorption of 2- to 4-fold. These observations are consistent with the well-documented PTH receptors found on osteoblasts and the characteristic responsiveness of these cells to PTH (Chambers, 1980; Rodan and Martin, 1981), whereas most (O'Grady and Cameron, 1971; Silve *et al.*, 1982; Rouleau *et al.*, 1986) but not all (Rao *et al.*, 1983) investigators detect no PTH receptors on osteoclasts.

Osteoblastic cells upon incubation with bone-resorbing hormones may release, into culture supernatants, osteoclast resorption-stimulating activity (ORSA) which directly stimulates resorption by osteoclasts disaggregated from bone (McSheehy and Chambers, 1986b, 1987; Thomson *et al.*, 1987b; Nicholson *et al.*, 1989). However, such activity is not always detectable in culture supernatants (Chambers, 1982; Chambers *et al.*, 1984c; Thomson *et al.*, 1986), even when taken from hormone-responsive cocultures of osteoblastic cells with osteoclasts (K. Fuller and T. J. Chambers, unpublished observations). Moreover, the activity is found only at high concentrations 50% or more of conditioned media; further dilution leads to loss of activity (K. Fuller and T. J. Chambers, unpublished observations). The low levels of ORSA release suggested by these observations, especially coupled with the tedious and poorly productive nature of the bone slice assay, have proved a major impediment to its identification.

The release of hemopoietic cell growth factors by liquid cultures of bone marrow cells may represent an analogous situation. Under circumstances where supernatants show no detectable growth factor activity, cytokine is found bound to GAGs of the ECM produced in culture by the bone marrow stromal cells (Gordon et al., 1987; Roberts et al., 1988). Only when the binding sites in the stroma become saturated does the cytokine become detectable in the culture supernatant (Heard et al., 1982; Gualtieri et al., 1984; Lipschitz et al., 1987). GAGs show a high affinity for a number of other growth factors of manifold biological activity (Gospodarowicz et al., 1984; Maciag et al., 1984; Schreiber et al., 1985; Hauschka et al., 1986). The retention of ORSA by GAGs or other ECM components produced by osteoblasts (Rodan and Rodan, 1984; Ecarot-Charrier and Broekhuyse, 1987) would explain why stimulation of bone resorption is reproducibly seen in cocultures of osteoclasts and osteoblasts, but not often detected in incubations of osteoclasts with osteoblast-conditioned medium.

In addition to the ionic interactions that bind some cytokines to GAGs as previously mentioned, cytokines may be bound to the cells or matrix that line bone surfaces through lectin-like interactions (Springer and Lasky, 1991), or may be integral cell membrane proteins (see, e.g., Brachmann et al., 1989; Nishihara et al., 1989; Wong et al., 1989). These three types of interaction represent a hierarchy encompassing increasing dependence upon close contact for interaction, and increasing potential for control over cytokine localization. Either cytokine or ECM may be bound to lectin-like, and the degree of specificity in such interactions may enable a cell or group of cells that emits such a factor to establish a gradient of the factor on the surface of emitting and adjacent cells. The requirement for a binding partner would allow the gradient to be limited to those cells in a sheet that express the partner, with binding proportional to factor-concentration and partner-density. Such a system might enable complex domains and gradients of ORSA to be established on the bone surface, and would seem to be well suited to the regulation of the migratory and resorptive activity of osteoclasts.

Because ORSA is difficult to detect even with a detection system that is otherwise extremely sensitive, only small amounts of ORSA are likely to exist in osteoblast-conditioned supernatants. This fact, together with the relative inefficiency of the bioassay, makes identification of ORSA through analysis of osteoblastic supernatants unpromising. An alternative approach is to screen agents known to stimulate bone resorption in organ culture for a direct effect on osteoclasts. This is potentially productive, since several such cytokines are produced by osteoblasts, often in increased amounts in response to resorbing hormones. Any agent produced by osteoblastic cells in response to bone-resorbing hormones that stimulates resorption in organ culture would be a strong candidate as an osteoblast-derived mediator of osteoclastic stimulation.

There are many such agents, including interleukin 1 (IL-1) (Hanazawa et al., 1985, 1987; Lorenzo et al., 1990), TGFβ (Centrella and Canalis, 1985; Robey et al., 1987; Canalis et al., 1988), PDGF (Valentin-Opran et al., 1987), M-CSF (Felix et al., 1988; Horowitz et al., 1989), G-CSF (Felix et al., 1988), M-CSF (Sato et al., 1986; Elford et al., 1987) and DIF/LIF (Shiina-Ishimi et al., 1986; Abe et al., 1988). The very number of agents of this sort represents a caveat which extends to still unidentified osteoblastic products that may similarly cause bone resorption in organ culture (Perry et al., 1987; Meghji et al., 1988; Perry et al., 1989; Morris et al., 1990).

On the other hand, we have been struck by the long list of cytokine candidates we have tested that have proved inert as activators of isolated osteoclasts in the bone slice assay. This experience holds despite testing a wide range of doses and adding heparin where appropriate. There was a theoretical basis for the suggestion that systemic hormones such as PTH were unlikely to act directly on osteoclasts (Chambers, 1980), but no basis for extending this prediction to agents that did not act systemically; on the contrary, an osteoblast-generated local messenger is integral to the model. Many of these cytokines are multifunctional, produced by and acting on many cells, and owing specificity as much to localization of production as to structure. For some at least, the osteoclast clearly lacks receptors, but it is difficult to think of another cell so devoid of cytokine responsiveness, and surprising that so many hormone-responsive, osteoblast-derived cytokines that stimulate bone resorption in intact bone fail to affect isolated osteoclasts. Perhaps due to its role in the dissolution of substrate that accumulates so many cytokines (see, e.g., Hauschka et al., 1986) by adsorption onto hydroxyapatite during bone formation, regulation is best effected through a membrane-bound or -inserted form of cytokine, a possibility also favored by the essentially contact-dependent mechanism by which PTH and other agents stimulate osteoclasts.

Another potential explanation can be posed from a different perspective. The number of cytokines to which osteoclasts respond directly is strikingly low, but the list is replete with such factors that stimulate osteoclasts in proximity to osteoblasts. Indeed, the extent of the latter list is about what one would expect as products of osteoblasts and other cells acting directly on osteoclasts. Perhaps such cytokines do not directly induce osteoblasts to stimulate osteoclasts, as generally assumed, but rather facilitate the direct response of osteoclasts.

REFERENCES

Abe, E., Ishimi, Y., Takahashi, N., Akatsu, T., Ozawa, H., Yamana, H., Yoshiki, S., and Suda, T. (1988). A differentiation-inducing factor produced by the osteoblastic cell line MC3T3-E1 stimulates bone resorption by promoting osteoclast formation. *J. Bone Miner. Res.* **3**, 635–645.

Akatsu, T., Takahashi, N., Debari, K., Morita, I., Murota, S., Nagata, N., Takatani, O., and Suda, T. (1989). Prostaglandins promote osteoclast like cell formation by a mechanism involving cyclic adenosine 3',5'-monophosphate in mouse bone marrow cell cultures. *J. Bone Miner. Res.* **4**, 29–35.

Akisaka, T., Yamamoto, T., and Gay, C. V. (1988). Ultracytochemical investigation of calcium-activated adenosine triphosphatase (Ca^{2+}-ATPase) in chick tibia. *J. Bone Miner. Res.* **3**, 19–25.

Anderson, R. E., Woodbury, D. M., and Jee, W. S. S. (1986). Humoral and ionic regulation of osteoclast acidity. *Calcif. Tissue Int.* **39**, 252–258.

Arnett, T. R., and Dempster, D. W. (1986). Effect of pH on bone resorption by rat osteoclasts *in vitro. Endocrinology (Baltimore)* **119**, 119–124.

Arnett, T. R., and Dempster, D. W. (1987). A comparative study of disaggregated chick and rat osteoclasts *in vitro:* effects of calcitonin and prostaglandins. *Endocrinology (Baltimore)* **120**, 602–608.

Arnett, T. R., and Dempster, D. W. (1990). Perspectives: Protons and osteoclasts. *J. Bone Miner. Res.* **5**, 1099–1103.

Ashton, B. A., Allen, T. D., Howlett, C. R., Eaglesom, C. C., Hattori, A., and Owen, M. (1980). Formation of bone and cartilage by marrow stromal cells in diffusion chambers *in vivo. Clin. Orthop.* **151**, 294.

Bagi, C. M., and Miller, S. C. (1989). Osteoclast features of cells that resorb demineralized and mineral-containing bone implants in rats. *Scanning Microsc.* **3**, 963–970.

Baron, R. (1989). Molecular mechanisms of bone resorption by the osteoclast. *Anat. Rec.* **224**, 317–324.

Baron, R., and Vignery, A. (1981). Behaviour of osteoclasts during a rapid change in their number induced by high doses of parathyroid hormone or calcitonin in intact rats. *Metab. Bone Dis. Relat. Res.* **2**, 339–346.

Baron, R., Neff, L., Louvard, D., and Courtoy, P. J. (1985). Cell-mediated extracellular acidification and bone resorption: evidence for a low pH in resorbing lacunae and localization of a 100kD lysosomal membrane protein at the osteoclast ruffled border. *J. Cell Biol.* **101**, 2210–2222.

Baron, R., Neff, L., Roy, C., Boisvert, A., and Caplan, M. (1986). Evidence for a high and specific concentration of (Na/K)ATPase in the plasma membrane of the osteoclast. *Cell* **46**, 311–320.

Baron, R., Neff, L., Courtoy, P. J., Louvard, D., and Farquhar, M. G. (1988). Polarized secretion of lysosomal enzymes: Co-distribution of cation-independent mannose-6-phosphate receptors and lysosomal enzymes along the osteoclast exocytic pathway. *J. Cell Biol.* **106,** 1863–1872.

Bartocci, A., Mastrogiannis, D. S., Migliorati, G., Stockert, R. J., Wolkoff, A. W., and Stanley, E. R. (1987). Macrophages specifically regulate the concentration of their own growth factor in the circulation. *Proc. Natl. Acad. Sci. U.S.A.* **84,** 6179–6183.

Bianco, P., Costantini, M., Dearden, L. C., and Bonucci, E. (1987). Expression of tartrate-resistant acid phosphatase in bone marrow macrophages. *Basic Appl. Histochem.* **31,** 433–440.

Blair, H. C., Kahn, A. J., Crouch, E. C., Jeffrey, J.J., and Teitelbaum, S. L. (1986). Isolated osteoclasts resorb the organic and inorganic components of bone. *J. Cell Biol.* **102,** 1164–1172.

Blair, H. C., Teitelbaum, S. L., Ghiselli, R., and Gluck, S. (1989a). Osteoclastic bone resorption by a polarized vacuolar proton pump. *Science* **245,** 855–857.

Blair, H., Korziol, C., Mead, R., Gluck, S., Teitelbaum, S., and Schlesinger, P. (1989b). Osteoclast ruffled membranes contain proton pump that is tightly coupled to anion (Cl^-) permeability. *J. Bone Miner. Res.* **4,** Suppl. 1, Abstr. No. 584.

Bowman, E. J., Siebers, A., and Altendorf, K. (1988). Bafilomycins: A class of inhibitors of membrane ATPases from microorganisms, animal cells, and plant cells. *Proc. Natl. Acad. Sci. U.S.A.* **85,** 7972–7976.

Boyde, A. (1972). Scanning electron microscopy studies of bone. *In* "The Biochemistry and Physiology of Bone" (G. H. Bourne, ed.), Vol. 1, pp. 259–310. Academic Press, New York.

Boyde, A., Hobdell, M. H. (1969). Scanning electron microscopy of lamellar bone. *Z. Zellforsch Mikrosk. Anat.* **93,** 213–231.

Brachmann, R., Lindquist, P. B., Nagashima, M., Kohr, W., Lipari, T., Napier, M., and Derynck, R. (1989). Transmembrane TGF-α precursors activate EGF/EGFα receptors. *Cell* **56,** 691–700.

Burstone, M. S. (1958). Histochemical demonstration of acid phosphatases with naphthol AS-phosphate. *J. Natl. Cancer Inst.* **21,** 423–539.

Cabantchik, Z. I., Knauf, P. A., and Rothstein, A. (1978). The anion transport of the red blood cell. *Biochim. Biophys. Acta* **515,** 239–302.

Canalis, E., McCarthy, J., and Centrella, M. (1988). Isolation of growth factors from adult bovine bone. *Calcif. Tissue Int.* **43,** 346–351.

Cao, H., and Gay, C. V. (1985). Effects of parathyroid hormone and calcitonin on carbonic anhydrase location in osteoclasts of cultured embryonic chick bone. *Experientia* **41,** 1472.

Centrella, M., and Canalis, E. (1985). Transforming and non-transforming growth factors are present in the medium conditioned by fetal rat calvaria. *Proc. Natl. Acad. Sci. U.S.A.* **82,** 7335–7339.

Chambers, T. J. (1978). Multinucleate giant cells. *J. Pathol.* **126,** 125–148.

Chambers, T. J. (1980). The cellular basis of bone resorption. *Clin. Orthop. Relat. Res.* **151,** 283–293.

Chambers, T. J. (1982). Osteoblasts release osteoclasts from calcitonin-induced quiescence. *J. Cell Sci.* **57,** 247–260.

Chambers, T. J. (1985). The pathobiology of the osteoclast. *J. Clin. Pathol.* **38,** 241–252.

Chambers, T. J. (1989). The origin of the osteoclast. *In* "Bone and Mineral Research Annual" (W. Peck, ed.), Vol. 6, pp. 1–25. Elsevier, Amsterdam.

Chambers, T. J., and Fuller, K. (1985). Bone cells predispose bone surfaces to resorption by exposure of mineral to osteoclastic contact. *J. Cell Sci.* **76,** 155–165.

Chambers, T. J., and Magnus, C. J. (1982). Calcitonin alters behaviour of isolated osteoclasts. *J. Pathol.* **136**, 27–39.

Chambers, T. J., and Moore, A. (1983). The sensitivity of isolated osteoclasts to morphological transformation by calcitonin. *J. Clin. Endocrinol. Metab.* **57**, 819–824.

Chambers, T. J., Revell, P. A., Fuller, K., and Athanasou, N. A. (1984a). Resorption of bone by isolated rabbit osteoclasts. *J. Cell Sci.* **66**, 383–399.

Chambers, T. J., Thomson, B. M., and Fuller, K. (1984b). Effect of substrate composition on bone resorption by rabbit osteoclasts. *J. Cell Sci.* **70**, 61–71.

Chambers, T. J., Athanasou, N. A., and Fuller, K. (1984c). The effect of parathyroid hormone and calcitonin on the cytoplasmic spreading of isolated osteoclasts. *J. Endocrinol.* **102**, 281–286.

Chambers, T. J., McSheehy, P. M. J., Thomson, B. M., and Fuller, K. (1985a). The effect of calcium-regulating hormones and prostaglandins on bone resorption by osteoclasts disaggregated from neonatal rabbit bones. *Endocrinology (Baltimore)* **116**, 234–239.

Chambers, T. J., Darby, J. A., and Fuller, K. (1985b). Mammalian collagenase predisposes bone surfaces to osteoclastic resorption. *Cell Tissue Res.* **241**, 671–675.

Chambers, T. J., Fuller, K., Darby, J. A., Pringle, J. A. S., and Horton, M. A. (1986). Monoclonal antibodies against osteoclasts inhibit bone resorption *in vitro. Bone Miner.* **1**, 127–135.

Chambers, T. J., Fuller, K., and Darby, J. A. (1987). Hormonal regulation of acid phosphatase release by osteoclasts disaggregated from neonatal rat bone. *J. Cell Physiol.* **132**, 90–96.

Chenu, C., Pfeilschifter, J., Mundy, G. R., and Roodman, G. D. (1988). Transforming growth factor β inhibits formation of osteoclast-like cells in long-term human marrow cultures. *Proc. Natl. Acad. Sci. U.S.A.* **85**, 5683–5687.

Chenu, C., Kurihara, N., Mundy, G. R., and Roodman, G. D. (1990). Prostaglandin E_2 inhibits formation of osteoclast-like cells in long-term human marrow cultures but is not a mediator of the inhibitory effects of transforming growth factor β. *J. Bone Miner. Res.* **5**, 677–687.

Chow, J., and Chambers, T. J. (1991). An assessment of the prevalence of organic material on bone surfaces. *Calcif. Tissue Int.* (in press).

Collins, D. A., and Chambers, T. J. (1991). Effect of prostaglandins E_1, E_2 and $F_{2\alpha}$ on osteoclast formation in mouse bone marrow cultures. *J. Bone Miner. Res.* **6**, 157–164.

Conaway, H. H., Waite, L. C., and Kenny, A. D. (1973). Immobilization and bone mass in rats: Effects of parathyroidectomy and acetazolamide. *Calcif. Tissue Res.* **11**, 323–330.

Crocker, P. R., and Gordon, S. (1985). Isolation and characterisation of resident stromal macrophages and hemopoietic cell clusters from mouse bone marrow. *J. Exp. Med.* **162**, 993.

Davies, J., Warwick, J., Tutty, N., Philip, R., Helfrich, M., and Horton, M. (1989). The osteoclast functional antigen, implicated in the regulation of bone resorption, is biochemically related to the vitronectin receptor. *J. Cell Biol.* **109**, 1817–1826.

Delaisse, J.-M., Eeckhout, Y., and Vaes, G. (1984). *In vivo* and *in vitro* evidence for the involvement of cysteine proteinases in bone resorption. *Biochem. Biophys. Res. Commun.* **125**, 441–447.

Delaisse, J. M., Eeckhout, Y., Sear, C., Galloway, A., McCullagh, K., and Vaes, G. (1985). A new synthetic inhibitor of mammalian tissue collagenase inhibits bone resorption in culture. *Biochem. Biophys. Res. Commun.* **133**, 483–490.

Delaisse, J. M., Boyde, A., Maconnachie, E., Ali, N. N., Sear, C., Eeckhout, Y., Vaes, G., and Jones, S. J. (1987). The effects of inhibitors of cysteine-proteinases and collagenase on the resorptive activity of isolated osteoclasts. *Bone* **8**, 305–313.

Delaisse, J. M., Eeckhout, Y., and Vaes, L. G. (1988). Bone-resorbing agents affect the production and distribution of procollagenase as well as the activity of collagens in bone tissue. *Endocrinology (Baltimore)* **123**, 264–276.

de Vernejoul, M.-C., Horowitz, M., Dernignon, J., Neff, L., and Baron, R. (1988). Bone resorption by isolated chick osteoclasts in culture is stimulated by murine spleen cell supernatant fluids (osteoclast-activating factor) and inhibited by calcitonin and prostaglandin E_2. *J. Bone Miner. Res.* **3**, 69–80.

Ecarot-Charrier, B., and Broekhuyse, H. (1987). Proteoglycans synthesized by cultured mouse osteoblasts. *J. Biol. Chem.* **262**, 5345–5352.

Eeckhout, Y., Delaisse, J. M., and Vaes, G. (1986). Direct extraction and assay of bone tissue collagenase and its relation to parathyroid-hormone-induced bone resorption. *Biochem. J.* **239**, 793–796.

Eeckhout, Y., Delaisse, J. M., Ledent, P., and Vaes, G. (1988). The proteinases of bone resorption. *In* "The Control of Tissue Damage" (A. M. Glauert, ed.), pp. 297–313. Elsevier, Amsterdam.

Elford, P. R., Felix, R., Cecchini, M., Trechsel, U., and Fleisch, H. (1987). Murine osteoblast-like cells and the osteogenic cell MC3T3-E1 release a macrophage colony-stimulating activity in culture. *Calcif. Tissue Int.* **41**, 151–156.

Eliam, M. C., Baslé, M., Bouizar, Z., Bielakoff, J., Moukhtar, M., and de Vernejoul, M. C. (1988). Influence of blood calcium on calcitonin receptors in isolated chick osteoclasts. *J. Endocrinol.* **119**, 243–248.

Felix, R., Elford, P. R., Stoerckle, M., Cecchini, M., Wetterwald, A., Trechsel, U., Fleisch, H., and Stradler, B. M. (1988). Production of haemopoietic growth factors by bone tissue and bone cells in culture. *J. Bone Miner. Res.* **3**, 27–36.

Felix, F., Cecchini, M. G., and Fleisch, H. (1990a). Macrophage colony stimulating factor restores *in vivo* bone resorption in the op/op mouse. *Endocrinology (Baltimore)* **127**, 2592–2594.

Felix, R., Cecchini, M. G., Hofstetter, W., Elford, P. R., Stutzer, A., and Fleisch, H. (1990b). Impairment of macrophage colony-stimulating factor production and lack of resident bone marrow macrophages in the osteopetrotic op/op mouse. *J. Bone Miner. Res.* **5**, 781–789.

Flanagan, A. M., Chambers, T. J., Helfrich, M., Horton, M. A., Evely, R. S., and Martin, T. J. (1991). An assessment of the ability of human bone marrow cultures to generate osteoclasts. Submitted.

Fornasier, V. L. (1977). Osteoid: An ultrastructural study. *Hum. Pathol.* **8**, 243–254.

Fornasier, V. L. (1980). Transmission electron microscopy studies of osteoid maturation. *Metab. Bone Dis. Relat. Res.* **25**, 103–108.

Fuller, K., and Chambers, T. J. (1987). Generation of osteoclasts in cultures of rabbit bone marrow and spleen cells. *J. Cell. Physiol.* **132**, 441–452.

Gay, C. V., and Mueller, W. J. (1974). Carbonic anhydrase and osteoclasts: Localization by labeled inhibitor autoradiography. *Science* **183**, 432–434.

Gay, C. V., Schraer, H., Anderson, R. E., and Cao, H. (1984). Current studies on the location of carbonic anhydrase in osteoclasts. *Ann. N.Y. Acad. Sci.* **429**, 473–478.

Geiger, B. (1983). Membrane–cytoskeleton interaction. *Biochim. Biophys. Acta* **737**, 305–341.

Glimcher, M. J., and Kenzora, J. E. (1979). The biology of osteonecrosis of the human femoral head and its clinical implications. *Clin. Orthop.* **138**, 284.

Glowacki, J., and Cox, K. A. (1986). Osteoclast features of cells that resorb bone implants in rats. *Calcif. Tissue Int.* **39,** 97–103.

Glowacki, J., Jasty, M., and Goldring, S. (1986). Comparison of multinucleated cells elicited in rats by particulate bone, polyethylene, of polymethylmethacrylate. *J. Bone Miner. Res.* **1,** 327–331.

Goldhaber, P., and Rabadjija, L. (1987). H^+ stimulation of cell-mediated bone resorption in tissue culture. *Am. J. Physiol.* **253,** E90–E98.

Goldring, S. R., Roelke, M., and Glowacki, J. (1988). Multinucleated cells elicited in response to implants of devitalized bone particles possess receptors for calcitonin. *J. Bone Miner. Res.* **1,** 117–120.

Gordon, M. Y., Riley, G. P., Watt, S. M., and Greaves, M. F. (1987). Compartmentalization of a haemopoietic growth factor (GM-CSF) by glycosaminoglycans in the bone marrow microenvironment. *Nature (London)* **326,** 403–405.

Gospodarowicz, D., Cheng, J., Lui, G.-M., Baird, A., and Böhlent, P. (1984). Isolation of brain fibroblast growth factor by heparin-Sepharose affinity chromatography: identity with pituitary fibroblast growth factor. *Proc. Natl. Acad. Sci. U.S.A.* **81,** 6963–6967.

Grigoriadis, A. E., Heersche, J. N. M., and Aubin, J. E. (1988). Differentiation of muscle, fat, cartilage, and bone from progenitor cells present in a bone-derived clonal cell population: effect of dexamethasone. *J. Cell Biol.* **106,** 2139.

Grills, B. L., Gallagher, J. A., Allan, E. H., Yumita, S., and Martin, T. J. (1990). Identification of plasminogen activator in osteoclasts. *J. Bone Miner. Res.* **5,** 499–505.

Gualtieri, R. J., Shadduck, R. K., Baker, D. G., and Queensberry, P. J. (1984). Hematopoietic regulatory factors produced in long-term murine bone marrow cultures and the effect of *in vitro* irradiation. *Blood* **64,** 516–525.

Hagenaars, C. E., Van der Kraan, A. A. M., Kawilarang-de Haas, E. W. M., Visser, J. W. M., and Nijweide, P. J. (1989). Osteoclast formation from cloned pluripotent haemopoietic stem cells. *Bone Miner.* **6,** 187–190.

Hall, G. E., and Kenny, A. D. (1986). Bone resorption induced by parathyroid hormone and dibutryl cyclic AMP: Role of carbonic anhydrase. *J. Pharmacol. Exp. Ther.* **238,** 778–782.

Hall, T. J., and Chambers, T. J. (1989). Optimal bone resorption by isolated rat osteoclasts requires chloride/bicarbonate exchange. *Calcif. Tissue Int.* **45,** 378–380.

Hall, T. J., and Chambers, T. J. (1990). Na^+/H^+ Antiporter is the primary proton transport system used by osteoclasts during bone resorption. *J. Cell Physiol.* **142,** 420–424.

Hall, T. J., Higgins, W., Tardif, C., and Chambers, T. J. (1991). A comparison of the effects of inhibitors of carbonic anhydrase on osteoclastic bone resorption and purified carbonic anhydrase isozyme II. *Calcif. Tissue Int.* (in press).

Ham, A. W., and Harris, W. R. (1972). In "The Biochemistry and Physiology of Bone" (G. H. Bourne, ed.), Vol. 1, pp. 337. Academic Press, New York.

Hamilton, J. A., Lingelback, S. R., Partridge, N. C., and Martin, T. J. (1984). Stimulation of plasminogen activator in osteoblast-like cells by bone-resorbing hormones. *Biochem. Biophys. Res. Commun.* **122,** 230–236.

Hanazawa, S., Ohmori, Y., Amano, S., Miyoshi, T., Kumegawa, M., and Kitano, S. (1985). Spontaneous production of interleukin-1-like cytokine from a mouse osteoblastic cell line. *Biochem. Biophys. Res. Commun.* **131,** 774–779.

Hanazawa, S., Amano, S., Nakada, K., Ohmori, Y., Miyoshi, T., Hirose, K., and Kitano, S. (1987) Biological characterization of interleukin-1-like cytokine produced by cultured bone cells from newborn mouse calvaria. *Calcif. Tissue Int.* **41,** 31–37.

Hattersley, G., and Chambers, T. J. (1989a). Calcitonin receptors as markers for osteoclastic differentiation: correlation between generation of bone resorptive cells and cells that express calcitonin receptors in mouse bone marrow cultures. *Endocrinology (Baltimore)* **125,** 1606–1612.

Hattersley, G., and Chambers, T. J. (1989b). Generation of osteoclastic function in mouse bone marrow cultures: multinuclearity and tartrate-resistant acid phosphatase are unreliable markers for osteoclastic differentiation. *Endocrinology (Baltimore)* **124,** 1689–1696.

Hattersley, G., and Chambers, T. J. (1989c). Generation of osteoclasts from hemopoietic cells and a multipotential cell line *in vitro. J. Cell. Physiol.* **140,** 478–482.

Hattersley, G., and Chambers, T. J. (1990a). Effects of interleukin 3 and of granulocyte-macrophage and macrophage colony stimulating factors on osteoclast differentiation from mouse hemopoietic tissue. *J. Cell Physiol.* **142,** 201–209.

Hattersley, G., and Chambers, T. J. (1990b). The role of bone marrow stroma in induction of osteoclastic differentiation. *In* "Calcium Regulation and Bone Metabolism: Basic and Clinical Aspects" (D. V. Cohn, F. H. Glorieux, and T. J. Martin, eds.), Vol. 10, pp. 439–442. Elsevier, Amsterdam.

Hauschka, P. V., Mavrakos, A. E., Iafrati, M. D., Doleman, S. E., and Klagsbrun, M. (1986). Growth factors in bone matrix. Isolation of multiple types by affinity chromatography on heparin-Sepharose. *J. Biol. Chem.* **261,** 12665–12674.

Heard, J.-M., Fichelson, S., and Varet, B. (1982). Role of colony-stimulating activity in murine long-term bone marrow cultures: evidence for its production and consumption by the adherent cells. *Blood* **59,** 761–767.

Heath, J. K., Atkinson, S. J., Meikle, M. C., and Reynolds, J. J. (1984). Mouse osteoblasts synthesize collagenase in response to bone resorbing agents. *Biochim. Biophys. Acta* **802,** 151–154.

Horowitz, M. C., Coleman, D. L., Ryaby, J. T., and Einhorn, T. A. (1989). Osteotropic agents induce the differential secretion of granulocyte-macrophage colony-stimulating factor by the osteoblast cell line MC3T3-E1. *J. Bone Miner. Res.* **4,** 911–921.

Horton, J. E., Wezeman, F. H., and Kuettner, K. E. (1978). Inhibition of bone resorption *in vitro* by a cartilage-derived anticollagenase factor. *Science,* **199,** 1342–1344.

Horton, M. A., and Davies, J. (1989). Perspectives: Adhesion receptors in bone. *J. Bone Miner. Res.* **4,** 803–808.

Horton, M. A., Lewis, D., McNulty, K., Pringle, J. A. S., and Chambers, T. J. (1985). Monoclonal antibodies to osteoclastomas (giant cell bone tumours): definition of osteoclast-specific cellular antigens. *Cancer Res.* **45,** 5663–5669.

Hughes, D. E., MacDonald, B. R., Russell, R. G. G., and Gowen, M. (1989). Inhibition of osteoclast-like cell formation by biphosphonates in long-term cultures of human bone marrow. *J. Clin. Invest.* **83,** 1930–1935.

Hunter, S. J., Schraer, H., and Gay, C. V. (1988). Characterization of isolated and cultured chick osteoclasts: The effects of acetazolamide, calcitonin, and parathyroid hormone on acid production. *J. Bone Miner. Res.* **3,** 297–303.

Hynes, R. O. (1987). Integrins: A family of cell surface receptors. *Cell* **48,** 549–554.

Jaworski, Z. F. G., Duck, B., and Sekaly, G. (1981). Kinetics of osteoclasts and their nuclei in evolving secondary Haversian systems. *J. Anat.* **133,** 397–405.

Jilka, R. L., and Cohn, D. V. (1983). A collagenolytic response to parathormone, 1,25 dihydroxycholecalciferol D_3 and prostaglandin E_2 in bone of osteoporotic (mi/mi) mice. *Endocrinology (Baltimore)* **112,** 945–950.

Jilka, R. L., and Hamilton, J. W. (1985). Evidence for two pathways for stimulation of collagenolysis in bone. *Calcif. Tissue Int.* **37,** 300–306.

Jones, S. J., Boyde, A., Ali, N. N., and Maconnachie, E. (1985). A review of bone cell and substratum interactions: an illustration of the role of scanning electron microscopy. *Scanning* **7**, 5–24.

Jones, S. J., Boyde, A., and Ali, N. N. (1986). The interface of cells and their matrices in mineralized tissues: A review. *Scanning Electron Microsc.* **4**, 1555–1565.

Kaye, M. (1984). When is it an osteoclast? *J. Clin. Pathol.* **37**, 398–400.

Kellokumpu, S., Neff, L., Jamsa-Kellokumpu, S., Kopito, R., and Baron, R. (1988). A 115-kD polypeptide immunologically related to erythrocyte band 3 is present in golgi membranes. *Science* **242**, 1308–1311.

Kenny, A. D. (1985). Role of carbonic anhydrase in bone: Partial inhibition of disuse atrophy of bone by parenteral acetazolamide. *Calcif. Tissue Int.* **37**, 126–133.

Ketcham, C. M., Baumbach, G. A., Bazer, F. W., and Roberts, R. M. (1985). The type 5 acid phosphatase from spleen of humans with hair cell leukaemia. *J. Biol. Chem.* **260**, 5768–5776.

Klein-Nulend, J., and Raisz, L. G. (1989). Effects of two inhibitors of anion transport on bone resorption in organ culture. *Endocrinology (Baltimore)* **125**, 1019–1024.

Kodama, H., Izuka, M., Tomiyama, T., Yoshida, K., Seki, M., Suda, T., and Nishikawa, S.-i. (1991a). Response of newly established mouse myeloid leukemic cell lines to MC3T3-G2/PA6 preadipocytes and hematopoietic factors. *Blood* **1**, 49–54.

Kodama, H., Yamasaki, A., Nose, M., Niida, S., Ohgame, Y., Abe, M., Kumegawa, M., and Suda, T. (1991b). Congenital osteoclast deficiency in osteopetrotic (op/op) mice is cured by injections of macrophage colony-stimulating factor. *J. Exp. Med.* **173**, 269–272.

Krieger, N. S., and Tashjian, A. H. (1980). Parathyroid hormone stimulates bone resorption via a Na–Ca exchange mechanism. *Nature (London)* **287**, 843–845.

Kukita, T., and Roodman, G. D. (1989). Development of a monoclonal antibody to osteoclasts formed *in vitro* which recognizes mononuclear osteoclast precursors in the marrow. *Endocrinology (Baltimore)* **125**, 630–637.

Kukita, T., McManus, L. M., Civin, C., and Roodman, G. D. (1989). Osteoclast-like cells formed in long-term human bone marrow cultures express a similar surface phenotype as authentic osteoclasts. *Lab. Invest.* **60**, 532–538.

Kukita, A., Bouewald, L., Rosen, D., Seyedin, S., Mundy, G. R., and Roodman, G. D. (1990a). Osteoinductive factor inhibits formation of human osteoclast-like cells. *Proc. Natl. Acad. Sci. U.S.A.* **87**, 3023–3026.

Kukita, A., Chenu, C., McManus, L. M., Mundy, G. R., and Roodman, G. D. (1990b). Atypical multinucleated cells form in long-term marrow cultures from patients with Paget's disease. *J. Clin. Invest.* **85**, 1280–1286.

Kurihara, N., Bertolini, D., Suda, T., Akayama, Y., and Roodman, G. D. (1990a). IL-6 stimulated osteoclast-like multinucleated cell formation in long-term human cultures by inducing Il-1 release. *J. Immunol.* **144**, 4226–4230.

Kurihara, N., Chenu, C., Miller, M., Civin, C., and Roodman, G. D. (1990b). Identification of committed mononuclear precursors for osteoclast-like cells formed in long term human marrow cultures. *Endocrinology (Baltimore)* **126**, 2733–2741.

Kurihara, N., Gluck, S., and Roodman, G. D. (1990c). Sequential expression of phenotype markers for osteoclasts during differentiation of precursors for multinucleated cells formed in long term human marrow cultures. *Endocrinology (Baltimore)* **127**, 3215–3221.

Lian, J. B., Tissinari, M., and Glowacki, J. (1984). Resorption of implanted bone prepared from normal and warfarin-treated rats. *J. Clin. Invest.* **73**, 1223.

Lindberg, P., Brandstrom, A., and Wallmark, B. (1987). Structure-activity relationships of omeprazole analogues and their mechanisms of action. *Trends Pharmacol. Sci.* **8**, 399–402.

Lipschitz, D. A., Udupa, K. B., Taylor, J. M., Shadduck, R. K., and Waheed, A. (1987). Role of colony-stimulating factor in myelopoiesis in murine long-term bone marrow cultures. *Blood* **69**, 1211–1217.

Lorenzo, J. A., Sousa, S. L., Van Den Brink-Webb, S. E., and Korn, J. H. (1990). Production of both interleukin-1α and β by newborn mouse calvarial cultures. *J. Bone Miner. Res.* **5**, 77–83.

Loutit, J. F., and Nisbet, N. W. (1979). Resorption of bone. *Lancet* **ii**, 26–28.

Loutit, J. F., and Nisbet, N. W. (1982). The origin of the osteoclast. *Immunobiology* **161**, 193–203.

Loutit, J. F., and Townsend, K. M. S. (1982). Longevity of osteoclasts in radiation chimeras of osteopetrotic beige and normal mice. *B. J. Exp. Pathol.* **63**, 221–223.

Luk, S. C., Nopajaroonsri, C., and Simon, G. T. (1974). The ultrastructure of endosteum: a topographic study in young adult rabbits. *J. Ultrastruct. Res.* **46**, 165–183.

MacDonald, B. R., Mundy, G. R., Clark, S., Wang, E. A., Kuehl, T. J., Stanley, E. R., and Roodman, G. D. (1986). Effects of human recombinant CSF-GM and highly purified CSF-1 on the formation of multinucleated cells with osteoclast characteristics in long-term bone marrow cultures. *J. Bone Miner. Res.* **1**, 227–233.

MacDonald, B. R., Takahashi, N., McManus, L. M., Holahan, J., Mundy, G. R., and Roodman, G. D. (1987). Formation of multinucleated cells that respond to osteotropic hormones in long-term human bone marrow cultures. *Endocrinology (Baltimore)* **120**, 2326–2333.

Maciag, I., Mehlman, T., Friesel, R., and Schreiber, A. B. (1984). Heparin binds endothelial cell growth factor, the principal endothelial cell mitogen in bovine brain. *Science* **225**, 932–935.

Malgaroli, A., Meldolesi, J., Zambonin-Zallone, A., and Teti, A. (1989). Control of cytosolic free calcium in rat and chicken osteoclasts. *J. Biol. Chem.* **264**, 14342–14347.

Malone, J. D., Teitelbaum, S., Griffin, G. L., Senior, R. M., and Kahn, A. J. (1982). Recruitment of osteoclast precursors by purified bone matrix constituents. *J. Cell Biol.* **92**, 227.

Marchisio, P. C., Cirillo, D., Laldini, L., Primavera, M. V., Teti, A., and Zambonin-Zallone, A. (1984). Cell–substratum interaction of cultured avian osteoclasts is mediated by specific adhesion structures. *J. Cell Biol.* **99**, 1696–1705.

Maren, T. H. (1960). A simplified micromethod for the determination of carbonic anhydrase and its inhibitors. *J. Pharmacol. Exp. Ther.* **130**, 26–29.

Maren, T. H. (1984). Carbonic anhydrase: The middle years, 1945–1960, and introduction to pharmacology of sulfonamides. *Ann. N.Y. Acad. Sci.* **429**, 10–17.

Maren, T. H. and Sanyal, G. (1983). The activity of sulfonamides and anions against the carbonic anhydrases of animals, plants, and bacteria. *Annu. Rev. Pharmacol. Toxicol.* **23**, 439–459.

Marks, S. C., Jr., and Chambers, T. J. (1991). The giant cells recruited by subcutaneous implants of mineralized bone particles and slices in rabbits are not osteoclasts. *J. Bone Miner. Res.* **6**, 395–400.

Marks, S. C., and Lane, P. W. (1976). Osteopetrosis, a new recessive skeletal mutation on chromosome 12 of the mouse. *J. Hered.* **67**, 11–18.

Marks, S. C., and Popoff, S. N. (1988). Bone cell biology: The regulation of development, structure and function in the skeleton. *Am. J. Anat.* **183**, 1–44.

Marks, S. C., Jr., and Schneider, G. B. (1982). Transformation of osteoclast phenotype in rats cured of congenital osteopetrosis. *J. Morphol.* **174**, 141–147.

Marks, S. C., Seifert, M. F., and McGuire, J. L. (1984). Congenitally osteopetrotic (op/op) mice are not cured by transplants of spleen or bone marrow cells from normal littermates. *Metab. Bone Dis. Relat. Res.* **5**, 183–186.

McSheehy, P. M. J., and Chambers, T. J. (1986a). Osteoblastic cells mediate osteoclastic responsiveness to parathyroid hormone. *Endocrinology (Baltimore)* **118**, 824–828.

McSheehy, P. M. J., and Chambers, T. J. (1986b). Osteoblast-like cells in the presence of parathyroid hormone release soluble factor that stimulates osteoclastic bone resorption. *Endocrinology (Baltimore)* **119**, 1654–1659.

McSheehy, P. M. J., and Chambers, T. J. (1987). 1,25-Dihydroxyvitamin D_3 stimulates rat osteoblastic cells to release a soluble factor that increases osteoclastic bone resorption. *J. Clin. Invest.* **80**, 425–429.

Meghji, S., Sandy, J. R., Scutt, A. M., Harvey, W., and Harris, M. (1988). Heterogeneity of bone resorbing factors produced by unstimulated murine osteoblasts *in vitro* and in response to stimulation by parathyroid hormone and mononuclear cell factors. *Arch. Oral Biol.* **33**, 773–778.

Metcalf, D. (1988). "The Molecular Control of Blood Cells." Harvard Univ. Press, Cambridge, Massachusetts.

Miller, S. C., and Jee, W. S. S. (1987). The bone lining cell: a distinct phenotype? *Calcif. Tissue Int.* **41**, 1–5.

Miller, S. C., Bowman, B. M., Smith, J. M., and Jee, W. S. S. (1980). Characterization of endosteal bone-lining cells from fatty marrow bone sites in adult beagle. *Anat. Rec.* **198**, 163–173.

Miller, S. C., de Saint-George, L., Bowman, B. M., and Jee, W. S. S. (1989). Bone lining cells: structure and function. *Scanning Microsc.* **3**, 953–961.

Minkin, C., and Jennings, J. M. (1972). Carbonic anhydrase and bone remodeling: Sulfonamide inhibition of bone resorption in organ culture. *Science* **176**, 1031–1033.

Miyauchi, A., Hruska, K. A., Greenfield, E. M., Duncan, R., Alvarez, J., Baratollo, R., Colucci, S., Zambonin-Zallone, A., Teitelbaum, S. L., and Teti, A. (1990). Osteoclast cytosolic calcium, regulated by voltage-gated calcium channels and extracellular calcium, controls podosome assembly and bone resorption. *J. Cell Biol.* **111**, 2543–2552.

Moolenaar, W. H. (1986). Regulation of cytoplasmic pH by Na/H exchange. *Trends Biochem. Sci.* **11**, 141–143.

Moore, M. A. S., Broxmeyer, H. E., Sheridan, A. P., Meyers, P. A., Jacobsen, N., and Winchester, R. J. (1980). Continuous human bone marrow culture: Ia antigen characterisation of probable pluripotential stem cells. *Blood* **55**, 682–690.

Morris, C. A., Mitnick, M. E., Weir, E. C., Horowitz, M., Kreider, B. L., and Insogna, K. L. (1990). The parathyroid hormone-related protein stimulates human osteoblast-like cells to secrete a 9,000 dalton bone-resorbing protein. *Endocrinology (Baltimore)* **126**, 1783–1785.

Mundy, G. R., and Poser, J. W. (1983). Chemotactic activity of the γ-carboxyglutamic acid containing protein in bone. *Calcif. Tissue Int.* **35**, 164.

Mundy, G. R., Varani, J., Orr, W., Gondek, M. D., and Ward, P. A. (1978). Resorbing bone is chemotactic for monocytes. *Nature (London)* **275**, 132.

Murrills, R. J., and Dempster, D. W. (1990). The effects of stimulators of intracellular cyclic AMP on rat and chick osteoclasts *in vitro:* validation of a simplified light microscope assay of bone resorption. *Bone* **11**, 333–344.

Neuman, W. F., Mulryan, B. J., and Martin, G. R. (1960). A chemical view of osteoclasts based on studies with Yttrium. *Clin. Orthop.* **17**, 124–134.

Nicholson, G. C., Moseley, J. M., Sexton, P. M., Mendelsohn, F. A. O., and Martin, T. J.

(1986a). Abundant calcitonin receptors in isolated rat osteoclasts. *J. Clin. Invest.* **78,** 355–360.

Nicholson, G. C., Livesey, S. A., Moseley, J. M., and Martin, T. J. (1986b). Actions of calcitonin, parathyroid hormone, and prostaglandin E_2 on cyclic AMP formation in chicken and rat osteoclasts. *J. Cell. Biochem.* **31,** 229–241.

Nicholson, G. C., Moseley, J. M. Sexton, P. M., and Martin, T. J. (1987). Chicken osteoclasts do not possess calcitonin receptors. *J. Bone Miner. Res.* **2,** 53–59.

Nicholson, G. C., Yumita, S., Moseley, J. M., Yates, A. J. P., and Martin, T. J. (1988). Forskolin augments the effects of calcitonin on cytoplasmic spreading of isolated rat osteoclasts and plasma calcium levels in the rat. *J. Bone Miner. Res.* **3,** 181–184.

Nicholson, G. C., Kent, G. N., Rowe, D. J., Cronin, B. J., Evely, R. S., and Moseley, J. M. (1989). PTH acts indirectly on isolated rat osteoclasts to increase resorption pit number. *J. Bone Miner. Res.* **4,** Suppl. 1, S210.

Nijweide, P. J., Burger, E. H., and Feyen, J. H. M. (1986). Cells of bone: Proliferation, differentiation, and hormonal regulation. *Physiol. Rev.* **66,** 855–886.

Nishihara, T., Ishihara, Y., Noguchi, T., and Koga, T. (1989). Membrane Il-1 induces bone resorption in organ culture. *J. Immunol.* **143,** 1881–1886.

Noda, M., and Rodan, G. A. (1989). Transcriptional regulation of osteopontin production in rat osteoblast-like cells by parathyroid hormone. *J. Cell Biol.* **108,** 713–718.

Nong, Y.-H., Titus, R. G., Ribeiro, J. M. C., and Remold, H. G. (1989). Peptides encoded by the calcitonin gene inhibit macrophage function. *J. Immunol.* **143,** 45–49.

O'Grady, R. L., and Cameron, D. A. (1971). Demonstration of binding sites of parathyroid hormone in bone cells. *Endocrinol. 1971: Proc. Int. Symp., 3rd* pp. 374–379.

Oldberg, A., Franzen, A., and Heinegard D. (1986). Cloning and sequence analysis of rat bone sialoprotein (osteopontin) cDNA reveals an Arg-Gly-Asp cell-binding sequence. *Proc. Natl. Acad. Sci. U.S.A.* **83,** 8819–8823.

Owen, M. (1985). Lineage of osteogenic cells and their relationship to the stromal system. *In* "Bone and Mineral Research" (W. A. Peck, ed.), Vol. 3, pp. 1–25. Elsevier, Amsterdam.

Parfitt, A. M. (1984). The cellular basis of bone remodeling: the quantum concept reexamined in light of recent advances in the cell biology of bone. *Calcif. Tissue Int.* **36,** Suppl., S37–S45.

Peignoux-Deville, J., Bordat, C., and Vidal, B. (1989). Demonstration of bone resorbing cells in elasmobranchs; Comparison with osteoclasts. *Tissue Cell* **21,** 925–933.

Perry, H. M., Skogen, W., Chappel, J. C., Wilner, G. D., Kahn, A. J., and Teitelbaum, S. L. (1987). Conditioned medium from osteoblast-like cells mediates parathyroid hormone induced bone resorption. *Calcif. Tissue Int.* **40,** 298–300.

Perry, H. M., Skogen, W., Chappel, J., Kahn, A. J., Wilner, G., and Teitelbaum, S. L. (1989). Partial characterization of a parathyroid hormone-stimulated resorption factor(s) from osteoblast-like cells. *Endocrinology (Baltimore)* **125,** 2075–2082.

Pfeilschifter, J., Erdmann, J., Schmidt, W., Naumann, A., Minne, H. W., and Ziegler, R. (1990). Differential regulation of plasminogen activator and plasminogen activator inhibitor by osteotropic factors in primary cultures of mature osteoblasts and osteoblast precursors. *Endocrinology (Baltimore)* **126,** 703–711.

Pollard, J. W., Bartocci, A., Arceci, R., Orlofsky, A., Ladner, M. B., and Stanley, E. R. (1987). Apparent role of the macrophage growth factor, CSF-1, in placental development. *Nature (London)* **330,** 485–486.

Popoff, S. N., and Marks, S. C. J. (1986). Ultrastructure of the giant cell infiltrate of subcutaneously implanted bone particles in rats and mice. *Am. J. Anat.* **177,** 491–503.

Raina, V. (1972). Normal osteoid tissue. *J. Clin. Pathol.* **25**, 229–232.

Raisz, L. G., Simmons, H. A., Thompson, W. J., Shepard, K. L., Anderson, P. S., and Rodan, G. A. (1988). Effects of a potent carbonic anhydrase inhibitor on bone resorption in organ culture. *Endocrinology (Baltimore)* **122**, 1083–1086.

Ransjö, M., Lerner, U. H., and Heersche, J. N. M. (1988). Calcitonin-like effects of forskolin and choleratoxin on surface area of motility of isolated rabbit osteoclasts. *J. Bone Miner. Res.* **3**, 611–619.

Rao, L. G., Heersche, J. M. N., Marchu, L. L., and Sturtridge, W. (1981). Immunohistochemical demonstration of calcitonin binding to specific cell types in fixed rat bone tissue. *Endocrinology (Baltimore)* **108**, 1982–1992.

Rao, L. G., Murray, T. M., and Heersche, T. N. M. (1983). Immunohistochemical demonstration of parathyroid hormone binding to specific cell types in fixed rat bone tissue. *Endocrinology (Baltimore)* **113**, 805–810.

Redhead, C. R., and Baker, P. F. (1988). Control of intracellular pH in rat calvarial osteoblasts: Coexistence of both chloride-bicarbonate and sodium-hydrogen exchange. *Calcif. Tissue Int.* **42**, 237–242.

Regenstreif, L. J., and Rossant, J. (1989). Expression of the c-fms protooncogene and of the cytokine, CSF-1, during mouse embryogenesis. *Dev. Biol.* **133**, 284–294.

Reinholt, F. P., Hultenby, K., Oldberg, A., and Heinegard, R. (1990). Osteopontin—a possible anchor of osteoclasts to bone. *Proc. Natl. Acad. Sci. U.S.A.* **87**, 4473–4475.

Rifas, L., Halstead, L. R., Peck, W. A., Avioli, L. V., and Welgus, H. G. (1989). Human osteoblasts *in vitro* secrete tissue inhibitor of metalloproteinases and gelatinase but not interstitial collagenase as major cellular products. *J. Clin. Invest.* **84**, 686–694.

Rifkin, B. R., Auszmann, J. M., Kleckner, A. P., Vernillo, A. T., and Fine, A. S. (1988). Calcitonin stimulates cAMP accumulation in chicken osteoclasts. *Life Sci.* **42**, 799–804.

Roberts, R. A., Spooner, E., Parkinson, E. K., Lord, B. I., Allen, T. D., and Dexter, T. M. (1987). Metabolically inactive 3T3 cells can substitute for marrow stromal cells to promote the proliferation and development of multipotent haemopoietic stem cells. *J. Cell. Physiol.* **132**, 203–214.

Roberts, R. A., Gallagher, J., Spooner, E., Allen, T. D., Bloomfield, F., and Dexter, T. M. (1988). Heparan sulphate bound growth factors: a mechanism for stromal cell mediated haemopoiesis. *Nature (London)* **332**, 376–378.

Robey, P. G., Young, M. F., Flanders, K. C., Roche, N. S., Kondaiah, P., Reddi, A., Termine, J. D., Sporn, M. B., and Roberts, A. N. (1987). Osteoblasts synthesize and respond to transforming growth factor-type β (TGF β). *J. Cell Biol.* **105**, 457–463.

Rodan, G. A., and Martin T. J. (1981). The role of osteoblasts in hormonal control of bone resorption. *Calcif. Tissue Int.* **33**, 349–351.

Rodan, G. A., and Rodan, S. B. (1984). Expression of the osteoblastic phenotype. *In* "Advances in Bone and Mineral Research Annual" (W. A. Peck, ed.), Vol. 2, pp. 244–285. Elsevier, Amsterdam.

Rouleau, M. F., Warshawsky, H., and Goltzman, D. (1986). Parathyroid hormone binding *in vivo* to renal, hepatic and skeletal tissues of the rat using a radioautographic technique. *Endocrinology (Baltimore)* **118**, 919–931.

Ruoslahti, E., and Pierschbacher, M. D. (1986). Arg-Gly-Asp: A versatile cell recognition signal. *Cell* **44**, 517–518.

Sakamoto, S., and Sakamoto, M. (1984). Osteoblast collagenase: collagenase synthesis by clonally-derived mouse osteogenic cells. *Biochem. Int.* **9**, 51–59.

Sakamoto, S., and Sakamoto, M. (1985). On the possibility that bone matrix collagen is removed prior to bone mineral during cell-mediated bone resorption. *In* "Current

Advances in Skeletogenesis" (A. Ornoy, A. Harell, and J. Sela, eds.), pp. 65–70. Elsevier, Amsterdam.

Sakamoto, S., and Sakamoto, M. (1986). Bone collagenase, osteoblasts, and cell mediated bone resorption. *In* "Bone and Mineral Research Annual" (W. A. Peck, ed.), Vol. 4, pp. 49–102. Elsevier, Amsterdam.

Sato, K., Fujii, Y., Asano, S., Ohtsuki, T., Kawakami, M., Kasono, K., Tsushima, T., and Shizume, K. (1986). Recombinant human interleukin 1α and β stimulate mouse osteoblast-like cells (MC3T3-E1) to produce macrophage-colony stimulating activity and prostaglandin E_2. *Biochem. Biophys. Res. Commun.* **141**, 285–291.

Scherft, J. P. (1972). The lamina limitations of the organic matrix of calcified cartilage and bone. *J. Ultrastruct. Res.* **38**, 318–331.

Scheven, B. A. A., Visser, J. W. M., and Nijweide, P. J. (1986). *In vitro* osteoclast generation from different bone marrow fractions, including a highly enriched haemopoietic stem cell population. *Nature (London)* **321**, 79–81.

Schneider, G. B., and Byrnes, J. E. (1983). The cellular specificity of the cure for neonatal osteopetrosis in the ia rat. *Exp. Cell Biol.* **51**, 44–50.

Schneider, G. B., and Relfson, M. (1988). The effects of transplantation of granulocyte-macrophage progenitors on bone resorption in osteopetrotic rats. *J. Bone Miner. Res.* **3**, 225–232.

Schreiber, A. B., Kenney, J., Kowalski, W. J., Friesel, R., Mehlman, T., and Maciag, T. (1985). Interaction of endothelial cell growth factor with heparin: characterization by receptor and antibody recognition. *Proc. Natl. Acad. Sci. U.S.A.* **82**, 6138–6142.

Scott, B. L. (1967). Thymidine-^{3}H electron microscope radioautography of osteogenic cells in the fetal rat. *J. Cell Biol.* **35**, 115.

Shen, V., Kohler, G., Jeffrey, J. J., and Peck, W. A. (1988). Bone-resorbing agents promote and interferon-γ inhibits bone cell collagenase production. *J. Bone Miner. Res.* **3**, 657–666.

Shiina-Ishimi, Y., Abe, E., Tanaka, H., and Suda, T. (1986). Synthesis of colony-stimulating factor (CSF) and differentiation-inducing factor (D-factor) by osteoblastic cell, clone MC3T3-E1. *Biochem. Biophys. Res. Commun.* **134**, 400–406.

Shinar, D. M., Sato, M., and Rodan, G. A. (1990). The effect of hemopoietic growth factors on the generation of osteoclast-like cells in mouse bone marrow cultures. *Endocrinology (Baltimore)* **126**, 1728–1735.

Silve, C. M., Hradek, G. T., Jones, A. L., and Arnaud, C. D. (1982). Parathyroid hormone receptor in intact embryonic chicken bone: charcterisation and cellular localisation. *J. Cell Biol.* **94**, 379–386.

Silver, I. A., Murrills, R. J., and Etherington, D. J. (1988). Microelectrode studies on the acid microenvironment beneath adherent macrophages and osteoclasts. *Exp. Cell Res.* **175**, 266–276.

Silverton, S. F., Dodgson, S. J., Fallon, M. D., and Forster, R. E. (1987). Carbonic anhydrase activity of chick osteoclasts is increased by parathyroid hormone. *Am. J. Physiol.* **253**, E670–E674.

Simpson, A., and Horton, M. A. (1989). Expression of the vitronectin receptor during embryonic development: An immunohistological study of the ontogeny of the osteoclast in the rabbit. *Br. J. Exp. Pathol.* **70**, 257–265.

Sly, W. S., Hewett-Emmett, D., Whyte, M. P., Yu, Y.-S. L., and Tashjian, R. E. (1983). Carbonic anhydrase II deficiency identified as the primary defect in the autosomal recessive syndrome of osteopetrosis with renal tubular acidosis and cerebral calcification. *Proc. Natl. Acad. Sci. U.S.A.* **80**, 2752–2756.

Snipes, R. G., Lam, K. W., Dodd, R. C., Gray, T. K., and Cohen, M. S. (1986). Acid phosphatase in mononuclear phagocytes and the U937 cell line: monocyte-derived macrophages express tartrate-resistant acid phosphatase. *Blood* **67**, 729–734.

Springer, T. A., and Lasky, L. A. (1991). Sticky sugars for selectins. *Nature (London)* **349**, 196–197.

Sundquist, K. T., Leppilampi, M., Jarvelin, K., Kumpulainen, T., and Vaanenen, H. K. (1987). Carbonic anhydrase isozymes in isolated rat peripheral monocytes, tissue macrophages, and osteoclasts. *Bone* **8**, 33–38.

Sundquist, K. T., Lakkakorpi, P., Wallmark, B., and Vaananen, K. (1990). Inhibition of osteoclast proton transport by bafilomycin in A_1 abolishes bone resorption. *Biochem. Biophys. Res. Commun.* **168**, 309–313.

Takahashi, N., Yamama, H., Yoshiki, S., Roodman, D. G., Mundy, G. R., Jones, S. J., Boyde, A., and Suda, T. (1988). Osteoclast-like cell formation and its regulation by osteotropic hormones in mouse marrow cultures. *Endocrinology (Baltimore)* **122**, 1373–1382.

Takahashi, N., Kukita, T., MacDonald, B. R., Bird, A., Mundy, G. R., McManus, L. M., Miller, M., Boyde, A., Jones, S. J., and Roodman, G. D. (1989). Osteoclast-like cells form in long-term human bone marrow but not in peripheral blood. *J. Clin. Invest.* **84**, 543–550.

Tashjian, R. E. (1989). The carbonic anhydrases: Widening perspectives on their evolution, expression and function. *Bioessays* **10**, 186–192.

Taylor, L. M., Tertinegg, I., Okuda, A., and Heersche, J. N. M. (1989). Expression of calcitonin receptors during osteoclast differentiation in mouse metatarsals. *J. Bone Miner. Res.* **4**, 751–758.

Teti, A., Blair, H. C., Schlesinger, P., Grano, M., Zambonin-Zallone, A., Kahn, A. J., Teitelbaum, S. L., and Hruska, K. A. (1989a). Extracellular protons acidify osteoclasts, reduce cytosolic calcium, and promote expression of cell-matrix attachment structures. *J. Clin. Invest.* **84**, 773–780.

Teti, A., Blair, H. C., Teitelbaum, S. L., Kahn, A. J., Koziol, C., Konsek, J., Zambonin-Zallone, A., and Schlesinger, P. H. (1989b). Cytoplasmic pH regulation and chloride/bicarbonate exchange in avian osteoclasts. *J. Clin. Invest.* **83**, 227–233.

Thavarajah, M., Evans, D. B., Binderup, L., and Kanis, J. A. (1990). 1,25(OH)$_2$D$_3$ and calcipotriol (MC903) have similar effects on the induction of osteoclast-like cell formation in human bone marrow cultures. *Endocrinology (Baltimore)* **125**, 630–637.

Thomson, B. M., Saklatvala, J., and Chambers, T. J. (1986). Osteoblasts mediate interleukin 1 stimulation of bone resorption by rat osteoclasts. *J. Exp. Med.* **164**, 104–112.

Thomson, B. M., Atkinson, S. J., Reynolds, J. J., and Meickle, M. C. (1987a). Degradation of type I collagen fibres by mouse osteoblasts is stimulated by 1,25 dihydroxyvitamin D$_3$ and inhibited by human recombinant TIMP. *Biochem. Biophys. Res. Commun.* **148**, 596–602.

Thomson, B. M., Mundy, G. R., and Chambers, T. J. (1987b). Tumor necrosis factors α and β induce osteoblastic cells to stimulate osteoclastic bone resorption. *J. Immunol.* **138**, 775–779.

Tuukkanen, J., and Vaananen, H. K. (1986). Omeprazole, a specific inhibitor of H$^+$, K$^+$-ATPase, inhibits bone resorption *in vitro*. *Calcif. Tissue Int.* **38**, 123–125.

Udagawa, N., Takahashi, N., Akatsu, T., Sasaki, T., Yamaguchi, A., Kodama, H., Martin, T. J., and Suda, T. (1989). The bone marrow-derived stromal cell lines MC3T3-G2/PA6 and ST2 support osteoclast-like cell differentiation in co-cultures with mouse spleen cells. *Endocrinology (Baltimore)* **125**, 1805–1813.

Udagawa, N., Takahashi, N., Akatsu, T., Tanaka, H., Sasaki, T., Nishihara, T., Koga, T., Martin, T. J., and Suda, T. (1990). Origin of osteoclasts: mature monocytes and macrophages are capable of differentiating into osteoclasts under a suitable microenvironment prepared by bone marrow-derived stromal cells. *Proc. Natl. Acad. Sci. U.S.A.* **87,** 7260–7264.

Vaananen, H. K. (1984). Immunohistochemical localization of carbonic anhydrase isoenzymes I and II in human bone, cartilage and giant cell tumor. *Histochemistry* **81,** 485–487.

Vaananen, H. K., and Parvinen, E. K. (1983). Highly active isozyme of carbonic anhydrase in the rat calvarial osteoclasts. Immunohistochemical study. *Histochemistry* **81,** 485–487.

Vaananen, J. K., Karhukorpi, E. K., Sundquist, K., Wallmark, B., Hentunen, T., Tuukanen, J., and Lakkakorpi, P. (1990). Evidence for the presence of a proton pump of the vacuolar H^+-ATPase type in the ruffled borders of osteoclasts. *J. Cell Biol.* **111,** 1305–1311.

Vaes, G. (1965). Excretion of acid and of lysosomal acid hydrolases during bone resorption induced in tissue culture by parathyroid extract. *Exp. Cell Res.* **39,** 470–474.

Vaes, G. (1968). On the mechanisms of bone resorption. The action of parathyroid hormone on the secretion and synthesis of lysosomal enzymes and on the extracellular release of acid by bone cells. *J. Cell Biol.* **39,** 676–697.

Vaes, G. (1980). Collagenase, lysosomes and osteoclastic bone resorption. *In* "Collagenase in Normal and Pathological Connective Tissue" (D. E. Woolley and J. M. Evanson, eds.), pp. 185–207. Wiley, New York.

Vaes, G. (1988). Cellular biology and biochemical mechanism of bone resorption. *Clin. Orthop.* **231,** 239–271.

Valentin-Opran, A., Delgado, R., Valente, T., Mundy, G. R., and Graves, D. T. (1987). Autocrine production of platelet-derived growth factor (PDGF)-like peptides by cultured normal human bone cells. *J. Bone Miner. Res.* **2,** Suppl. 1, Abstr. No. 254.

Vanderwiel, C. J. (1980). An ultrastructural study of the components which make up the resting surface of bone. *Metab. Bone Dis. Relat. Res.* **2S,** 109–116.

Van Tran, P., Vignery, A., and Baron, A. (1982). Cellular kinetics of the bone remodeling sequence in the rat. *Anat. Rec.* **202,** 445–451.

Vigne, P., Frelin, C., Cragoe, E. J., and Lazdunski, M. (1984). Structure–activity relationships of amiloride and certain of its analogues in relation to the blockade of the Na/H exchange system. *Mol. Pharmacol.* **25,** 131–136.

Waite, L. C. (1972). Carbonic anhydrase inhibitors, parathyroid hormone, and calcium metabolism. *Endocrinology (Baltimore)* **91,** 1160–1165.

Waite, L. C., Volkert, W. A., and Kenny, A. D. (1970). Inhibition of bone resorption by acetazolamide in the rat. *Endocrinology (Baltimore)* **87,** 1129–1139.

Walters, L. M., and Schneider, G. B. (1987). Cellular response to ectopically implanted silk sutures and osteopetrotic bone. *Cell Tissue Res.* **248,** 79–88.

Walters, L. M., and Schneider, G. B. (1988). Tartrate-resistant acid phosphatase activity in tibial osteoclasts and cells elicited by ectopic bone and suture implants in normal and osteopetrotic rats. *Bone Miner.* **4,** 49–62.

Warshawsky, J., Goltzman, D., Rouleau, M. F., and Bergeron, J. J. M. (1980). Direct *in-vivo* demonstration by autoradiography of specific binding sites for calcitonin in skeletal and renal tissues of the rat. *J. Cell Biol.* **85,** 682–694.

Wiktor-Jedrzejczak, W., Ahmed, A., Szczylik, C., and Skelly, R. R. (1982). Hematological characterization of congenital osteopetrosis in *op/op* mouse. *J. Exp. Med.* **156,** 1516–1527.

Wiktor-Jedrzejczak, W., Bartocci, A., Ferrante, A. W., Ahmed-Ansari, A., Sell, K. W., Pollard, J. W., and Stanley, E. R. (1990). Total absence of colony-stimulating factor 1 in the macrophage-deficient osteopetrotic (op/op) mouse. *Proc. Natl. Acad. Sci. U.S.A.* **87**, 4828–4832.

Wong, S. T., Winchell, L. F., McCune, B. K., Earp. H. S., Teixido, J., Massague, J., Herman, B., and Lee, D. C. (1989). The TGF-α precursor expressed on the cell surface binds to the EGF receptor on adjacent cells, leading to signal transduction. *Cell* **56**, 495–506.

Yan, L. T., Li, C. Y., and Finkel, H. E. (1972). Leukemic reticuloendotheliosis. The role of tartrate-resistant acid phosphatase in diagnosis and splenectomy in treatment. *Arach. Intern. Med.* **130**, 248–256.

Yoon, K., Buenaga, R., and Rodan, G. A. (1987). Tissue specificity and developmental expression of rat osteopontin. *Biochem. Biophys. Res. Commun.* **148**, 1129–1136.

Yoshida, H., Hayashi, S.-I., Kunisada, T., Ogawa, M., Nishikawa, S., Okamura, H., Sudo, T., Shultz, L. D., and Nishikawa, S.-I. (1990). The murine mutation osteopetrosis is in the coding region of the macrophage colony stimulating factor gene. *Nature (London)* **345**, 442–444.

Zaidi, M., Fuller, K., Bevis, P. J. R., GainesDas, R. E., Chambers, T. J., and MacIntyre, I. (1987). Calcitonin gene-related peptide inhibits osteoclastic bone resorption: a comparative study. *Calcif. Tissue Int.* **40**, 149–154.

Zaidi, M., Datta, H. K., Patchell, A., Moonga, B., and MacIntyre, I. (1989). Calcium-inactivated intracellular calcium elevation: a novel mechanism of osteoclast regulation. *Biochem. Biophys. Res. Commun.* **163**, 1461–1465.

Zaidi, M., Datta, H. K., Bevis, P. J. R., Wimalawansa, S. J., and MacIntyre, I. (1990). Amylin-Amide: a new bone conserving peptide from the pancreas. *Exp. Physiol.* (in press).

Zambonin-Zallone, A., Teti, A., Carano, A., and Marchisio, P. C. (1988). The distribution of podosomes in osteoclasts cultured on bone laminae: Effect of retinol. *J. Bone Miner. Res.* **3**, 517–523.

Zambonin-Zallone, A., Teti, A., Grano, M., Rubinacci, A., Abbadini, M., Gaboli, M., and Marchisio, P. C. (1989). Immunocytochemical distribution of extracellular matrix receptors in human osteoclasts: A B$_3$ integrin is colocalized with vinculin and talin in the podosomes of osteoclastoma giant cells. *Exp. Cell Res.* **182**, 645–652.

Zeidel, M. L., Silva, P., and Seifter, J. L. (1986). Intracellular pH regulation in rabbit renal medullary collecting duct cells. Role of chloride–bicarbonate exchange. *J. Clin. Invest.* **77**, 1682–1688.

VITAMINS AND HORMONES, VOL. 46

Expression and Function of the Calcitonin Gene Products

MONE ZAIDI*, BALJIT S. MOONGA*, PETER J. R. BEVIS*, A. S. M. TOWHIDUL ALAM*, STEPHEN LEGON†, SUNIL WIMALAWANSA†, IAIN MacINTYRE†, AND LARS H. BREIMER**

*Department of Cellular and Molecular Sciences
St. George's Hospital Medical School
London SW17 ORE, England
†Departments of Medicine and Chemical Pathology
Hammersmith Hospital
London W12 ONN, England
**Institute of Cancer Research
Chester Beatty Laboratories
London SW7, England

I. Molecular Biology

A. Gene Organization

The starting point for the study of the calcitonin genes was the isolation and characterization of clones representing calcitonin

87

mRNA. This was achieved by several groups (Amara *et al.*, 1980; Jacobs *et al.*, 1981; Allison *et al.*, 1981) and was made possible by the availability of suitable antibodies and cell-free protein synthesis systems which allowed the selection of coding sequences from clone libraries. This work with either rat or human sequences showed that calcitonin mRNA is about 1000 bases in length and encodes a precursor protein of 136 (rat) or 141 (human) amino acids. The amino-terminus of this protein is a short hydrophobic signal peptide, typical of secreted proteins. The remainder of the precursor (procalcitonin) contains calcitonin itself and the amino- and carboxyl-terminal flanking peptides. This type of organization is frequently seen in the precursors of small regulatory peptides and the active peptides are released by cleavage of the precursor at runs of two to four dibasic amino acids (lysine or arginine). Such cleavage should release a 33-amino acid peptide from procalcitonin, and elimination of its carboxyl-terminal glycine residue converts this to the mature calcitonin peptide with a carboxyl-terminal amide group.

The interesting information that comes from these studies is the sequence of the two flanking peptides. This would have been difficult to obtain by sequencing of procalcitonin itself, as this is not found in large amounts. The question that is immediately raised by these studies concerns the possible function of these two peptides. The most exciting possibility would, of course, be that they were themselves regulatory peptides with potential therapeutic or diagnostic uses. Other possibilities are that these are required for the correct processing of procalcitonin or simply that they are vestigial features of the genes having no function at present. There is little that the molecular biologist can do to determine whether or not a predicted peptide might have a paracrine or endocrine function, but it is perhaps surprising that more attention has not been given to the other possibilities. It is possible to construct mutant genes to see whether changes in the flanking peptides interfere with the processing of the prohormone when the construct is reintroduced into the appropriate cells. It is also possible to infer from evolutionary stability of sequences whether or not they might have important functions which would be conserved between species.

Calcitonin was by no means the first regulatory peptide sequence to be cloned and the previous considerations would apply to many other such genes. What distinguishes calcitonin from others is that this has proved to be only the first chapter in a continuing story that has led to the discovery of several further regulatory peptides. The crucial discovery was made by Rosenfeld *et al.* (1981), working with serially transplanted cells from a rat medullary carcinoma of the thyroid. These cells occasionally lose their ability to produce calcitonin. This is accompanied by a slight increase in the size of the mRNA detected by calcitonin cDNA probes. Such an observation would well have been dismissed as an aberration to be expected in a transplanted tumor. However, these findings were pursued by cloning the altered mRNA and locating its sequence on the map of the calcitonin gene (Amara *et al.*, 1982). Our present understanding of the organization of the gene is illustrated in Fig. 1. The sequence of the calcitonin mRNA is represented in the genome by four exons separated by short intron sequences. Exon I is noncoding, exon II encodes the signal peptide, exon III the major part of the amino-terminal flanking peptide, and exon IV, the last seven amino acids of this peptide, the whole of calcitonin itself and its carboxyl-terminal flanking peptide. When cells switch from producing calcitonin, the longer mRNA detected with calcitonin probes is produced by splicing together the first three exons of the calcitonin gene, with the next two exons (V and VI), which are located further downstream. Translation of this new mRNA leads to the production of

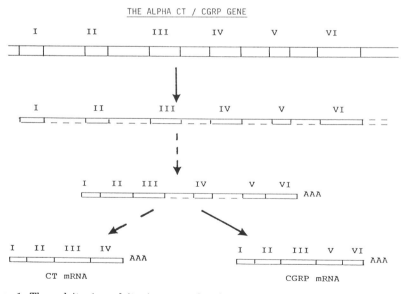

FIG. 1. The calcitonin–calcitonin gene-related peptide (CGRP) gene. The gene (top line) is made up of six exons and is transcribed to give a primary transcript terminating beyond exon VI. This is processed to give a common intermediate which may be spliced and polyadenylated to give either calcitonin or CGRP messenger RNAs. CT, calcitonin.

a polypeptide comprising the signal peptide and the amino-terminal flanking peptide of preprocalcitonin, and a further sequence encoded by exon V, exon VI being noncoding. Cleavage of this predicted polypeptide at its paired dibasic amino acids releases a 37-amino acid peptide, called the calcitonin gene-related peptide (CGRP).

The production of CGRP mRNA was shown to be a normal feature of calcitonin gene transcription. Calcitonin gene-related peptide mRNA is present in normal thyroid and medullary thyroid carcinoma at about 5–10% of the level of calcitonin mRNA, and is widely distributed in neural tissues where calcitonin mRNA is not found (for detailed review see Zaidi *et al.*, 1987a). Utilizing the predicted rat CGRP, Morris *et al.* (1984) isolated and sequenced a closely related peptide from human medullary thyroid carcinoma; the same organization of sequences in the genome was found (Steenbergh *et al.*, 1984; Edbrooke *et al.*, 1985; Kimura *et al.*, 1987). Thus, by judicious combination of molecular biology and peptide chemistry, it proved possible to progress from calcitonin itself to the new peptide, CGRP.

B. ALTERNATIVE SPLICING

As the physiological effects of the two peptides are quite different and the ratio of the two mRNAs varies dramatically in different tissues, there must be some mechanism for regulating the levels of the two mRNAs. Since the calcitonin-coding sequence is not eliminated or otherwise modified in CGRP-producing cells, the control must be at the level of transcription, processing, or stability of mRNAs. One way to approach this problem is to study the precursor RNAs found in cells producing one or the other mRNA. Such work is often undertaken, but is beset by technical difficulties that often make interpretation difficult. A keen student of literature may find evidence presented in favor of a number of competing models explaining how tissue-specific control is achieved. There is, however, agreement that the primary transcript of the calcitonin–CGRP gene extends from the beginning of exon I to a point some distance beyond the end of exon VI, even in cells producing a preponderance of calcitonin. The debate has centered around which step is decisive in committing the cell to producing calcitonin or CGRP. Clearly, if the transcript is cleaved and polyadenylated at the end of exon IV, then CGRP cannot be produced. These two models make different predictions about the processing intermediates which would be expected in cells committed to one or the other pathway. However, the two models are difficult to distinguish in practice, as the intermediates are shortlived and not easy to resolve on standard gel systems. The situation is further confused because the order of the various splicing reactions is not rigidly determined (Bovenberg *et al.*, 1986), and the number of possible intermediates is therefore large.

The way out of this difficulty was recognized by Leff *et al.* (1987). In preliminary experiments, they established that the cloned calcitonin–CGRP gene could be introduced into a variety of tissue culture cells and was expressed in a characteristic fashion. Lymphocytes, for instance, produced only calcitonin while adrenal medullary carcinoma cells produce more than 90% CGRP. If cleavage and polyadenylation at the end of exon IV commits the cell to calcitonin production, then loss of necessary polyadenylation signals would cause the cell to produce CGRP by default. When appropriately mutated calcitonin–CGRP genes were introduced into lymphocytes, the lack of suitable polyadenylation signals prevented calcitonin production, but did not lead to the production of CGRP. It would appear that the lymphocyte does not have the necessary factor(s) to make the CGRP-specific splice joining exon III to exon V sequences. Further experiments demonstrated that cells which produce CGRP mRNA from the intact calcitonin–CGRP gene were in fact able to recognize the polyadenylation site at the end of exon IV when this was presented to them in a hybrid gene lacking exon III. It is clear, then, that CGRP is produced by cells because they are able to splice together exon III and exon V sequences and not because they are unable to recognize the polyadenylation site at the end of exon IV.

The reason why cells can or cannot splice two exons together appears to reside not in the nature of the two sequences to be joined, but rather in the structure formed by the sequences separating them. Further experiments with mutated calcitonin–CGRP genes showed that deletion of sequences between splice donor and acceptor could so alter the structure of the precursor as to allow lymphocytes to make the CGRP-specific splice between exon III and V RNAs. The "factor" that they lack may be something which interacts with precursor RNAs to alter their secondary structure and allow splicing to take place. It remains to be established what this factor is (a small RNA perhaps?) and how its synthesis is regulated in an appropriate fashion.

C. The Second CGRP and Calcitonin Sequences

The discovery of CGRP illustrates how evolution has operated to generate diversity by permitting the independent production of quite separate regulatory peptides from a single gene. However, a second mechanism, gene duplication, has also operated to extend the range of peptides which can be produced from the basic calcitonin–CGRP gene. With probes representing the calcitonin coding sequence in Southern blot analysis of genomic DNA, a single band appears, indicating that there is only one such sequence in the genome. If, however, the CGRP coding sequence is used as a probe, then two bands are seen. There are two sequences in the human or rat genomes which are so similar that they cannot be distinguished by blot hybridization techniques using the CGRP coding sequence as a probe. The second sequence was quickly cloned and sequenced, and shown to encode a potential second CGRP peptide in both rat and human. This sequence is expressed and is transcribed from a second gene. This is sometimes referred to as the "β" calcitonin—CGRP gene and sometimes as *CALC-II*. This gene has sequences having close homology with exons II, III, and V of the α gene, so the two predicted prepro-CGRPs are very similar. Perhaps the crucial difference lies in the calcitonin coding region. The β gene lacks a region of close homology with exon IV of the α gene, but two groups have identified a region having weak homology (Alevizaki *et al.,* 1986; Steenbergh *et al.,* 1986). This putative exon IV encodes a calcitonin-like peptide, but the sequence is immediately preceded by a chain termination codon and the "exon" does not have a suitable poly-adenylation signal at its 3' end. The β gene appears to be the result of a local gene duplication. Both genes are located on the short arm of chromosome 11 (Alevizaki *et al.,* 1986; Przepiorka *et al.,* 1984). Perhaps this duplication was advantageous because it provided a way for a cell to produce CGRP independently of calcitonin or of the supposed factors facilitating α-CGRP splicing.

D. NEW MEMBERS OF THE CALCITONIN–CGRP GENE PEPTIDE FAMILY

Although the cloning of the calcitonin genes has led to the discovery of more new and interesting information than almost any other similar gene, there are good reasons to believe that there is more to come. There have been a number of reports that there is a second type of calcitonin in human which is detectable with antisera raised against salmon calcitonin (Fischer *et al.,* 1983; Gropp *et al.,* 1985). The degree of homology between human and salmon calcitonins is low (19 out of 32 amino acids); one would not expect to detect this using hybridization techniques directly. However, if the gene exists, it is possible that it retains more homology in some other region. Alternatively, if the peptide can be characterized then its amino acid sequence can be used to generate suitable probes for cloning the gene. While the existence of further calcitonins remains in some doubt, there is undoubtedly a further member of the calcitonin–CGRP gene family. Two groups have characterized a CGRP-like peptide from pancreatic islet cells (Cooper *et al.,* 1987; Westermark *et al.,* 1987a). This has been termed islet amyloid polypeptide (IAPP) or diabetes-associated peptide (DAP), and now more popularly, *amylin.* Its sequence has 46% homology with the known CGRPs. This is likely to be too low for its gene to cross hybridize directly with CGRP-coding sequences.

E. Evolution of the Calcitonin–CGRP Genes

A study of the evolution of a gene can provide useful information about which parts of the gene are most important for its biological activity. Studies of single genes in several species generally show that active sites tend to be conserved while the other regions are less stable. When a gene becomes duplicated and the two genes come to have different activities, the pattern of changes seen in critical regions of the gene can then be correlated with changes in biological properties. Such natural experiments may have little practical relevance for small regulatory peptides, such as calcitonin or CGRP, since structure–function relationships can more readily be established by synthesizing and assaying variant sequences. However, the study of the calcitonin– CGRP genes has led to the prediction of a variety of new peptides whose significance is difficult to evaluate. In cases where there is no obvious clue as to the likely biological activity, it can be difficult to provide suitable biological assays. In such cases, a demonstration of the evolutionary stability of a predicted peptide may be a useful guide to its likely significance. It should be remembered, however, that when dealing with relatively short sequences such as the domains of a pro- hormone, chance may have a significant influence on the accumula- tion of base changes in the DNA.

There is a considerable amount of evidence for the existence of cal- citonin-like peptides in a number of invertebrates (Fritsch *et al.,* 1979, 1980; Girgis, 1980; Perez-Cano *et al.,* 1982a,b). Unfortunately, there are as yet no reported amino acid or DNA sequences from these orga- nisms, so this analysis will be concentrated on vertebrate sequences. The DNA sequences of clones representing calcitonin–CGRP genes or messenger RNAs have been compiled to provide information on seven different genes; two each, from rat and from human, and single gene sequences from salmon, cow, and chicken (Jacobs *et al.,* 1981; Amara *et al.,* 1985; Jonas *et al.,* 1985; Riley *et al.,* 1986; Le Moullec *et al.,* 1984; Steenbergh *et al.,* 1984, 1985, 1986; Edbrooke *et al.,* 1985; Alevizaki *et al.,* 1986; Poschl *et al.,* 1987; Minvielle *et al.,* 1986, 1987; Lasmoles *et al.*, 1985a,b). In addition, there is a third sequence in human, sometimes referred to as the "γ sequence" which has strong homology with exons II and III of the calcitonin–CGRP genes (Alevizaki *et al.*, 1987). This region has not been studied in detail and the nucleotide sequence is presented in Fig. 2. The strong homology with the beta-gene extends through the intron, dividing exons II and III, indicating that this region is probably the result of a recent duplication of this part of the β gene. The absence of an initiation codon and the presence of two deletions, each of two bases, alters the reading frame of this region making it unlikely that it could encode calcitonin or CGRP-like peptides in any subsequent exons. Furthermore, no significant homology with calcitonin or CGRP sequences can be detected using nonstringent hybridization procedures. As this region appears to be a "pseudogene," it will not be considered in the following comparisons of the seven gene sequences. These are presented in Table I, where the degree of homology with the human α sequence is shown for the various domains of the preprohormones. Further data are available in the form of amino acid sequences of calcitonins and CGRPs, and these are presented in Tables II and III, respectively.

1. *Signal Peptide*

The first domain to consider is the signal peptide which extends from the initiating methionine to the peptide bond joining two small neutral amino acids (Ala-Ala or Ala-Val) found between positions 23–24 and 26–27 in various species. The conservation of DNA and of amino acid sequences between species is not striking indicating that precise amino acid sequence is not crucial to the function of the signal peptide. The key feature of signal sequences is their hydrophobic character, rather than their specific amino acid sequence, and this can be seen as a conserved feature when hydropathy plots of the predicted proteins are compared (Fig. 3). The constraint imposed by the need to conserve the hydrophobic character of this region is sufficient to preserve homology between the closely related human and rodent genes, but the nonmammalian genes have drifted considerably.

2. *Amino-Terminal Flanking Peptides*

The amino-terminal flanking peptides of calcitonin and CGRP differ by only the six (calcitonin) or four (CGRP) amino acids encoded by exons IV or V, respectively. The degree of interspecies conservation of both DNA and amino acid sequence is similar to that seen with the signal peptide, indicating perhaps that the role of this region is similarly not dependent on its particular amino acid sequence, but perhaps

```
                                                              EXON II
ALPHA GENE  ...ggtttatctcattcttcccttgcag AGAGGTGTCATGGGCTTCCAAAAGTTCTCCCCCTTCCTGGCTCTCAGCATCTTG
                                             **   *****  ******   **   ****   ****** ***
GAMMA GENE  ...cggcatcatttttacttgttacatag       CAAACAAAGGCTCCCAGAAGTTCTCCCGCTTGCTGGCTCTCAG--TCTTG
                       *  *  * * ** *   **      **     ** *******  ***  ****** *******
BETA  GENE  ...tagtaacgtcatccttccttacag AGAGGCGGCATGGGTTTCCGGAAGTTCTCCCCCTTCCCGGCTCTCAGTATCTTG

                                      INTRON II
GTCCTGTTGCAGGCAGGCAGCCTCCATGCAGCAGCACCATTCAG gtaagacagcctgaa..... 857 b.p. ....cactgagtttgcttccc
*******  *******                *******  **                                 **  ******** *******
GTCCTGTGCCAGGCAGCAGCCTCCAGGCAGCAGCGCCATTCAG gtgagacagcttgga..... 216 b.p. ....cattgagtttgcttccc
*******  **  *******      *******                                            *  ******** ******
GTCCTGTACCAGGCGGGCAGCCTCCAGGCGGCGCCATTCAG gtgagacagcctgga..... 216 b.p. ....caaggagtttgcttccc

     EXON III
ctccacag GTCGGCCCTGGAGAGCAGCCCAGCAGCAGACCCGGCCACGCTCAGTGAGGACGAGAAGCGCGCCTCCTGCTGGCTGCACTGGTGCAGGAC
******** ***                 *******   ********************************************************
ctccacag GTCTCCCGTGGAGAGCAGCAGCCCA---GACCCGGCCACACTCAGTGAGGAGGAAGTGCGCCTCCTGCTGGCTGCACTGGTGCAGGAC
******** ****  **                     **  ****************************************************
ttccacag GTCTGCCCTGGAGAGCAGCAGCCCA---GACCCGGCCACACTCAGTAAAGAGGACGCGCGCCTCCTGCTGGCTGCACTGGTGCAGGAC

                                      INTRON III
TATGTGCAGATGAAGGCCAGTGAGCTGGAGCAGGAGCAAGAGAGAGAGGGCTCCAG gtgaggctcccaagcgctc.....    ALPHA
******************************  ****                        *****  *
TATGTGCAGATGAAGGCCAGTGAGCTGGAGCAGGAGCAGGAGACAGAG--CTCCAG gtgaggctcccaagcgccc.....    GAMMA
******************  ****  **                         ****** ****************  *
TATGTGCAGATGAAGGCCAGTGAGCTGAAGCAGGAGGACACAGGGCTCCAG gtgaggttccccaagcgccc.....    BETA
```

FIG. 2. Nucleotide sequence of human "γ-calcitonin–calcitonin gene-related peptide (CGRP)" sequence in the region homologous with exons II and III of the α and β genes. Strong homology with β gene extends through the intron region.

TABLE I
COMPARISON OF CT–CGRP mRNA AND PEPTIDE SEQUENCES[a]

	5'	SIG	NF	CT	CT-C	CT-3'	CGRP	CG-C	CG-3'
mRNA									
Human 1	100	100	100	100	100	100	100	100	100
Human 2	-	88	93	71	62	69	95	100	70
Rat 1	65	84	80	90	68	51	89	83	78
Rat 2	-	79	80	--	--	--	91	75	66
Bovine	-	-	-	67	70	58	85	83	-
Chicken	-	63	65	68	48	53	81	50	-
Salmon	-	56	64	61	40	50	-	-	-
Peptide									
Human 1	--	100	100	100	100	--	100	100	--
Human 2	--	84	82	45	39	--	92	100	--
Rat 1	--	68	71	94	44	--	89	100	--
Rat 2	--	68	73	--	--	--	92	50	--
Bovine	--	-	-	45	52	--	82	75	--
Chicken	--	48	54	48	14	--	89	25	--
Salmon	--	35	51	52	11	--	-	-	--

[a]Nucleotide sequence data from the sources documented in the text and our own partial bovine sequence (K. Collyear, unpublished ovservations) was analyzed for homology with the human α-calcitonin–CGRP sequence using the IBI/Pustell analysis programs. Values represent percentage homologies scoring insertions and deletions as one mismatch, regardless of length. Domains analyzed are $-5':5'$ noncoding sequence. SIG, Signal peptide; NF amino-terminal flanking peptide (for CGRP, except in the case of salmon); CT, calcitonin; CT-C, carboxyl-terminal flanking peptide for calcitonin; CT-3', 3' noncoding sequence from calcitonin mRNA; CGRP, calcitonin gene-related peptide; CG-C, carboxyl-terminal flanking peptide for CGRP; and CG-3, 3' noncoding sequence from CGRP mRNA. Analysis is not possible for some regions (--) and data is not yet available for others (-).

more on the tertiary structure it adopts. The hydropathy plot (Fig. 3) shows a characteristic pattern of hydrophilic and hydrophobic regions, particularly in the latter half of the domain, ending with a long hydrophilic region next to the calcitonin or CGRP domain. The amino-terminal flanking peptides have not been seen as potential regulatory peptides, as they are not believed to be exported and are commonly assumed to have a role in the processing of the prohormone. In this respect it is likely that the hydrophilic domain at the carboxyl-terminus would ensure that the calcitonin or CGRP sequence was not buried within the tertiary structure of the prohormone. Interestingly, paired dibasic amino acids, the usual signal for excision of regulatory pep-

TABLE II
Comparison of Calcitonin Peptides[a]

	*			*	*	*	*		*							
Human 1	C	G	N	L	S	T	C	M	L	G	T	Y	T	Q	D	F
Rat	C	G	N	L	S	T	C	M	L	G	T	Y	T	Q	D	L
Pig	C	S	N	L	S	T	C	V	L	S	A	Y	W	R	N	L
Cow	C	S	N	L	S	T	C	V	L	S	A	Y	W	K	D	L
Sheep	C	S	N	L	S	T	C	V	L	S	A	Y	W	K	D	L
Salmon 1	C	S	N	L	S	T	C	V	L	G	K	L	S	Q	E	L
Salmon 2	C	S	N	L	S	T	C	M	L	G	K	L	S	Q	D	L
Salmon 3	C	S	N	L	S	T	C	V	L	G	K	L	S	Q	D	L
Eel	C	S	N	L	S	T	C	V	L	G	K	L	S	Q	E	L
Chicken	C	A	S	L	S	T	C	V	L	G	K	L	S	Q	E	L
Human 2	Y	S	N	L	S	T	C	L	Q	G	T	Y	L	Q	Y	L

												*				*	*
Human 1	N	K	F	H	T	F	P	Q	T	A	I	G	V	G	A	P	G
Rat	N	K	F	H	T	F	P	Q	T	S	I	G	V	G	A	P	G
Pig	N	N	F	H	R	F	S	G	M	G	F	G	P	E	T	P	G
Cow	N	N	Y	H	R	F	S	G	M	G	F	G	P	E	T	P	G
Sheep	N	N	Y	H	R	Y	P	G	M	G	F	G	P	E	T	P	G
Salmon 1	H	K	L	Q	T	Y	P	R	T	N	T	G	S	G	T	P	G
Salmon 2	H	K	L	Q	T	F	P	R	T	N	T	G	A	G	V	P	G
Salmon 3	H	K	L	Q	T	F	P	R	T	N	T	G	A	G	V	P	G
Eel	H	K	L	Q	T	Y	P	R	T	D	V	G	A	G	T	P	G
Chicken	H	K	L	Q	T	Y	S	R	T	D	V	G	A	E	T	P	G
Human 2	K	N	F	H	M	F	P	G	I	N	F	G	P	Q	I	P	G

[a]Calcitonins are grouped according to three known types (human, bovine, and salmon types). With the putative coding sequence from the second (β) human gene. (*) denote residues conserved in all authentic calcitonins.

tides from their precursor proteins, occur twice within this region of the rat β-calcitonin–CGRP gene and once in the salmon gene, allowing for the possibility that one or two short peptides might be released during maturation of the prohormone. However, the other genes lack this feature, making it unlikely that these are actually regulatory peptides.

3. *Calcitonin*

The calcitonin peptides are separated from their amino-terminal flanking peptides by a pair of dibasic amino acids, and from their carboxyl-terminal flanking peptides by three dibasic amino acids in all seven genes. Calcitonin itself is a 32-amino acid single-chain polypeptide with a carboxyl-terminal amide derived from a glycine residue.

TABLE III
THE CGRP–DAP (IAPP) PEPTIDE FAMILY[a]

Block 1 (positions 1–13)

	1	2	3	4	5	6	7	8	9	10	11	12	13
		*		*	*	*	*	*	*	*	*	*	*
Human 1	A	C	D	T	A	T	C	V	T	H	R	L	A
Human 2	A	C	N	T	A	T	C	V	T	H	R	L	A
Rat 1	S	C	N	T	A	T	C	V	T	H	R	L	A
Rat 2	S	C	N	T	A	T	C	V	T	H	R	L	A
Cow	S	C	N	T	A	T	C	V	T	H	R	L	A
Pig	S	C	N	T	A	T	C	V	T	H	R	L	A
Chicken	A	C	N	T	A	T	C	V	T	H	R	L	A
		*	*	*	*	*	*		*		*	*	*
Human DAP	K	C	N	T	A	T	C	A	T	Q	R	L	A
Cat DAP	K		N	T	A	T		A	T	Q	R	L	A
		*		*	*	*	*		*		*	*	*
Sal CT1	C	S	N	L	S	T	C	V	L	G	K	L	S
			*			*	*	*			+	*	

Block 2 (positions 1–13)

	1	2	3	4	5	6	7	8	9	10	11	12	13
			*	*	*	*	*	*			*		
Human 1	G	L	L	S	R	S	G	G	V	V	K	N	N
Human 2	G	L	L	S	R	S	G	G	M	V	K	S	N
Rat 1	G	L	L	S	R	S	G	G	V	V	K	D	N
Rat 2	G	L	L	S	R	S	G	G	V	V	K	D	N
Cow	G	L	L	S	R	S	G	G	V	V	K	E	H
Pig	G	L	L	S	R	S	G	G	M	V	K	S	N
Chicken	D	F	L	S	R	S	G	G	V	G	K	N	N
			*		*	*							
Human DAP	N	F	L	V	H	S	S	N	N	F	G	A	I
Cat DAP	N	F	L	I	R	S	S	N	N	L	G	A	I
Sal CT1	Q	E	L	H	K						L	Q	T
	+		*		+							+	

Block 3 (positions 1–12)

	1	2	3	4	5	6	7	8	9	10	11	12
	*	*	*	*		*				*	*	*
Human 1	F	V	P	T	N	V	G	S	K	A	F	G
Human 2	F	V	P	T	N	V	G	S	K	A	F	G
Rat 1	F	V	P	T	N	V	G	S	E	A	F	G
Rat 2	F	V	P	T	N	V	G	S	K	A	F	G
Cow	F	V	P	T	N	V	R	T	E	A	F	G
Pig	F	V	P	T	D	V	G	S	E	A	F	G
Chicken	F	V	P	T	N	V	G	S	K	A	F	G
				*	*	*	*	*				
Human DAP	L	S	S	T	N	V	G	S	N	T	Y	
Cat DAP	L											
			P	R		*			*			
Sal CT1	Y			T	N	T	G	S	G	T	P	G
	+			*	*		*	*		*		*

[a] Comparison of calcitonin gene-related peptide (CGRP)-like peptides. Upper sequences are known as CGTPs with diabetic-associated peptide (DAP or amylin) sequences beneath. The salmon calcitonin sequence is shown with a gap introduced to maximize homology. Asterisks above the CGRPs denote conserved residues in CGRP, those between are common to some CGRPs and DAPs, and those beneath the DAPs are common to all CGRPs and DAPs. Lower row of asterisks denote residues which are common to the salmon calcitonin and some of the CGRP or DAP sequences with (+) representing strongly homologous matches (lys-arg, glu-asp, gln-asn, tyr-phe).

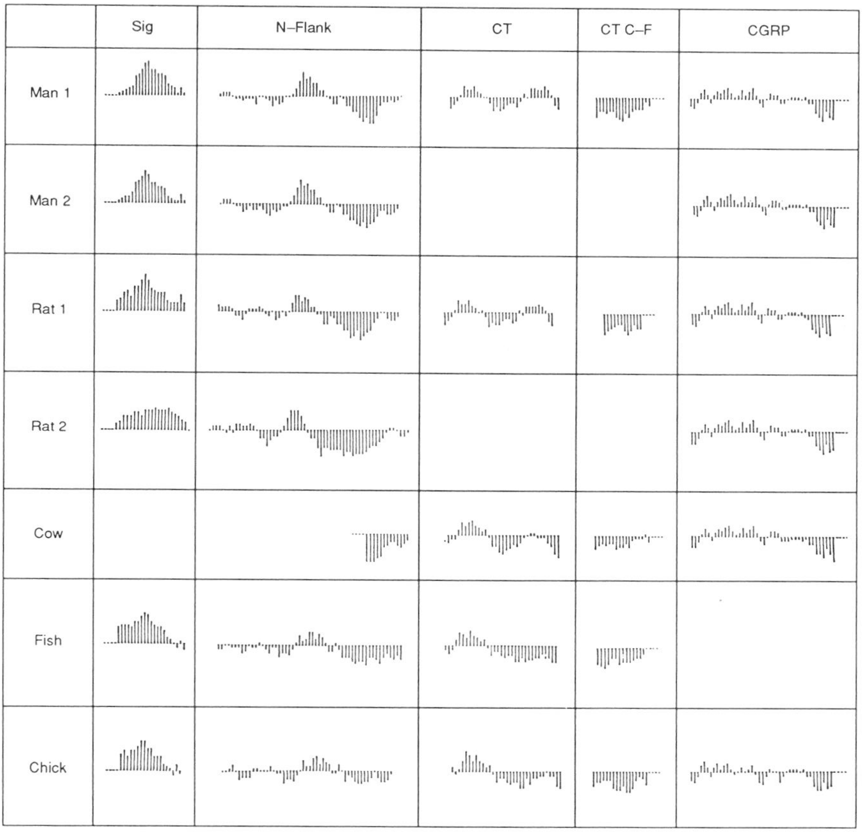

	Sig	N–Flank	CT	CT C–F	CGRP
Man 1					
Man 2					
Rat 1					
Rat 2					
Cow					
Fish					
Chick					

FIG. 3. Hydropathy plots of peptides encoded by the calcitonin–calcitonin gene-related peptide genes. Data obtained from the analysis of nucleotide sequences summarized in Table I using the IBI/Pustell program averaging values over nine residues. Hydrophilic regions appear above the line, hydrophobic regions below the line. SIG, Signal peptide; N-FLANK, amino-terminal flanking peptide (for CGRP except in the case of fish sequence); CT C-F, carboxyl-terminal flanking peptide of calcitonin; CGRP, calcitonin gene-related peptide region including carboxyl-terminal dibasic residues and flanking tetrapeptide.

Table II lists the amino acid sequence of nine calcitonins and a calcitonin-like sequence found in the human β-CGRP gene (Alevizaki *et al.*, 1986; Steenberg *et al.*, 1986). The known calcitonins fall into three classes typified by the human, bovine, and salmon sequences. Within any one class there is a high degree of sequence conservation, but between classes the divergence is more than 50%, with only nine resi-

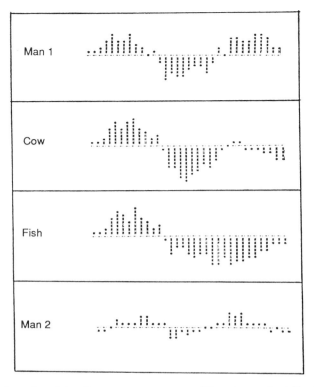

Fig. 4. Hydropathy plots of consensus sequences of four types of calcitonin peptides. As the program averages values over nine residues, the first and last five residues cannot normally be analyzed. Sequences were therefore flanked by five glycine residues for this analysis. Where a clear consensus could not be estimated, amino acids matching the consensus in another group were chosen, and where this was not possible, the prototype sequence was chosen, i.e., human, bovine, and salmon I. Data from Table II.

dues being conserved. These peptides have been isolated, sequenced, and synthesized (for review see Breimer *et al.,* 1988). The hydropathy plots (Fig. 4) show that the overall character of the calcitonins is conserved in the amino-terminal half of the peptides, but they differ considerably toward the carboxyl terminus.

The exception to this is the human "β-calcitonin" sequence where, despite a similar degree of sequence conservation, the conserved amino-terminal hydropathy profile has been lost. There is no possibility of this peptide being expressed in the present day human genome, as it is preceded by chain termination triplets, but it has been interesting to speculate that it might be a recent descendant of an active gene sequence and consequently might retain some useful biological activity. It is not particularly close in sequence to any one of the three classes containing features of each of them, and might thus represent a fourth class of active peptide. However, its sequence has diverged from the α sequence at the same rate as has the 3' noncoding sequence (Table I). It is also interesting to note that two of the eight conserved residues have also undergone change. This, coupled with the loss of the typical hydropathy profile, indicates a lack of selective pressure on this sequence for a considerable period of time.

4. CGRP and Amylin

In contrast with the highly variable calcitonin amino acid sequence, the CGRP sequence is well conserved between species (Table III). This is generally taken as an indication of the importance of CGRP as a vasoactive peptide. The second class of peptide, known as IAPP, DAP, or amylin has 46% homology with the CGRPs, and should be considered as a member of the same family (Westermark et al., 1987b; Cooper et al., 1987). The conservation of sequence between cat and human may be taken as an indication of the importance of this peptide. The hydropathy plots of the two classes of peptide (Fig. 5) show little evidence of a family resemblance—clearly the two branches of the family have been separated for a considerable time. Also shown in Table III, is the sequence of salmon calcitonin-1 aligned with the CGRP and amylin sequences to achieve maximum homology. There is a total of 12 perfect matches and a further 5 conservative substitutions between the CGRP and amylin sequences and this calcitonin, indicating perhaps an ancient duplication of a common ancestral coding sequence.

5. Carboxyl-Terminal Flanking Peptide

The final domain of the prohormone to consider is the carboxyl-terminal flanking peptide. In human, the carboxyl-terminal flanking peptide of calcitonin is cosecreted with calcitonin (Hillyard et al., 1983). The sequences of the various calcitonin flanking peptides are shown in Table IV. The sequences initially available for comparison (rat and human) gave little support to the idea that this might be a new regulatory peptide. The degree of sequence conservation is unremarkable and the rat peptide is five amino acids shorter. The human sequence appears to be closer to the ancestral form, as both the bovine and chicken peptides are also 21 amino acids in length. The gene sequence of bovine calcitonin predicts a peptide with 11 residues in common with the human sequence. This homology (52%) is greater

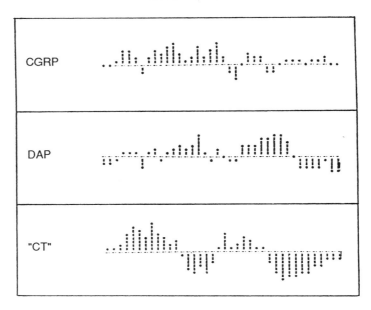

F𝗂𝗀. 5. Hydropathy plots of consensus calcitonin gene-related peptide-like peptides. Consensus sequences for calcitonin gene-related peptide (CGRP) and diabetes-associated peptide (amylin) were analyzed in Fig. 4. The salmon calcitonin sequence ("CT") is the sequence shown in Table III with the gap introduced to maximize homology with CGRPs being filled in with authentic CGRP residues.

than that seen with the corresponding calcitonins (45%) and raises again the possibility that this domain may have some more specific function in these species. The salmon and chicken sequences have little in common with the mammalian sequences, although they have an interesting region of homology with each other. The carboxyl-terminal flanking peptide associated with CGRP is four amino acids in length. It shows strong conservation between mammalian species, which could indicate an important role for this peptide. As the sequences are short, it would be rash to make judgements as to the significance of this degree of conservation.

Based on this analysis of available sequence information it is possible to speculate on how the calcitonin–CGRP genes may have evolved. Two very ancient events may be identified: an exon duplication giving rise to CGRP and calcitonin exons, and a gene duplication giving rise to CGRP and amylin genes. The "salmon-type" calcitonin–CGRP gene is seen at present in dog fishes and has also been inherited by birds. During the evolution of the mammals, radical changes oc-

TABLE IV

Comparison of Carboxyl-Terminal Flanking Peptides of Calcitonin and Calcitonin Gene-Related Peptides[a]

Calcitonin C-Terminal Flanking Peptides[b]

Rat	D	M	A	K	D	L	E	T	N	H	H	P	Y	F	G	N					
	*			*	*	*	*		*	*		*									
Human	D	M	S	S	D	L	E	R	D	H	R	P	H	V	S	M	P	Q	N	A	N
	*				*	*	*	*	*	*	*		*				*		*		*
Cow	D	V	A	N	S	L	E	R	D	H	S	F	H	F	G	V	P	Q	D	A	N
	*		*			*									*			*			*
Chicken	N	V	L	N	D	L	D	H	E	R	Y	A	N	Y	G	E	T	L	G	N	
			*						*	*		*	*	*		*					
Salmon					L	P	E	S	N	R	Y	A	S	Y	G	D	S	Y	D	G	I

CGRP Flanking Peptides[c]

Human 1	D	L	Q	A
	*	*	*	*
Human 2	D	L	Q	A
	*	*	*	*
Rat 1	D	L	Q	A
	*	*	*	
Rat 2	D	L	R	V
	*	*		
Cow	D	L	Q	D
			*	
Chicken	S	V	Q	I

[a] An asterisk indicates a conservation of residues in adjacent sequences.

[b] C-Terminal, Carboxyl-terminal.

[c] CGRP, Calcitonin gene-related peptide.

curred in the calcitonin-coding exon, giving rise to two new forms of calcitonin; the bovine form, seen in cows, pigs, and sheep, and the human form, seen in humans and rats. At about the time the primate and rodent lines separated, there was a duplication of the calcitonin–CGRP gene, giving rise to the α and β genes seen in present day human and rat. Most recently of all, there appears to have been a further duplication affecting exons II and III of the human β gene, giving rise to the "γ sequence."

There are, however, a number of observations that seem to contradict this simple model of the evolution of the calcitonin-CGRP genes, and suggest that human-type and salmon-type genes have coexisted throughout evolution. The calcitonin-like immunoreactivity detected in invertebrates (Fritsch *et al.*, 1979, 1980; Girgis, 1980; Perez-Cano *et al.*, 1982) and frogs (Perez-Cano *et al.*, 1981, 1982a) is of a human-type rather than salmon. Furthermore, there are reports indicating that a salmon-type calcitonin can be detected in man either by radioimmunoassay (Fischer *et al.*, 1983; Gropp *et al.*, 1985) or by hybridization with a chicken (i.e., salmon-type) DNA probe (Lasmoles *et al.*, 1985a). It should be stressed, however, that in neither case is this evidence supported by the amino acid sequence of the peptide or the DNA sequence of a cloned gene.

II. Chemistry

A. Primary Structure

1. *Calcitonin*

Several mammalian and submammalian calcitonins have been isolated, sequenced, and synthesized. These include porcine (from normal thyroid; Baghdiantz *et al.*, 1964; Potts *et al.*, 1968; Rittel *et al.*, 1968), human (from medullary thyroid carcinoma tissue; Riniker *et al.*, 1968; Neher *et al.*, 1968), bovine (from normal thyroid; Brewer and Ronan, 1969), ovine (from normal thyroid; Potts *et al.*, 1970), salmon (from ultimobranchial bodies; O'Dor *et al.*, 1969; Niall *et al.*, 1969), eel (from ultimobranchial bodies; Otani *et al.*, 1976; Morikawa *et al.*, 1976), and rat (from normal rat thyroid; Raulias *et al.*, 1976; from medullary thyroid carcinoma tissue; Byfield *et al.*, 1976a,b). The calcitonin sequences display considerable differences in amino acid composition, ranging from 2 (between rat and human) to 19 (between human and ovine) amino acid substitutions.

The successful determination of the primary structure of calcitonin molecules was followed by studies designed to evaluate the effect of structural modifications on biological function. Some of the earliest studies (see, e.g., Byfield *et al.*, 1972) predicted that the two ends of the calcitonin molecule were important for bioactivity. This would be obvious from the high level of conservation observed at the termini (Table II). It was suggested correctly at the time that these highly conserved termini are juxtaposed in spatial configuration, and that the variable middle portion of the molecule (positions 10–27) controlled the potency and duration of action of the peptide.

Another major advancement was the determination of elements in the primary structure of the molecule that were essential for biological activity. Rigorous studies using calcitonin fragments and chemically modified analogues showed that the carboxyl-terminus and its proline–amide residue, the disulphide bond between positions 2 and 7 (Rittel *et al.*, 1976), and the methionine residue at position 8 in human calcitonin (Seiber *et al.*, 1970) were necessary prerequisites for biological activity. Surprisingly, oxidation of the methionine residue at position 25 in the porcine, bovine, and ovine calcitonin did not lead to a loss of biological activity. Generally, it was observed that replacement modifications that tended to increase homology with salmon calcitonin enhanced biological potency (Maier *et al.*, 1974). However, more recent studies on the tertiary structure and molecular flexibility of calcitonin have questioned some of these conclusions.

2. Calcitonin Gene-Related Peptide

Studies on the structure–activity relationship of CGRP are somewhat more preliminary than those on calcitonin. Apart from minor differences, we found that the four CGRP sequences behave similarly (Tippins *et al.*, 1986; Zaidi *et al.*, 1987b, 1990g). At similar molar concentrations the four peptides cause an equivalent elevation of blood flow in the rabbit skin and enhance the contractility of the rat atrium to a similar extent (Tippins *et al.*, 1986; Brain *et al.*, 1986; Zaidi *et al.*, 1990g). Second, the four CGRP peptides also share some of the effects of calcitonin on the osteoclast and renal calcitonin receptor at several hundredfold molar concentrations than calcitonin, but with identical potencies (Zaidi *et al.*, 1987b,c, 1988a).

A study of the effect of enzymic digest fragments and chemically modified products was carried out using three biological assays (Zaidi *et al.*, 1990g). In one of these, the osteoclast bone resorption assay, the activity of CGRP is mediated via calcitonin receptors (Zaidi *et al.*, 1987b,c, 1988a), while in the other two, the blood flow and edema assays, the effect is mediated via CGRP receptors. The results clearly indicate that the intact CGRP molecule is required for its full biological activity. None of the fragments produced by either trypsin- or chymotrypsin-catalyzed hydrolysis of specific peptide bonds showed a significant effect in any of the three assay systems used, with the only exception of fragment Ala[1]Lys[35], which exhibited a reduced activity in the blood flow and bone resorption assays. The reduced potency shown by amino-acetylated CGRP and the complete destruction of biological activity upon either oxidation or reduction followed by methylation seemed to indicate that the amino-terminal region of the peptide, and in particular the Cys[2] Cys[7] disulphide bridge play an important part in the interaction of the molecule with the CGRP or calcitonin receptor. However, the lack of biological activity of the amino-terminal fragments Ala[1] Arg[11], Ala[1] Ser[16] and Ala[1] Arg[18] suggested that the remaining part of the molecule is probably necessary for the peptide to assume the right conformation, and therefore to ensure a correct interaction with the receptor. The fact that partial modifications such as acetylation of Lys[24] or Lys[35] or substitution, in β-CGRP of Val[22] and Asn[25] with Met and Ser, respectively, did not cause relevant changes in biological activity, corroborates the hypothesis of this secondary, but nevertheless important role played by the carboxyl-terminal region of the peptide.

These findings have been supported by a report of the CGRP receptor antagonist activity of human CGRPVal[8]Phe[37] (Chiba et al., 1989). This fragment was found to be essential for the binding of intact CGRP to its receptor; nevertheless, without the amino-terminal disulphide bridge and ring structure this carboxyl-terminal fragment was unable to induce the subsequent intracellular signal transduction event. The fragment was, however, able to promote adenylate cyclase activity in renal cells, which indicates an action on calcitonin receptors (Wohlwend et al., 1985). Chiba and colleagues (1989) concluded that the carboxyl-terminal of calcitonin is more important than the amino-terminal in binding to the calcitonin receptor, which may have a broad specificity in recognizing the carboxyl-terminal portions of binding agonists. From their results it might have been expected that our tests on carboxyl-terminal fragments would show some agonist activity in the osteoclast assay and antagonist activity in the blood flow and edema assays. This was not the case, possibly because the carboxyl-terminal fragments that we tested were much shorter than that reported by Chiba and co-workers. Nevertheless, the results described demonstrated that similar structural prerequisites were required for the interaction of CGRP with receptors in vessels and bone. The present suggestion that the amino-terminal region of the peptide is essential for the binding of CGRP to its receptor, and that the carboxyl-terminal region also has an important role, is clearly relevant to further studies aimed at developing chemically different vasodilatory agents acting via the CGRP receptor.

3. *Amylin*

Amylin is a 37-amino acid polypeptide first isolated as "islet amyloid polypeptide" from an insulinoma and from the islet amyloid of a diabetic cat (Westermark *et al.*, 1987a), and also as "diabetic associated peptide" from the amyloid deposit of human Type II diabetes (Westermark *et al.*, 1986; Cooper *et al.*, 1987). Its amino acid sequence resembles that of the CGRP (Westermark *et al.*, 1986). There is a disulphide bridge between positions 2 and 7, and although the reported sequence lacks a carboxyl-terminal amide (Westermark *et al.*, 1987a,b, Cooper *et al.*, 1987), the circulating peptide appears to be almost certainly carboxyamidated. Amylin and its amide are both highly hydrophobic molecules and are often difficult to dissolve or maintain in solution.

We have shown that amylin and amylin-amide have powerful osteoclast-inhibitory and plasma calcium lowering actions similar to calcitonin (Datta *et al.*, 1989a; Zaidi *et al.*, 1990f). Amylin-amide is only about 30 times less potent than calcitonin in lowering plasma calcium. This is quite surprising. Despite the lack of close homology of primary structure (typically $< 13\%$) (Westermark *et al.*, 1987a,b; Cooper *et al.*, 1987), the two peptides are not too distant in their ability to interact with the osteoclast. This is in clear contrast with CGRP, that has about 30% sequence homology with calcitonin (for reviews see Zaidi *et al.*, 1987a; Breimer *et al.*, 1988), but is approximately 1000-fold less potent than the latter peptide in lowering plasma calcium (Zaidi *et al.*, 1988a) or inhibiting osteoclastic bone resorption (Zaidi *et al.*, 1987b,c, 1988a).

Interestingly, the amidated and unamidated forms of the amylin peptide were found to be active both *in vivo* and *in vitro*. This finding is in sharp contrast to calcitonin and CGRP, where deamidation leads to the abolition of biological activity. The unamidated peptide has also been shown to be active in significantly reducing glucose incorporation into glycogen in the rat skeletal muscle. Nevertheless, only the amidated form was found to possess agonist activity in stimulating cyclic AMP (cAMP) accumulation in human umbilical endothelial cells (J. McEwan *et al.*, unpublished observations). These cells are known to have high affinity binding sites for CGRP. Clearly, amidation of amylin is not a necessary prerequisite for its hypocalcemic and anti-insulin actions, but appears to be vital when the peptide mimics (probably via structurally homology) the vascular action of CGRP. Further studies are required to elucidate the nature of amylin interaction with known or novel receptors in target organs.

B. TERTIARY STRUCTURE

1. *Molecular Flexibility*

There has been no obviously convincing explanation until recently as to why ultimobranchial (salmon and eel) calcitonins are most potent both *in vivo* and *in vitro* (Galante *et al.*, 1971). Two possibilities have been debated: a greater affinity for the receptor (Marx *et al.*, 1972) and/or greater resistance to metabolic degradation (Habener *et al.*, 1971; deLuise *et al.*, 1970). However, it has become clear that one cannot reliably predict biological activity from information based solely on primary structure. Molecules with relatively little sequence homology could have similar conformational interactions with receptor–membrane complexes (Kaiser and Kezdi, 1984). Epand *et al.* (1986) were the first to suggest that "conformational flexibility" of the calcitonin molecule could significantly effect its biological activity. The flexibility theory suggests that a more "flexible" molecule is able to attain a larger number of conformations at the receptor–membrane complex. The degree of molecular flexibility depends on the bulkiness of its amino acid side chain (glycine is the least bulky) and thus, upon its tendency to form rigid helices (Kaiser and Kezdi, 1984). In both ultimobranchial calcitonins, salmon and eel, three glycine residues are highly conserved. Both peptides therefore possess a remarkably low helix-forming potential. This either allows the molecules a more energetically favorable access to the receptor–membrane complex, or allows them to escape a less active, though stable, conformation (Epand *et al.*, 1986). Although it appears that the valine residue at position 27 might induce conformational rigidity due to its bulky side chain, the effect is effectively cancelled by the presence of an alanine residue at position 29. More convincing evidence has come from experiments where amino acids having bulky side chains have been replaced with side chains that are less bulky. For example, the replacement substitution of valine with glycine at position 8 or leucine with alanine at position 16 have been shown to produce more potent analogues, again due to an increasingly flexible molecule.

2. *Other Conformational Interactions*

Nevertheless, it is clear that the consideration of conformational flexibility is often not enough to predict the relative activity of certain calcitonin analogues; neither is the consideration of any single factor, such as hydrophobic moment or overall peptide hydrophobicity. Peptides such as des-Leu[16]-sCT and human calcitonin have less helix-forming potential and are consequently more flexible than salmon calcitonin, but are much less potent (Epand et al., 1985). In addition, conformational coupling within the various regions of the molecule makes it more difficult to predict the potency of analogues. This is due to long range (with respect to the amino acid sequence) interactions between the amino and carboxyl regions of the molecules, at least in the receptor-bound form (Pless et al., 1971). It is also possible that the binding of calcitonin to its receptor is coupled to cooperative conformational interactions in different regions of the peptide in a manner analogous to that proposed for the binding of substrate to enzymes (Tanuichi, 1984).

3. The Disulphide Bridge

Some studies have even questioned the importance of the stereo-chemical arrangement of the amino-terminal residues produced by the formation of the disulphide bridge. An analogue of salmon calcitonin (des-ser[2]-sCT) with fewer amino acids at the amino-terminus is fully biologically active (Epand et al., 1986), and the replacement of the disulphide bridge in a carba-type analogue of eel calcitonin (eel-asu[1–7]-CT) also allows full retention of biological activity (Morikawa et al., 1976; Zaidi et al., 1990g). Orlowski et al. (1987) have shown that the opening of the disulphide bridge between positions 1 and 7 of salmon calcitonin and its replacement by an S-acetamido-methylcysteinyl linkage does not abolish the hypocalcemic or renal cAMP-stimulating activity of the peptide. Nevertheless, a similar modification in the human calcitonin molecule leads to the selective loss of the hypocalcemic effect and retention only of the renal effect. The authors have, however, stated that in a lipid-bound form, residues 1 and 7, when bound by a disulphide bridge, promote the formation of a helical structure in other regions of the molecule. Similarly, it has been clearly demonstrated that an intact hexapeptide ring structure is not essential for the binding of antagonistic arginine vasopressin (AVP) analogues to vasopressor or antidiuretic AVP receptors (Manning et al., 1987). These discoveries raise the possibility that other cyclic peptides, such as somatostatin, may also not require a ring structure for activity, and that modifications of this type may form the basis for the design of linear analogues of cyclic peptides as pharmacological probes and for therapeutic use.

III. ENDOCRINOLOGY

A. SECRETION

1. *Calcitonin*

The origin of plasma calcitonin from parafollicular C-cells of the thyroid was established (Foster *et al.*, 1969) soon after the discovery of the hormone (Copp and Cheney, 1962; Kumar *et al.*, 1963). The peptide is cosecreted in equimolar concentrations with its carboxyl-terminal flanking peptide, katacalcin, from the same granules in C-cells (for reviews see MacIntyre, 1988; MacIntyre *et al.*, 1987a; Zaidi *et al.*, 1987a, 1989f). Calcitonin gene-related peptide is also found in C-cells of normal thyroid tissue, although it is most evident in tumor cells in medullary thyroid carcinoma. Here it is frequently costored with calcitonin (Sikri *et al.*, 1985; for detailed review see Zaidi *et al.*, 1987a), but there are some cells containing the common amino-terminal peptide of CGRP that do not stain with calcitonin antisera. The common amino-terminal precursor to both peptides does not circulate in intact form in human subjects, but is processed and cleaved before secretion. It is not known how the two precursors or their cleavage products are packaged in the granules of Golgi. It seems likely that only some of the processing is completed before packaging in secretion granules, and that final clevage steps occur within granules, before secretion (MacIntyre *et al.*, 1987b). It is uncertain whether calcitonin is all secreted in monomer form or whether a significant proportion is secreted as a calcitonin–katacalcin complex to be processed peripherally.

The early work showing increased release of calcitonin with hypercalcemia (Copp and Cheney, 1962; Kumar *et al.*, 1963) remains the best evidence that calcium controls secretion. Plasma calcitonin levels increase as plasma calcium rises, and decreases as it falls. The elevation of the extracellular calcium concentration in steps as small as 0.1 mM has been shown to stimulate the secretion of calcitonin (Nemeth, 1987; Fried and Tashijan, 1986; Haller-Brem *et al.*, 1987). This is accompanied with the elevation of intracellular free calcium (Fried and Tashijan, 1986). Calcitonin gene-related peptide is also released in parallel with calcitonin (Haller-Brem *et al.*, 1987; Muff *et al.*, 1988) as the two peptides are costored, sometimes, within the same granule of a C-cell. It has also been demonstrated that ionomycin causes a 17-fold elevation of calcitonin and CGRP secretion in cloned human medullary thyroid carcinoma (TT) cells, suggesting that the secretion of the two peptides from C-cells is, at least in part, modulatable by changes in the intracellular calcium concentration (Haller-Brem *et al.*, 1987).

It is evident, however, that there are other factors regulating the release of calcitonin from C-cells. Receptors for 1,25-dihydroxy-vitamin D_3 have been identified on C-cells (Freake and MacIntyre, 1982), and it is possible that the hormonal form of vitamin D may have a direct effect on calcitonin secretion. Furthermore, chronic estrogen administration to women after the menopause elevates plasma calcitonin levels (Stevenson *et al.*, 1983), but it is not clear whether this is a direct or indirect effect. There is also evidence that gastrin and cholecystokinin induce calcitonin secretion (Care, 1970; Cooper *et al.*, 1971). It has been postulated that calcitonin has a special role after eating: its secretion, induced by gastrointestinal peptides, results in greater skeletal retention of calcium than would normally occur.

2. *Calcitonin Gene-Related Peptide*

Unlike calcitonin, CGRP is a vasodilator neuropeptide (for review see Zaidi *et al.*, 1987a). Normally the thyroid does not contribute to circulating CGRP in either human or rat, and whereas thyroidectomy in animals abolishes circulating calcitonin, no such effect on CGRP has been noted (Zaidi *et al.*, 1986a). Calcitonin gene-related peptide, however is released into the circulation from hyperplastic and malignant C-cells, although the plasma levels of the two peptides are widely discordant (Zaidi *et al.*, 1986a; Emson and Zaidi, 1989). We have demonstrated that blockade of axonal transport of the peptide by colchicine abolishes circulating CGRP (Zaidi *et al.*, 1985; Emson and Zaidi, 1989), and depolarization of nerve endings by capsaicin leads to a dramatic 15-fold elevation of plasma levels (Zaidi *et al.*, 1985; Diez Guerra *et al.*, 1987; Emson and Zaidi, 1989), and thus remain convinced that circulating peptide is derived mainly from perivascular and cardiac nerve terminals (Fig. 6) (Bevis *et al.*, 1986a,b). This conclusion is based on extensive experimental evidence, the details of which are beyond the scope of this chapter. However, at present, we are not certain whether CGRP has a true hormonal role in blood flow regulation, or whether circulating levels merely represent peptide that is split from nerve clefts when released to promote vasodilation. The second possibility appears more likely.

B. PLASMA LEVELS

1. *Calcitonin*

Plasma calcitonin immunoreactivity is heterogeneous, and by analogy with parathyroid hormone, it would not be surprising were a mixture of different forms of calcitonin secreted from the C-cells.

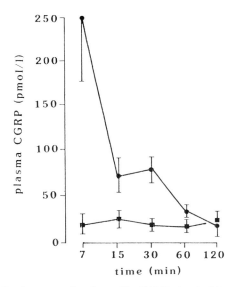

FIG. 6. Plasma calcitonin gene-related peptide (CGRP) levels following the injection of capsaicin (●) (10 mg/kg) or vehicle to adult 40-day-old rats. (■), Control.

Radioimmunoassay has been the method of choice for the routine determination of calcitonin in biological fluids, mainly due to its precision, sensitivity, and ability to handle a large number of samples. Nevertheless, the limitations in specificity of conventional radioimmunoassays are too well known to need enumeration here (for review see Heath *et al.*, 1984).

Radioimmunoassays of calcitonin are now being replaced by two-site immunometric or sandwich assays using either purified polyclonal antisera or monoclonal antibodies against defined antigenic epitopes. The assays are therefore based on the simultaneous detection of at least two epitopes that must be joined on the same molecule. It must be emphasized that such assays which require the presence of an intact molecule for signal generation do not detect calcitonin fragments. To improve assay sensitivity the antibody can be labeled with alkaline phosphatase, an enzyme that can activate a signal-regenerating calorimetric enzyme amplification system (Self, 1985). Briefly, the surface-bound conjugate is determined by its ability to dephosphorylate NADP to NAD, which activates a highly NAD-specific redox cycle to produce an intense color (Self, 1985; Seth *et al.*, 1988; Zaidi *et al.*, 1990c). One satisfactory type has been described by Seth *et al.* (1988) (Fig. 7). In principle, therefore, one can construct a rapid, nonisotopic

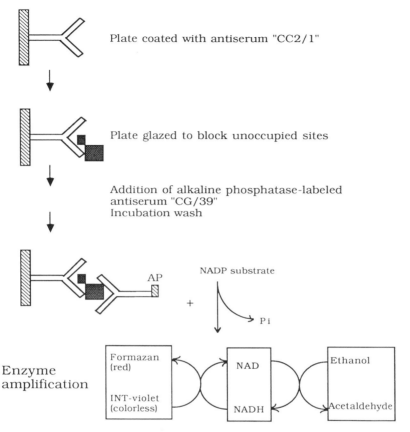

Plate coated with antiserum "CC2/1"

Plate glazed to block unoccupied sites

Addition of alkaline phosphatase-labeled
antiserum "CG/39"
Incubation wash

Fig. 7. Schematic representation of the enzymeimmunometric assay (EIA) of calcitonin gene-related peptide (CGRP). A two-site format is used to improve specificity,
and application of an alkaline phosphatase (AP)-based regenerating amplification system enhances sensitivity.

immunometric assay with improved specificity by employing the enzyme amplification system together with either high affinity polyclonal antisera or monoclonal antibodies. The assays are, in general,
more convenient in that the enzyme-labeled antiserum can be prepared with ease and is stable for more than 1 year. The microtiter
format adds to this convenience, as up to 30 samples, in duplicate per
plate may be easily loaded using multichannel pipettes, and the developed plates read quickly using readily available plate readers. The
assays provide an attractive alternative to the conventional
radioimmunoassay.

Immunometric assays are now being combined with sensitive bioassays applicable to plasma based on the exquisite hormonal sensitivity of isolated osteoclasts (for review see MacIntyre and Zaidi, 1990). A combination of these methods should resolve the differences in interpretation which have impeded progress in this field. Until very recently, bioassays for calcitonin based on whole animals or organ cultures of bone have been remarkably insensitive. Hence, best approximations of circulating bioactive calcitonin have been made using receptor assays (Ham et al., 1979) that might not truly represent biological function. Bearing in mind that the major physiological effect of calcitonin is on the osteoclast, bioassays based on the exquisite sensitivity of this cell to calcitonin can be very useful. Moreover, the morphological response of osteoclasts to calcitonin is sufficiently reproducible that it can be used as a bioassay of the hormone. We and others have developed ultrasensitive and highly specific bioassays for calcitonin based on calcitonin-induced inhibition of cell spreading, motility, enzyme secretion, and bone resorptive activity (Chambers and Moore, 1983; Chambers et al., 1987; Zaidi et al., 1988c, 1990d,h). We have found, using this approach that osteoclasts respond to calcitonin as a very uniform population, with a narrow dose–response range. Our assays lay down a whole new potential for calcitonin determination in biological fluids, being the only available methods sensitive enough to measure bioactive plasma levels (Zaidi et al., 1986b). Contrary to previous reports, suggesting that the calcitonin monomer was the only biologically active species found in plasma (Heath and Sizemore, 1983), we find that intact biological activity can also be readily detected in other, larger protein fractions (Zaidi et al., 1990h). We are not certain whether the high molecular weight bioactive calcitonin simply represents calcitonin that is loosely bound to protein, or is an authentic "big" molecule (Seth et al., 1989). Further work is required to reliably apply these assays to clinical usage, but we envisage that this should lead to the establishment of a normal reference range for bioactive circulating calcitonin.

2. Calcitonin Gene-Related Peptide

At present, the assay of circulating CGRP is of no clinical value apart from some suggestions that it may be a useful alternative or an adjunct to the diagnostic calcitonin assay for medullary thyroid carcinoma. Two-site immunometric assays for CGRP have been developed and are now being used to answer important questions relating to the physiology and pharmacology of this new peptide (Seth et al., 1988; Zaidi et al., 1990c). Immunoassays have utilized antibodies against rat or human α-CGRP, and these do not distinguish between the α and β forms of the peptide (Zaidi *et al.*, 1988b). As with calcitonin, radioimmunoassays comparing different antisera used in conjunction with gel filtration have suggested that immunoreactive CGRP is polymorphic and includes precursors and degradation products (Zaidi *et al.*, 1990h). An alternative and faster method of determining CGRP is the radioreceptor assay (for review see MacIntyre and Zaidi, 1990).

IV. Pharmacology

A. Clinical Pharmacology

1. *Calcitonin*

In order to predict the biological effect of a hormone, at least the following information is required: reliable and specific assays; site and identity of target cells and detailed receptor characteristics; the concentration and time course of the biologically active peptide in the receptor compartment; and the nature of post-receptor effects. In this section, we will discuss a model for the distribution of calcitonin within various receptor compartments (MacIntyre *et al.*, 1990). This is shown in Fig. 8. Monomeric calcitonin released from C-cells or injected into the plasma is in direct or indirect communication with a number of other compartments, A, B, and C. The transfer coefficients into these compartments are unknown but are likely to be different. One compartment may be assumed to be that of the osteoclast receptor. However, the other compartments of calcitonin that may be involved in other biological actions are presently unknown. A further complication exists when one considers the effect of plasma protein binding on circulating peptides. This effect may be reversible, but the rates of association and dissociation are unknown. Thus, the measurement of plasma levels at a particular point in time may reflect the amount of biologically active peptide in one compartment but not another. It is impossible to extrapolate from changing plasma levels measured at one time point only to effects at receptor level. With all of these problems it is surprising that any firm conclusions can be drawn from immunoassayable levels of plasma calcitonin. However, it is widely accepted that assays of circulating calcitonin provide a sound basis for the diagnosis and subsequent management of medullary thyroid carcinoma.

The prediction of biological effect from one plasma level is clearly

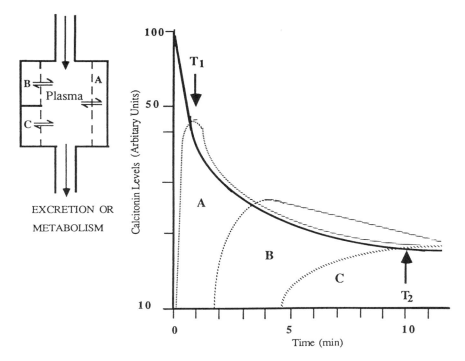

FIG. 8. Mammillary system showing the distribution of calcitonin within various compartments.

impossible. It must be emphasized that the biological effect of any peptide depends on the interaction between plasma levels of biologically active hormone, transfer coefficients into relevant receptor compartments, receptor binding and complex post-receptor factors, some of which are almost completely unknown for calcitonin. It is worthwhile mentioning that in the light of present knowledge, there is only one way to demonstrate a therapeutic effect of calcitonin—this is to carry out a randomized, preferably double-blind study using a range of doses and employing different routes of administration.

2. *Calcitonin Gene-Related Peptide*

It is unclear whether CGRP has a true hormonal role, but it is likely that the circulating peptide follows a similar compartmentalization pattern as that of calcitonin. Some investigations have focused on studying its phamacokinetic properties, and notable conclusions have emerged. First, CGRP appears to be protected from plasma peptidases (Brain and Williams, 1985), and there is no diminution of activity after 24 hours of incubation in human plasma. Second, infused CGRP shows a biexponential elimination curve, and after correction for the second slower phase, its half-life in plasma is in the region of 6–8 minutes (Kraenzlin et al., 1985; Struthers et al., 1986). This must be interpreted with caution as the data are derived from radioimmunoassay, which would indeed measure fragments as well as the intact molecule. Finally, it is interesting that the cardiovascular effects of CGRP infusion persist for a long time after the plasma levels have fallen to normal (Brain et al., 1986; Struthers et al., 1986; Benjamin et al., 1987). This might suggest that a substantial proportion of circulating CGRP moves into the receptor compartment to account for a prolonged biological half-life of about 20 minutes.

B. RECEPTOR DISTRIBUTION AND PHARMACOLOGY

1. Calcitonin

Marx et al. (1972) were the first to demonstrate the presence of calcitonin receptors in bone. This was followed by a number of confirmatory reports demonstrating high-affinity binding sites for the peptide on whole bone sections (Warshawsky et al., 1980) and on "osteoclast-rich" cultures (Luben et al., 1976). Finally, calcitonin receptors were characterized on isolated osteoclasts (Nicholson et al., 1986). Osteoclasts are the effectors of bone resorption and are the physiological target cells of the hormone. The binding of radiolabeled calcitonin to rat osteoclasts has been found to be saturable, highly specific, and incompletely reversible. A receptor component having a relative molecular weight of approximately 80,000 has been identified, being in good agreement with that observed on a breast cancer cell line (Moseley et al., 1982). Osteoclasts have a very high density (10^6), per cell, of calcitonin receptors (Nicholson et al., 1986), and it is notable that this is comparable only to the receptor number reported for epidermal growth factor receptors found on epidermal carcinoma cells (Wrann and Fox, 1979).

Calcitonin receptors are not confined to osteoclasts. Between 5000 and 30,000 receptors per cell have been identified on a variety of normal and malignant tissues, most importantly on the kidney (Marx et al., 1972, 1973; Goldring et al., 1978). Among normal tissues, the mammalian brain (Tschopp et al., 1985; Rizzo and Goltzman, 1981) and testes (Chausmer et al., 1982), pig lung (Fouchereau-Peron et al., 1981a), fish gill (Fouchereau-Peron et al., 1981b), and a variety of lymphoid cell lines (Marx et al., 1974; Moran et al., 1978) possess receptors for calcitonin. Malignant cells, such as lung and breast cancer cells (Hunt et al., 1977; Martin et al., 1980; Moseley et al., 1982, 1983; Lamp et al., 1981; Findlay et al., 1980a,b, 1981a, 1982; Ng et al., 1983), also express the calcitonin receptor. Attempts at isolating and sequencing the receptor protein using tumor cells have not yet been successful, partly because of the small receptor number per cell, and partly because of the hydrophobicity of the membrane domains. Nevertheless, some fundamentally important phenomena associated with calcitonin receptor stimulation have been uncovered. These include calcitonin-induced receptor loss (Tashijan et al., 1978; Findlay et al., 1981b, 1984), down-regulation (Roos et al., 1986), and desensitization (Findlay et al., 1981b, 1984), as well as persistent activation of adenylate cyclase in response to calcitonin (Lamp et al., 1981; Michelangeli et al., 1983).

The functional significance of "ectopic" or "inappropriately expressed" calcitonin receptors on tumor cells still remains unclear. In tumors associated with elevated calcitonin levels, these may trap circulating peptides, and perhaps alter tumor behavior (for review see Martin et al., 1980). Such cancers may also be subject to calcitonin treatment (Martin et al., 1981). In particular, it has been suggested that the effect of calcitonin in hypercalcemia associated with lung and breast cancers may at least, in part, be due to the effect of the peptide on the production of osteoclast-stimulating factors from tumor cells. There is also no obvious explanation for the occurrence of calcitonin, or indeed, CGRP receptors (Findlay et al., 1980a) on calcitonin- or CGRP-producing cancer cells (Zajac et al., 1985; Zaidi et al., 1987a,d, 1989a,c). It would be interesting to determine whether the calcitonin-like product can act on the producer cell to modify its growth or function (an autocrine effect?) (Ng et al., 1983).

2. Calcitonin Gene-Related Peptide

Although CGRP can stimulate adenylate cyclase activity by acting at the calcitonin receptor in more than one tissue (Wohlwend et al., 1985; Zaidi et al., 1988b), specific high-affinity binding sites for CGRP have been extensively mapped throughout the nervous and cardiovascular systems of both human and rat, using both biochemical and autoradiographic methods (Goltzman and Mitchell, 1985; Skofitsch and Jacobowitz, 1985; Tschopp et al., 1985; Inagaki et al.,

1986; Wimalawansa et al., 1987). The highest number of high-affinity CGRP-specific binding sites have been found in the cerebellum (molecular and Purkinje layers) and spinal cord (mainly substantia gelatinosa), in addition to other brain regions, including vessels and pia mater. There is considerable overlap between the distribution of CGRP-immunoreactive structures and binding sites (Tschopp et al., 1985), suggesting a widespread involvement of CGRP in a variety of brain functions. A second class of highly specific CGRP receptors linked to cAMP that have no cross-reactivity with the calcitonins, these have been identified in the intima and media of coronary, superior mesenteric, femoral, distal limb, and other visceral arteries (Sigrist et al., 1986; Kubota et al., 1985; Wimalawansa et al., 1987), as well as in the atria and ventricles of the heart (Sigrist et al., 1986). Finally, acinar cells of the pancreas also express CGRP-binding sites (Seifert et al., 1985). The interaction of CGRP with this receptor causes the release of amylase, and it is thought that the peptide may be released into the insuloacinar circulation from the islets of Langerhans, to stimulate enzyme secretion via a cAMP-mediated system.

Another class of binding sites found in the central nervous system are those that are specific for salmon calcitonin, and show very little cross-reactivity with human calcitonin and CGRP. These have been particularly found in the dorsomedial and anterior hypothalamus. It is interesting to note that tissues containing CGRP-binding sites, including cerebellum, medial geniculate body, mammilary body, and lateral hypothalamic and vestibular nuclei lack the salmon calcitonin receptors. The relative ability of CGRP and human calcitonin to act on the salmon calcitonin receptor may suggest that CGRP could serve as an endogenous ligand for the salmon calcitonin receptor in the central nervous system (Goltzman and Mitchell, 1985). Interestingly, in contrast to calcitonin receptors found in bone, these receptors do not seem to be linked to adenylate cyclase.

C. BIOLOGICAL ACTION

1. *Bone*

a. In Vivo Effects. Calcitonin administered acutely to experimental animals with a high bone turnover, or into human subjects with Paget's bone disease, causes a marked fall of plasma calcium (Robinson et al., 1967; Woodhouse et al., 1971). Plasma calcium falls because the inhibition of osteoclastic activity markedly diminishes the flow of calcium from bone to blood. The basis of this effect is a direct inhibitory effect on the osteoclast. Besides the acute effect of inhibitory calcitonin there are some less well-understood effects of the peptide on bone. Calcitonin induces a rapid decrease in osteoclast numbers (Baron and Vignery, 1981; Hedland et al., 1983). When calcitonin is administered over several months to patients with Paget's disease, osteoclast numbers have been found to gradually decline (MacIntyre et al., 1987b).

b. In Vitro Effects. Calcitonin inhibits both normal and stimulated resorption of intact bone in organ culture (Milhaud et al., 1965; Friedman and Raisz, 1965; Robinson et al., 1967; Aliopoulious et al., 1965; Reynolds et al., 1968) and perfusion of isolated cat tibiae with calcitonin leads to increased calcium retention (MacIntyre et al., 1967). In addition, urinary hydroxyproline, a biochemical index of bone resorption, has been found to be markedly reduced following calcitonin administration (Martin et al., 1966; Aer, 1968).

At the cellular level it has been shown that osteoclasts rapidly lose ruffled borders when either normal or parathyroid hormone (PTH)-pretreated bones are incubated with calcitonin (Kallio et al., 1972; Holtrop et al., 1974). This is accompanied by the loss of cytoplasmic coating of the ruffled border plasmalemma, and the physical separation from underlying bone. The loss of ruffled borders of osteoclasts in response to calcitonin (Kallio et al., 1972) correlates temporally and qualitatively with the inhibition of ^{45}Ca release from organ cultures (Holtrop et al., 1974). These studies formed the basis of the earliest deductions that the osteoclast, the cell that resorbs bone, is the target for calcitonin. Nevertheless, it has been unclear until recently whether or not the morphological changes seen in fixed stained osteoclasts reflect a direct cellular effect, or whether these are produced as a consequence of the activation of another cellular target. These interpretational difficulties arose because of the lack of a suitable experimental system whereby osteoclasts could be studied in isolation from other bone cells.

c. Isolated Osteoclasts. i. Effect of calcitonin on osteoclast motility. Techniques have become available whereby osteoclasts can be isolated from mammalian bone and maintained for short periods in primary cultures (Chambers, 1982; Chambers et al., 1984). Using such preparations, Chambers and colleagues provided the first conclusive demonstration for a direct action of calcitonin on the osteoclast (Chambers and Magnus, 1982). The group was able to visualize an acute effect of calcitonin on freshly isolated osteoclasts in culture (Chambers and Magnus, 1982). The addition of femtomolar concentrations of salmon calcitonin to isolated populations of rat osteoclasts was followed by a complete cessation of cytoplasmic motility. Over the ensuing hours the cytoplasm gradually retracted and became irregular (Fig. 9). The rapidity of response to calcitonin in cultures of osteoclasts widely separated from other cells suggests that calcitonin acts directly on osteoclasts. This was, indeed, the first convincing evidence demonstrating that no other cells were involved in the action of calcitonin on osteoclasts. The predictability of the response, its specificity for osteoclasts, and the low near-physiological concentrations of calcitonin required clearly suggest that the phenomenon is of physiological significance. The acute effect of calcitonin on the osteoclast perhaps reflects a morphological expression of a cell that has also become incapable of resorbing bone. Indeed, one mechanism by which calcitonin may inhibit resorption is through the inhibition of motility-dependent processes in the resorbing cells, in particular activities such as enzyme extrusion.

We have developed methods to precisely quantitate calcitonin-induced changes in osteoclast motility. Until this time, such conclusions were based on subjective assessments of time-lapse video recordings. Our procedures depend on time-lapse image capture and video recording of a motile osteoclast and computer-assisted mathematical analysis of the digitized images (Zaidi et al., 1989d, 1990e). Motility of osteoclasts is expressed by a simple geometric transformation as described previously by Dunn and Brown (1986). We have found that calcitonin acutely inhibits all components of motility, including large amplitude, low frequency movements at the margin, namely retraction and protrusion; and movement of the center of gravity, or cell migration (Fig. 10).

ii. Effect of calcitonin on osteoclast secretory activity. Calcitonin also inhibits the release of acid hydrolases from both resorbing and unresorbing osteoclasts, and the inhibition of enzyme release correlates, both temporally and quantitatively with the inhibition of resorption (Chambers et al., 1987; Moonga et al., 1990). One such enzyme is acid phosphatase, the release of which leads to the breakdown of pyrophosphate, a natural inhibitor of bone resorption (Zaidi et al., 1989b; Moonga et al., 1989).

Calcitonin treatment also inhibits Na^+,K^+-ATPase activity (Akisaka and Gay, 1986), and alters carbonic anhydrase localization. In untreated osteoclasts the enzyme appears along the ruffled border, and in calcitonin-treated cells the enzyme appears in the adjacent cytosol (Anderson et al., 1982). These enzymes are believed to play an important role in acidification of the resorptive hemivacuole, and the inhibition of their activity may represent a mechanism whereby calcitonin exerts its effect on bone resorption.

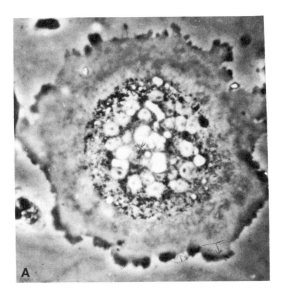

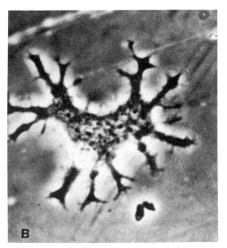

FIG. 9. An osteoclast 90 minutes following the exposure to vehicle (A) or calcitonin (B). Courtesy of Professor T. J. Chambers, Department of Histopathology, St. George's Hospital Medical School, London (with permission).

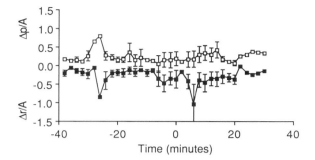

FIG. 10. Quantification of the motility of isolated rat osteoclasts. Retraction (Δr) and protrusion (Δp) of pseudopodia can be quantitated separately and expressed as the rate of change per unit cell area. (For reference to the method see Zaidi *et al.*, 1990e.)

iii. Effect of calcitonin on bone resorption. Osteoclasts, mechanically disaggregated from bone and sedimented onto slices of devitalized cortical bone, form excavations in bone within a few hours (Chambers and Magnus, 1982) (Fig. 11). This process is inhibited by very low concentrations of calcitonin (Chambers *et al.*, 1985a,b; Zaidi *et al.*, 1987b,c, 1988a, 1990d,h); salmon calcitonin is most potent, while porcine and human calcitonin show the same effects but at 30-fold higher molar concentrations. Clearly, osteoclasts are more sensitive to resorption-inhibition than to motility-inhibition; perhaps the motility potential required for bone resorption is much greater than that required for pseudopodial movement. Despite this, the relative potencies of the calcitonins as inhibitors of motility are very similar to their relative potencies as inhibitors of resorption (Chambers and Ali, 1983; Chambers and Moore, 1983; Chambers *et al.*, 1986; Zaidi *et al.*, 1990d). Although all known agents affecting osteoclast motility affect bone resorption (calcitonin and prostaglandins), the reverse is clearly not true. There are at least three such exceptions. First, agents that elevate free cytosolic calcium in osteoclasts inhibit not motility, but resorption. These agents include ionomycin (Datta *et al.*, 1989a), perchlorate (Zaidi *et al.*, 1990i), elevated extracellular calcium (Zaidi *et al.*, 1989e; Datta *et al.*, 1989b, 1990), and high micromolar concentrations of verapamil (Zaidi *et al.*, 1990b). Second, macrophage-colony stimulating factor (M-CSF) inhibits resorption in rodent osteoclasts without any observable effects on motility, suggesting that the intracellular pathway used for M-CSF is different from that used by calcitonin. Finally, prostaglandins inhibit resorption by chicken osteoclasts without "observable" effects on motility.

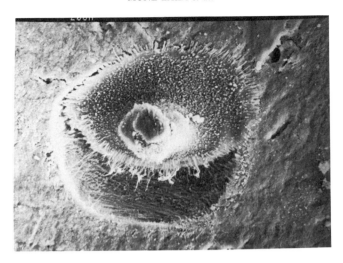

Fig. 11. Scanning electron micrograph of an osteoclastic excavation in a piece of devitalized human cortical bone substrate (× 1190) (Courtesy of Professor T. J. Chambers).

Several authors have found that, unlike rat osteoclasts, osteoclasts from chickens do not respond to calcitonin. Chicken osteoclasts do not possess calcitonin receptors, do not show cAMP generation, motility inhibition or cessation of bone resorption in response to calcitonin, even with chicken calcitonin (Arnett and Dempster, 1987; Dempster *et al.*, 1987). Others, however, have found calcitonin receptors (Rifkin *et al.*, 1988) and motility-inhibition (Cao and Gay, 1985), and the inhibition of resorption (de Vernejoul *et al.*, 1988) at similar molar concentrations of calcitonin. Workers finding no response, however, used normal chickens, whereas those who found effects used calcium-deficient animals. It is likely that the high circulating levels of calcitonin in normal animals (Kenney, 1971) had led to calcitonin receptor downregulation, whereas in chickens rendered calcium-deficient, circulating calcitonin was depressed and calcitonin responsiveness of osteoclasts was restored. It has been suggested that chicken must be maintained hypocalcemic for several weeks in order that a small number of functional calcitonin receptors become detectable.

  d. *Effects of Calcitonin on Other Cells of Bone.* The behavior of other bone cells changes after administration of pharmacological doses of calcitonin *in vivo* (Norimatsu *et al.*, 1978; Salmon *et al.*, 1983). For example, osteocytes are known to shrink in response to calcitonin. This effect has, however, not been confirmed *in vitro*. Cells of osteoblast

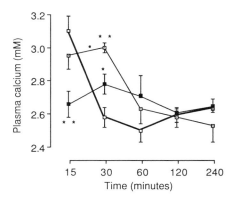

FIG. 12. Time course comparing the actions of human calcitonin gene-related peptide (α) (1000 pmol per chick) (■), bovine parathyroid hormone (1-84) (500 pmol per chick) (▣), and vehicle containing $CaCl_2$ (100 μmol/ml) (□) on plasma calcium levels (± SD) of 50–60 g chicks. Statistics by Student's t test compared to controls, $*p < .05$, $**p < .01$.

lineage, except in a late passage clone of osteosarcoma cells (UMR 106.06) (Gutierrez *et al.*, 1984; Forrest *et al.*, 1985) generally lack calcitonin receptors. In certain submammalian vertebrate species without a bony skeleton, such as the shark, calcitonin has a hypercalcemic effect (Glowacki *et al.*, 1985). This effect is thought to be mediated via calcium-transporting organs (kidney, intestine, or gill).

e. Effects of Calcitonin Gene-Related Peptide. Calcium gene-related peptide shares the acute effects of calcitonin at a 1000-fold higher molar concentration, suggesting that the effects on bone are probably exerted via the calcitonin receptor. Calcium gene-related peptide causes hypocalcemia (Tippins *et al.*, 1984; Roos *et al.*, 1986; Zaidi *et al.*, 1988a), stimulates cAMP formation in mouse calvaria (Zaidi *et al.*, 1988a), inhibits both basal and stimulated resorption of intact bone (D'Souza *et al.*, 1989; Roos *et al.*, 1986), and inhibits spreading (Chambers *et al.*, 1986), motility, and resorption of bone by isolated osteoclasts (Zaidi *et al.*, 1987b,c, 1988a). The *in vivo* effects of CGRP in the rabbit and chicken are different, and partly resemble those of PTH (Tippins *et al.*, 1984). Although in the rabbit, the peptide causes hypocalcemia. At doses comparable to those of calcitonin, at higher molar concentrations a sustained PTH-like response follows initial hypocalcemia. In the chicken, CGRP partially has a PTH-like effect (Fig. 12) (Bevis *et al.*, 1990). In human, systemic CGRP infusion gives no observable effect on plasma calcium (Struthers *et al.*, 1986). Nevertheless, the peptide causes a 40- to 50-fold rise of cAMP in normal human os-

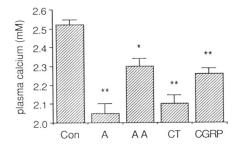

F IG. 13. The effect of intravenous injection of 500 pmol amylin (A) (Peninsula), amylin-amide (AA), asu[1//7]-eel calcitonin (CT) (ISF), human calcitonin gene-related peptide-α (CGRP) (Sandoz), or vehicle on plasma calcium levels in 50 g male Wistar rats ($n = 6$ per group). Statistics by Student's t test. *$p < .05$, **$p < .01$. Con, Control (With permission from *Biochemical and Biophysical Research Communications.*)

teoblasts (Crawford *et al.*, 1985). The presence of putative receptors for CGRP on osteoblasts may represent a second and more important effect of CGRP on bone cells, and a predominantly osteoblastic effect might account for the PTH-like response seen in rabbits and chickens.

f. Amylin and Bone. We have investigated the effects of amylin and its amidated homologue, amylin-amide, on calcium metabolism. We have demonstrated profound hypocalcemic and osteoclast-inhibitory effects of both peptides in the rat, rabbit, and in human (Fig. 13). (Gilby *et al.*, 1991). Taken together, these findings suggest that amylin has a primary role in the conservation of bone (Fig. 14).

Our studies on amylin have major implications. First, we have shown that amylin-amide is about 30 times less potent than calcitonin in lowering plasma calcium, while having a comparable duration of effect. In addition, like calcitonin, amylin-amide acts directly on the osteoclast to inhibit its resorptive activity. The peptide is undoubtedly the most potent non-calcitonin hypocalcemic substance so far identified. Indeed, these observations are not completely unexpected, since both amylin and calcitonin belong to the same family of peptides encoded by genes that have a common ancestral origin (Mosselman *et al.*, 1988). In decreasing order of hypocalcemic and anti-resorptive activity, the peptides can be placed as follows: asu(1–7)-CT $>$ hCT $>$ amylin/amylin-amide $>$ CGRP. This paradox suggests that the amylin peptides activate receptors on the osteoclast that are different from those activated by calcitonin, the putative "amylin receptors." Alternatively, the hypocalcemic effect of amylin may be due to activation of the osteoclast calcitonin receptor.

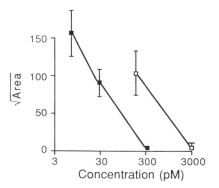

FIG. 14. The effect of a range of doses of human amylin-amide (A-A) (□) and the International Reference Preparation of human calcitonin (CT) (■) on the mean area of bone resorbed per slice (expressed as a √ area ± SEM). Six slices were used per dose. (With permission from the *Quarterly Journal of Experimental Physiology*.)

There is an important difference between the nature of responsiveness of plasma calcium levels to high doses of amylin and CGRP. In the rabbit, CGRP is known to produce hypocalcemia at low doses, but when infused at high doses, it is followed by a marked hypercalcemic response (Tippins *et al.*, 1986). In contrast, amylin infused at similarly high doses caused a prominent hypocalcemic response, without hypercalcemia (Datta *et al.*, 1989c). It would, therefore, be interesting to further study the mechanism of amylin action in these species.

At present we can only speculate on the possible role of amylin in extracellular calcium homeostasis. In this context it is notable that amylin-amide is as abundant in normal plasma (mean plasma levels, ± S.E.M., 20 ± 3 pM; Ghatei *et al.*, 1989) than calcitonin (normal range, 6–30 pM) (Stevenson *et al.*, 1979), and these findings taken together might suggest that amylin-amide is responsible for at least some of the plasma osteoclast-inhibiting activity formerly attributed solely to calcitonin.

g. Post-Receptor Regulation of the Calcitonin Effect. i. Cyclic AMP. Cyclic AMP generation has long been thought to be involved in the inhibition of osteoclasts by calcitonin. Calcitonin increases the cAMP content of bone (Murad *et al.*, 1970) and rat osteoclasts (Nicholson *et al.*, 1986), while purified preparations of primary cultures of osteoblasts lack an adenyl cyclase response to calcitonin. Second, cAMP itself, and analogues of cAMP, induce in rat osteoclasts a state of sustained immotility identical to that caused by calcitonin (Chambers

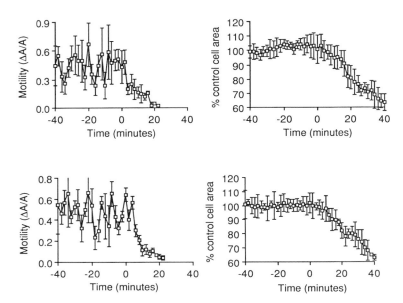

Fig. 15. Time-series analysis showing the effect of calcitonin (300 pmol/l) on rat osteoclast motility and spread area in the presence of physiological levels of extra-cellular calcium (1.26 mmol/l) (top panels) or calcium-free medium (bottom panels). Mean osteoclast motility is expressed as the rate of change of "shape area" (ΔA) per unit cell area (A); cell spread area is expressed as percent of the mean control cell area that has been computed from 20 sequential pretreatment recordings for each cell. Values are means ± SEM for (a) seven, (b) four and, (c) four cells. Time 0 corresponds to the time at which the compounds were added, and the negative time scale corresponds to pretreatment recordings. (With permission from the *Journal of Endocrinology.*)

and Ali, 1983; Zaidi *et al.*, 1990d). Finally, theophylline, an intra-cellular inhibitor of cAMP degradation potentiates calcitonin-induced osteoclastic quiescence, while imidazole, which increases cAMP degra-dation, reduces osteoclastic sensitivity to calcitonin (Chambers and Ali, 1983).

ii. G proteins. Before attempting to discuss studies on the proposed role of guanosine triphosphate (GTP)-binding proteins (G proteins) in mediating the calcitonin effect on the osteoclast, we must understand in detail the behavioral changes induced in osteoclasts by calcitonin (Zaidi *et al.*, 1990d). The calcitonin effect on the osteoclast can be resolved into at least two major components: quiescence ("Q" effect, half-life ~ 15 min) and retraction ("R" effect, half-life ~ 27 min) (Fig. 15). The more rapid component is the Q effect, characterized by a gradual slowing down of cell motility and finally the cessation of all

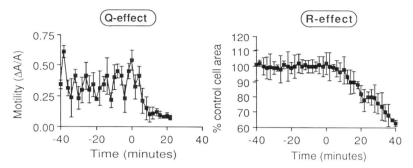

FIG. 16. Time-series analysis showing the effect of aluminum tetrafluoride anions (AlF_4^-) on osteoclast motility and spread area. Mean osteoclast motility is expressed as the rate of change of "shape area" (ΔA) per unit cell area (A); cell spread area is expressed as percent of the mean control cell area that has been computed from 20 sequential pretreatment recordings for each cell. Values are means ± SEM for four cells. Time 0 corresponds to the time at which AlF_4^- was added, and the negative time scale corresponds to pretreatment recordings. (With permission from the *Journal of Endocrinology*).

cellular motile processes. The R effect is characterized by gradual pseduopodial retraction leading to an absolute reduction of cell surface area. Both the Q and R effects appear to contribute to the inhibition of osteoclastic bone resorption by calcitonin, but it is clear that these two components are fundamentally different processes. Quiescence appears to be mediated by cAMP and is selectively mimicked by dibutyryl cAMP and forskolin. In contrast, osteoclastic retraction is a kinetically and qualitatively distinct cellular process which is selectively mimicked by a calcium ionophore, ionomycin, but not by dibutyryl cAMP. Thus, the full effect of calcitonin cannot be due to cAMP alone and there must be another second messenger, possibly calcium. Similar bifurcating intracellular pathways have been reported previously in a number of cell systems (see, e.g., Hishikawa *et al.*, 1985; Fleming *et al.*, 1989).

Most receptors which interact with effector systems to modulate intracellular levels of a second messenger such as cAMP do so via G proteins. This may also be true for calcitonin. A fundamental relationship between the calcitonin effect and G protein/s is implied by the demonstration that aluminum tetrafluoride ions, known to activate G proteins (Sternweis and Gilman, 1982), mimic both components (Q and R) of the calcitonin effect (Fig. 16). The abolition of the effects of calcitonin by lithium is further evidence of a linkage of the calcitonin response to G protein stimulation; lithium prevents the binding of guanine nucleotides to G proteins, thus functionally decoupling these proteins from membrane receptors. It has been demonstrated that lithium abolishes G protein-mediated activation of adenylate cyclase by adrenergic and cholinergic agonists (Avissar *et al.*, 1988). The anion abolishes the acute effects of calcitonin on osteoclast behavior (Q and R effects) and partially reverses the longer-term inhibitory effects of the peptide on bone resorption (Abeyasekera *et al.*, 1989; Zaidi *et al.*, 1989d, 1990d). Taken together, all our results with AlF_4^-, Li^+ and with cholera and pertussis toxin strongly imply that G proteins mediate the effect of calcitonin on the osteoclast.

The distinct effects of cholera toxin and pertussis toxin on osteoclast motility and spread area, respectively, suggest that at least two G proteins may be involved, each of which appear to modulate different intracellular pathway. The G protein family contains a relatively large number of closely related members (for review see Casey and Gilman, 1988), including the cholera toxin-sensitive G_s and pertussis toxin-sensitive G_i and G_o (Casey and Gilman, 1988). Nearly all G proteins possess an α subunit that has a site for NAD-dependent ADP-ribosylation by bacterial toxins (Neer and Clapham, 1988). Classically, ADP-ribosylation results in a characteristic alteration of G protein function; activation of G_S, in the case of modification by cholera toxin, and most often, an impaired ability to interact with the receptor in the case of pertussis toxin (Mulligan, 1988). The Q and R effects of calcitonin are selectively mimicked by cholera and pertussis toxin respectively (Fig. 17). Thus, it appears that the cAMP-mediated Q effect is dependent on the activation of a cholera toxin-sensitive G protein, whereas a pertussis toxin-sensitive G protein may mediate the cell retraction (R effect).

Certain conclusions follow that can be interpreted in terms of a dichotomous model of cell inhibition. The stimulation of the calcitonin receptor causes the activation of two G proteins (Fig. 18). One of these is G_s-like and is sensitive to stimulation by cholera toxin. This mediates the cAMP-dependent inhibition of cell motility (Q effect). The other appears to be a pertussis toxin-sensitive G protein mediating cell retraction (R effect), a process that mimics the ionomycin effect. We are uncertain of the identity of this latter G protein. It is possible that the protein may be a pertussis toxin-sensitive G_o, a protein known to be involved directly in calcium channel-gating in a variety of cell systems (Heschler *et al.*, 1987; Yatani, *et al.*, 1987). The second messenger for the R effect is calcium.

Finally, it is important to note that in view of the speculation that there is a separate receptor for amylin on the osteoclast (Datta *et al.*,

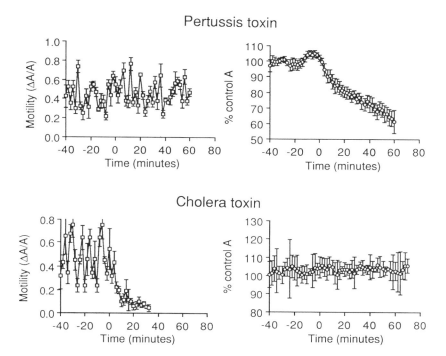

FIG. 17. Time-series analysis showing the effects of pertussis toxin (1 μg/l) and cholera toxin (1 μg/l) on rat osteoclast motility or spread cell area. Mean osteoclast motility is expressed as the rate of change of "shape area" (ΔA) per unit cell area (A); cell spread area is expressed as percent of the mean control cell area, computed from 20 sequential pretreatment recordings for each cell. Time 0 corresponds to the time at which the compounds were added, and the negative time scale corresponds to pretreatment recordings. Values are mean ± SEM for eight (pertussis toxin) or four (cholera toxin) cells. (With permission from the *Journal of Endocrinology*.)

1989c; Zaidi *et al.*, 1990f), the intracellular dichotomy observed with calcitonin might not reflect solely calcitonin receptor activation. Instead, this might represent a combination of effects of calcitonin on two receptor subtypes, the calcitonin subtype and the amylin subtype. Each of these could be linked to a distinct second messenger pathway via separate G proteins.

iii. Calcium. In order to convincingly establish a role for intracellular calcium in osteoclast regulation, we developed an indo 1-based microspectrofluorometric method for the measurement of intracellular calcium levels in isolated single osteoclasts. Calcitonin produces a biphasic intracellular calcium transient, consisting of a rapid

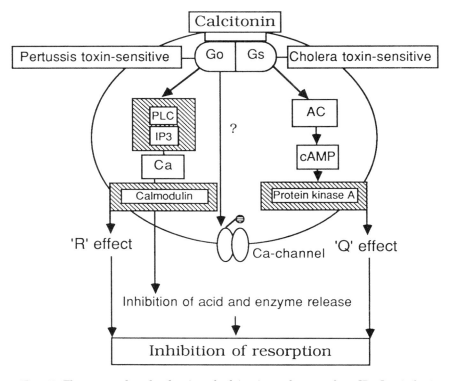

FIG. 18. The proposed mode of action of calcitonin on the osteoclast. IP$_3$, Inositol *tris*-phosphate; PLC, phospholipase C; cAMP, cyclic AMP; AC, adenylate cyclase. The shaded areas represent unconfirmed pathways.

initial spike followed by sustained elevation. It appears likely that the signaling process produced by calcitonin is at least partly due to calcium redistribution by a phospholipase C-inositol *tris*-phosphate (IP$_3$) mechanism, rather than solely calcium influx, because both the calcium-dependent R effect and the rapid calcium transient persist in calcium-free medium (Fig. 19).

2. Kidney

a. Calcitonin. Calcitonin may also act on the kidney to enhance the production of 1,25-dihydroxy-vitamin D$_3$ (Rasmussen *et al.,* 1972; Hass *et al.,* 1971). This might represent a true physiological effect of importance during pregnancy and childhood. The effects of PTH and calcitonin are exerted at different sites on the proximal straight tubule (Kawashima *et al.,* 1981); the calcitonin-sensitive site lacks cAMP (Ka-

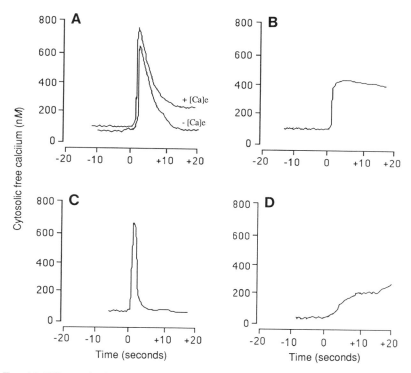

FIG. 19. Effects of calcitonin (1 nM) (A), elevated extracellular calcium (20 mM) (B), ionic perchlorate (10 μM) (C), and forskolin (20 μM) (D), on free cytosolic calcium levels in isolated rat osteoclasts measured by a single cell dual photon micro-spectrofluorimetric method described by Zaidi *et al.,* (1989e). (A), Calcitonin (1 lnM); (B), calcium (20 mM); (C), perchlorate (10 μM); (D), forskolin (20μM).

washima *et al.,* 1980; Horiuchi *et al.,* 1979; Zalups and Knox, 1983). This effect of calcitonin is probably mediated by prostaglandin E_2 (Yamada *et al.,* 1985). The other effects of calcitonin on the kidney are probably not of physiological importance, although they may be clinically relevant (for review see Agus *et al.,* 1981). At the distal nephron, the peptide acts by a cAMP-dependent mechanism (Marx *et al.,* 1972; Heersche *et al.,* 1974; Elalouf *et al.,* 1985), leading to naturesis and diuresis. More recently, it has been shown that calcitonin stimulates cAMP-dependent protein kinase activity and plasminogen activator production and inhibits cell multiplication in a cloned renal tubular cell line, LLC-PK1 (Goldring *et al.,* 1978).

b. Calcitonin Gene-Related Peptide. In mice intravenous CGRP infusion causes a sharp rise of renal cAMP levels; the peptide is 10 times less potent than calcitonin in this respect (Zaidi *et al.*, 1990a). The peptide also binds to the calcitonin receptor on the cloned LLC-PK1 cell line (Wohlwend *et al.*, 1985).

3. *Cardiovascular System*

The extensive distribution of CGRP in the cardiovascular system and its codistribution with the potent vasodilator, substance P, clearly points toward a possible function in cardiovascular regulation. Our understanding of the distribution of the peptide in the cardiovascular system comes from detailed immunochemical studies carried out in the rat and guinea pig.

a. Distribution. i. Heart. Interestingly, in the heart, the absolute amount of CGRP is lower than that found in the vascular system (Mulderry *et al.*, 1985a). Calcitonin gene-related peptide immunoreactivity is found in the pericardium and running around and parallel to the coronary arteries. The distribution pattern of CGRP in these areas also appears to parallel that of substance P (Wharton *et al.*, 1981), but differs from that of neuropeptide Y (Gu *et al.*, 1983). Fibers travel into the heart muscle itself, particularly into the papillary muscles. Many CGRP-immunoreactive fibers are seen within the nodes and traverse the conducting system, although no positive nerve cell bodies are seen in the ganglia of the sinoatrial node and atrioventricular nodes.

ii. Vessels. In blood vessels, varicose and smooth CGRP fibers are seen at the junction of the adventitia and media, and pass into the muscle layer. Dense perivascular networks are seen around the inferior vena cava, renal arteries, superior mesenteric arteries, femoral arteries, cerebral arteries, and carotid arteries (Mulderry *et al.*, 1985a; Wanaka *et al.*, 1987; McCulloch *et al.*, 1986). The innervation is often most marked at the origins of arteries, and the carotid and aortic bifurcations are particularly richly innervated with CGRP-containing fibers. At these sites, the association of CGRP-rich structures with VIP-, substance P-, and enkephalin-containing structures may point toward the involvement of the peptides in interoceptor-mediated cardiovascular control. In the venous system, dense CGRP-rich innervation has been noted in the inferior vena cava, and the renal and femoral veins, although there is a distal reduction of immunoreactivity. It is interesting to note that while in the mesenteric vasculature the distribution pattern of CGRP is quite similar to that reported for substance P, renal vessels exclusively contain CGRP, which is suggestive of a more specific role of the peptide in the control of renal blood flow. In the cerebral arterial system, the distribution pattern of CGRP appears to be more specific; there are either dense periadventitial fiber bands or fibers forming a meshwork in the adventitia. In the carotid arterial system, these arise from the trigeminal ganglia, whereas in the vertebrobasilar system, fibers originate from similar cells of the cervical root ganglia (McCulloch *et al.*, 1986; Wanaka *et al.*, 1987). Calcitonin gene-related peptide-containing fibers of the cerebral vascular system follow the same pattern as substance P-containing fibers, and in some fibers these two peptides are colocalized.

   b. Cardiac Effects. i. Conduction. The nodal innervation of CGRP might be of significance in the regulation of heart rate, and CGRP appears to be the only peptide that has a neurotransmitter role in cardioacceleration, via nonadrenergic noncholinergic (NANC) nerves to the sinus node. This response might be due to its specific action on pacemaker cells.

   ii. Contraction. Highly specific CGRP binding sites linked to cAMP have been demonstrated on membrane preparations of heart and muscle cells (Sigrist *et al.*, 1986; Holman *et al.*, 1986; Wimalawansa *et al.*, 1987). It appears likely that in an *in vivo* situation, CGRP, released locally from cardiac nerves, binds to specific functional receptors of the heart. There is also growing evidence that CGRP directly acts on the heart muscle in various experimental systems. The peptide has been shown to increase the rate and force of contraction both in the guinea pig perfused heart (Fisher *et al.*, 1983) and the rat isolated atrium (Tippins *et al.*, 1984), and in this respect the α form is more potent than the β-CGRP. These effects of CGRP do not appear to be mediated via adrenergic stimulation because a highly selective β-antagonist failed to inhibit the CGRP-induced chronotropic and ionotropic effects in guinea pig preparations. Surprisingly, this was foiund to be in direct contradiction to results from studies with the rat atrial preparations, where high micromolar concentrations of propanolol inhibited the effects of CGRP (Tippins *et al.*, 1984). This could be due to the known membrane stabilizing effect of propranolol at these rather high concentrations.

   c. Skin Microvasculature. The first recognition of the vasodilator action of CGRP was made by Brain *et al.* (1985) using preparations of microvessels (Fig. 20). The authors have found that the administration of femtomole doses of CGRP into the rabbit skin or its topical application onto a hamster cheek pouch preparation induces intense arteriolar dilatation with increased blood flow. When the peptide is injected intradermally into human volunteers there is a persistent flare that is quite unlike the typical histamine response. While histamine produces a wheel and flare, CGRP leads to intense port-wine reddening which persists several hours after the disappearance of the his-

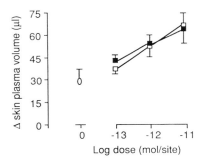

Fᴵɢ. 20. The effect of human calcitonin gene-related peptide (α) (□) and human calcitonin gene-related peptide (β) (■) on the potentiation of skin edema induced by bradykinin. The results are expressed as an increase of skin plasma volume. The peptides when injected without bradykinin did not cause edema formation at a concentration of 10^{-11} M. The open oval represents the effect of bradykinin on skin plasma volume. Results are mean ± SEM, $n = 4$ rabbits.

tamine response. In this respect, CGRP is similar in potency to prostaglandin E_2, and is several fold more potent than acetylcholine, ATP, ADP, adenosine, 5-hydroxytryptamine, substance P, isoprenaline, or VIP (Williams, 1982; Brain *et al.*, 1985). No difference has been noted in the responsiveness to α- or β-CGRP.

Calcitonin gene-related peptide, when injected alone, does not induce edema or protein extravasation (Gamse and Saria, 1985; Brain and Williams, 1985), but when administered to guinea pigs it potentiates edema induced by histamine, bradykinin, leucotriene B4, C5a-des-Arg, *N*-formyl methionyl leucyl phenylalanine, platelet-activating factor, and tachykinins (substance P, neurokinin A and B) (Brain and Williams, 1985) (Fig. 20). The potentiation of tissue edema by CGRP appears to be the consequence of arteriolar dilatation, causing an increased perfusion pressure at the level of the capillary and venule, where other edema mediators have already increased permeability (Williams, 1982; Brain and Williams, 1985). It is worthwhile mentioning that CGRP coexists with the tachykinins in single cells of sensory neurons (Lee *et al.*, 1985a), and it is likely that the peptides may interact to produce neurogenic inflammation or an axon-reflex flare reaction (Foreman *et al.*, 1983; Lembeck and Gamse, 1982; Brain and Williams, 1985). Interestingly, substance P together with CGRP produces edema in the rat, but not in the rabbit skin, suggesting that there may be intraspecies differences in the responsiveness to mediators.

d. Systemic Vasculature. i. In vitro effects. Calcitonin gene-related peptide dilates a variety of vascular preparations *in vitro,* including the coronary, cerebral, and systemic vasculature (McEwan *et al.,* 1987). This has been demonstrated in the rat aorta (Tippins *et al.,* 1984), cat cerebral vessels (Edvinsson *et al.,* 1985), cat, rabbit, and human pial vessels (Hanko *et al.,* 1985), human pulmonary, gastric, coronary, splenic, brachial, and transverse cervical arteries (Hughes *et al.,* 1985), and the mesenteric vasculature. In addition, the peptide has been shown to relax splenic strips precontracted with noradrenaline, by an action on cAMP-linked CGRP receptors of the red pulp of the spleen (Sigrist *et al.,* 1986).

Calcitonin gene-related peptide also dilates cerebral arteries. This effect is surprisingly more marked *in situ* than *in vitro.* It is also more potent in this respect than substance P. Chronic division of the trigeminal nerve has been found to deplete immunoreactive CGRP, and to lengthen the duration of, but not to alter the magnitude of, arteriolar responses to the microapplication of vasoconstrictor agents. Thus, the trigeminal nerve may provide the brain with a network of a reflex local and sustained response in emergency conditions, such as subarachnoid hemorrhage, where excessive vasoconstriction of larger arteries would threaten the survival of the nervous system. This clearly suggests that CGRP may have a primary role in preventing cerebral ischemia due to excessive vasoconstriction (McCulloch *et al.,* 1986).

The crucial question that still remains unanswered is whether or not vasodilation is dependent on the presence of the intact endothelium. In general, endothelial dependence is seen in, at least, major vessels (Brain *et al.,* 1985; Kubota *et al.,* 1985) such as in the rat aorta (Brain *et al.,* 1985), and in a wide variety of human large vessels (Hughes *et al.,* 1985). Vasorelaxation, that is independent of the endothelium, has been reported in cat cerebral vessels (Edvinsson *et al.,* 1985), cat, rabbit, and human pial and peripheral lingual arteries (Hanko *et al.,* 1985). The contrasting observations conceivably reflect interspecies and organ-specific differences in endothelial dependence.

ii. In vivo effects. Calcitonin gene-related peptide administered either intrarterially or intravenously causes marked vasodilation (Fisher *et al.,* 1983; Lundberg *et al.,* 1985). Systemic injection or infusion into healthy human volunteers leads to marked diastolic hypotension accompanied by tachycardia, intense skin flushing, a rise of skin temperature, and a reflex-mediated release of both catecholamines. Systemic levels of plasma immunoreactive CGRP as low as 56 pmol/l are sufficient to mediate this effect (Struthers *et al.,* 1986). These are only slightly above the normal mean circulating level of 25 pmol/l. However, circulating immunoreactivity is heterogeneous, biologically active levels of CGRP are probably much lower, and the infusion data may thus represent a response by pharmacological rather than physiological doses of the peptide. The local infusion of CGRP into the brachial artery in humans has confirmed both its potency at low doses (1.25–10 pmol/minute) and its long duration of action. The half-life of the biological effect has been estimated to be in the region of 19 minutes. This is in clear contrast to substance P, which, although an order of magnitude more potent than CGRP in producing equivalent vasodilatation (doses 0.25–1.25 pmol/minute), displays a shorter duration of action with a biological half-life of approximately 15 seconds. Furthermore, unlike the effect of substance P, that of CGRP is not accompanied by tachyphylaxis (Gennari and Fischer, 1985). Finally, there is yet another difference between the effect of CGRP and substance P. Calcitonin gene-related peptide appears to be a selective arterial dilator, since whereas substance P inhibits venoconstriction of superficial veins of the hand in response to norepinephrine infusion or a single deep breath, CGRP fails to affect these veins.

In humans, the local infusion of CGRP into normal or near-normal left anterior descending coronary arteries during routine coronary angiography produces marked dilatation of the epicardial coronaries. This is coupled with a dramatic decline of perfusion pressure (McEwan et al., 1986). In the pig open-chested model, dilatation of small cardiac resistance vessels by CGRP has been shown by reduction of the resistance of the coronary vascular bed and increased coronary blood flow observed after the local infusion of CGRP into the left anterior descending coronary artery (Greenwald et al., 1986). In neither humans nor pigs does the infusion of CGRP into the left anterior descending coronary artery cause a change in heart rate or blood pressure. An effect of CGRP on the coronary vasculature has also been shown using coronary arteries of isolated rat, rabbit, and pig heart preparations (Holman et al., 1986). Surprisingly, the potencies of rat and human CGRP peptides have been found to differ in this respect.

Interestingly, the in vivo effects of CGRP on systemic vessels can depend on the route of administration of the peptide. For example, intraventricular administration of CGRP or its microinjection into the central amygdaloid nucleus in experimental animals selectively stimulates noradrenergic outflow accompanied by intense tachycardia and hypertension (Fisher et al., 1983; Nguyen et al., 1986).

   e. Physiological Role. Though it has been established that CGRP is constantly released from perivascular and cardiac nerves, possibly in response to vasosensory stimuli (Zaidi et al., 1985, Diez Guerra et al., 1987; Emson and Zaidi, 1989), we are still not certain whether the peptide has a true hormonal role in blood flow regulation. It appears that plasma levels merely represent a spillover phenomenon when CGRP is released from nerve terminals to promote vasodilation.

4. Nervous System

a. Calcitonin. Calcitonin alleviates pain associated with bone disease by a central analgesic effect (Pecile *et al.*, 1975; Allan, 1983; Fraioli *et al.*, 1982). Intractable pain of advanced malignancy is also susceptible to relief by intramuscular or subarachnoid salmon calcitonin (Allan, 1983). There are many views on the mechanism of calcitonin-induced analgesia. These include effects of the peptide on serotonergic midbrain nuclei (Nakhla and Majumdar, 1978; Clementi *et al.*, 1984, 1985), opiate receptors (Barga *et al.*, 1978), and the prostaglandin–thromboxane system (Caserani *et al.*, 1979). Details of the proposed mechanisms are beyond the scope of this chapter.

Centrally administered calcitonin decreases food intake and gastric acid secretion and affects the pattern of intestinal movement (for review see Zaidi *et al.*, 1987a). Calcitonin appears to affect dopaminergic neurons in the hypothalamus (Clementi *et al.*, 1983) to produce profound pharmacological inhibitory effects on the release of prolactin (Oligiati *et al.*, 1981), leuteinizing hormone, thyrotropin, growth hormone, and thyrotropin-releasing hormone (Oligiati *et al.*, 1981; Mitsuma *et al.*, 1984). At pharmacological doses the peptide also affects avoidance behavior in experimental animals (Nicoletti *et al.*, 1982).

b. Calcitonin Gene-Related Peptide. The abundance of CGRP in the central nervous system (Kawai *et al.*, 1985) points toward a neurotransmitter or a neuromodulator role, particularly in the central regulation of visceral autonomic (cardiovascular, respiratory, taste, and sleep) and limbic functions, as well as in sensory and motor control (Zaidi *et al.*, 1987a). We will briefly review the distribution of the CGRP in important structures of the brain and spinal cord, and will speculate upon the potential modulatory role of the peptide in central neural regulation on the basis of other pharmacological evidence.

i. Distribution. Brain. Rosenfeld and colleagues had initially demonstrated that the facial, hypoglossal, peripenduncular, and parabrachial nuclei contained large amounts of CGRP mRNA (Rosenfeld *et al.*, 1983). A more extensive distribution of the peptide has since been revealed by extensive immunocytochemical studies. Specific CGRP-rich pathways have also been traced using retrograde tracing procedures. Three major CGRP-containing tracts have been shown to connect thalamic and hypothalamic nuclei to the limbic system (Kawai *et al.*, 1985): (1) from the insular cortex to the ventromedial thalamic nucleus (Shimada *et al.*, 1985a); (2) from the lateral septal area to the hypothalamus (Sakanaka *et al.*, 1985); and (3) from the ventral hypo-thalamic surface to the caudate nucleus to join a band of fibers that pass beneath the globus pallidus (Kawai *et al.*, 1985). Calcitonin gene-related peptide-rich fibers of the forebrain and diencephalon derive from the parabrachial area (Rosenfeld *et al.*, 1983; Shimada *et al.*, 1985b) and from the ventral surface of the hypothalamus (Sakanaka *et al.*, 1985). Two projections have been identified, one projecting between the dorsolateral hypothalamus and the ventromedial nucleus of the thalamus (the "lateral projection"), and the other originating from the ventral hypothalamus projecting to the red nucleus of the striae termi-nalis, central amygdaloid nucleus, and the far-lateral hypothalamus (the "ventral projection") (Shimada *et al.*, 1985b). In the lateral tract, CGRP is thought to be colocalized with cholecystokinin-like immu-noreactivity in single cells (Inagaki *et al.*, 1984). In single cells of the somatomotor and branchiomotor nuclei, especially those of the hypo-glossal and facial nerves, CGRP-like immunoreactivity is colocalized with acetylcholine single cells (Takami *et al.*, 1985a). The peptide is also localized with substance P in single cells whose fibers project from trigeminal and inferior ganglia, respectively to the spinal part of the trigeminal nerve and tractus solitarius (Lee *et al.*, 1985a; Wanaka *et al.*, 1987). It is likely that the corelease of peptides is mediated by a more central mechanism. Similarly, CGRP and γ-aminobutyric acid appear to coexist in Purkinje cells of the cerebellum (Kawai *et al.*, 1985).

Spinal cord. In the spinal cord, CGRP-rich structures are mainly confined to laminae I, II, V, and X of the dorsal horn, tract of Lissaeur, and small fibers throughout the gray matter. The pattern is somewhat similar to that of substance P, another predominantly sensory neuro-transmitter (Gibson *et al.*, 1981). Furthermore, as with substance P, these fibers have been shown to originate from the afferent fibers of the dorsal root ganglia (Gibson *et al.*, 1984a), and to a lesser extent from ventral afferents and supraspinal regions. In addition, CGRP-rich structures are found in the dorsolateral nucleus of the white mat-ter, fasciculus proprius, around intermediolateral cells of the thoracic region, and dense clusters in the sacral segment of the spinal cord around the parasympathetic nuclei and the spinal canal. A caudal increase of immunoreactivity has been found for a number of peptides (Anand *et al.*, 1983; Gibson *et al.*, 1984b,c). The interspecies distribu-tion, i.e., array of CGRP distribution in the spinal cord, is also fairly constant, suggesting that functional constraints may have led to the conservation of pattern.

Sensory nervous system. In sensory ganglia and primary afferents, it appears that together with substance P, CGRP-rich nerve fibers form a primary afferent neuron system comprising capsaicin-sensitive A(δ)- and C-fiber afferent nerves and medium-sized (type B) cells. In the dorsal root, nodose and trigeminal ganglia, 40% of all cells stain for CGRP, and barely half of these costore substance P (large- and medium-sized), while all cells positive for substance P are also positive for CGRP. The very large cells (diameter above 45 μm) only contain CGRP, and no substance P, and these are probably related to thermoceptor and mechanoceptor functions. Calcitonin gene-related peptide fibers are present in these ganglia at positions corresponding to those of substance P.

Motor neurons and nerves. Calcitonin gene-related peptide is also distributed in motor neurons of the ventral spinal cord (Gibson *et al.,* 1984a), motor nuclei of the cranial nerves, and in the caudal part of the nucleus ambiguus (Takami *et al.,* 1985a). The peptide is localized to vesicles (diameter 40–60 nm) in axon terminals within the synaptic trough of the neuromuscular junction (Takami *et al.,* 1985b) of the striated muscle of the tongue (with acetylcholine) (Lee *et al.,* 1985b) and esophagus (Rodrigo *et al.,* 1985).

Autonomic nervous system. In autonomic sympathetic ganglia (celiac and superior cervical), CGRP is only localized to fibers and not to cells. In the celiac ganglia, these are either "passing fibers" that form thick bundles and costore substance P, or are "terminating fibers" forming varicosities that do not costore substance P. The latter terminate in ganglia and possibly modulate ganglion function. Their number is markedly reduced in the superior cervical ganglia, where there are also no passing fibers. Clearly, CGRP-containing fibers outnumber those containing substance P in both ganglia. In parasympathetic ganglia, essentially the same distribution pattern is maintained in addition to the presence of cell bodies.

It is perhaps worth commenting on the extensive distribution network of CGRP in the gastrointestinal and urogenital tracts, supplying the organs and their vasculature (Mulderry *et al.,* 1985b; Ghatei *et al.,* 1984; Su *et al.,* 1986). In the mammalian esophagus, both sensory and motor fibers originating from the nodose and nucleus ambiguous respectively, form sub- and intraepithelial plexuses (known to be stretch sensitive; Robles Chillida *et al.,* 1983) and innervate the smooth and striated muscle (motor end plate). In contrast, less abundant substance P-containing fibers arise from the intramuscular ganglionic plexus and do not innervate the end plate (Leander *et al.,* 1982; Rodrigo *et al.,* 1985). In addition, high levels of CGRP occur in the pylorus descending colon and rectum, where CGRP-rich nerve fibers supply the circular muscle, submucosa, muscularis mucosa, and mucosa. In the urogenital system, CGRP-rich structures supply the vasculature, nonvascular smooth muscle of the ureter, bladder and uterus, squamous epithelium of the fallopian tubes, and connective tissue of the ovary, cervix, vagina, bladder, and ureter. The trigone of the bladder has the richest supply of CGRP-containing fibers. These fibers reach the urinary tract via the hypogastric and pelvic nerves that arise from lumbar and sacral dorsal root ganglia. The distribution pattern is similar to that of substance P.

ii. Central neuromodulation. There is growing pharmacological evidence suggesting that CGRP shares with calcitonin its profound effects on physiological, behavioral, and metabolic functions. This is in line with its distribution in the central nervous system. The basic mechanism of centrally administered CGRP or calcitonin appears to be the depression of neuronal excitability (Twery and Moss, 1985). In particular, it appears that CGRP is a central mediator of ingestive behavior, and as with calcitonin, the peptide suppresses feeding (Krahn *et al.*, 1984). This effect is exerted either via an action on the hypothalamic satiety center or by the inhibition of basal and stimulated gastric acid secretion (Lenz *et al.*, 1985). Calcitonin gene-related peptide also probably plays a role in the modulation of involuntary movements mediated by the basal ganglia.

iii. Peripheral neurotransmission. It is widely suggested that CGRP may modulate or transmit sensory impulses. The distribution of CGRP in the spinal cord, particularly in laminae containing neurons, responsive to noxious and innocuous stimuli and in ganglia giving rise to C and A(δ) afferent fibers its colocalization with the tachykinins, and its depletion following capsaicin (Zaidi *et al.*, 1985; Diez Guerra *et al.*, 1987; Emson and Zaidi, 1989) clearly falls in line with this suggestion. The possibility that CGRP is an autonomic neurotransmitter is based on its existence in autonomic ganglia and the diffuse CGRP-rich innervation of cardiovascular, gastrointestinal, urogenital, and special sensory systems.

There is also growing evidence from its distribution that CGRP functions in motor control. The peptide enhances diaphragmmatic contraction, presumably via its own receptor, and at high doses shows nonspecific inhibitory action on smooth muscle cells of the vas deferens. In addition, there is some evidence that CGRP acts on a presynaptic receptor, to inhibit noradrenaline release (Ohhashi and Jacobowitz, 1985).

Calcitonin gene-related peptide appears to have yet another novel neuromodulatory role. The peptide has been shown to increase the number of acetylcholine receptors on the surface of cultured myo-tubules (New and Mudge, 1986). The effect is also dose-dependent, is observable at physiological concentrations of CGRP, and the time course is similar to that of dibutyryl cAMP. In addition, CGRP en-hances the accumulation of cAMP in mouse diaphragm and cultured chick myotubules, suggesting that this effect is mediated by cAMP (Lauffer and Changeaux, 1987; Takami et al., 1986). Indeed, cAMP has long been suspected to play a role in the development of functional motor end plates (Carlsen, 1975), but it is unclear whether the poten-cies or the effects of the α and β forms of the peptide are different.

5. Special Sensory Functions

a. Ear. In the inner ear, CGRP-positive fibers are found in the in-traganglionic spiral bundle and hair cells of the Organ of Corti, and here the distribution simulates that of encephalin. These fibers seem to originate from the olivocochlear bundle (Kitajiri et al., 1985).

b. Eye. i. Distributions. Much more emphasis has been given to the role of CGRP in the eye. In the posterior chamber, CGRP is localized to stratified amacrine cells of the retina (Kiyama et al., 1985), and this pattern resembles that of tyrosine hydroxylase-containing cells, and of cells containing other neuropeptides (Stone et al., 1984; Palkama et al., 1986). In the anterior chamber of various species, including humans, CGRP-rich nerve fibers form a plexus over the iris, ciliary body, pupill-ary muscles, central choroid (all C-fibers; Lehtosalo et al., 1984) and uveal and choroidal blood vessels (Aδ-fibers) (Terenghi et al., 1985; Wahlestedt et al., 1985; Stone et al., 1986; Stone and McGlinn, 1988). Uveal fibers originate from the trigeminal ganglia and their distribu-tion resembles that of substance P (Miller et al., 1981). Calcitonin gene-related peptide fibers are extremely uncommon in the cornea, where they mainly occur subepithelially with a few epithelial nerve endings (Stone et al., 1986; Krootila, 1988).

ii. Functions. The functions of endogenous CGRP in the eye include vasorelaxatory and ciliary muscle control. It increases intraocular pressure and causes a disruption of the blood–aqueous barrier in ex-perimental animals (Unger et al., 1985; Wahlstedt et al., 1985, 1986; Oksala et al., 1986). This is thought to be the consequence of the marked increase of blood flow and capillary permeability in the ciliary process. Evidence suggests that the intracameral application of CGRP leads to a marked elevation in blood flow (Krootila et al., 1988), which correlates well with the distribution of peptide in the anterior chamber of the eye. Thus, a good case can be made for the involvement of CGRP in the irritative responses of the eye to noxious stimulation, a response that could be based on the presence of a sensory axon-reflex mechanism. This response could consist of miosis, a breakdown of the blood–aqueous barrier, anterior uveal vasodilatation, and an increased intraocular pressure (Perkins, 1957; Japmol *et al.*, 1976; Butler *et al.*, 1979). This is indeed an exciting possibility, as substance P has also been shown to produce some of these effects, especially miosis (Stjernschantz *et al.*, 1981), and that in low doses the latter peptide potentiates the effects of CGRP on the eye (Wahlestedt *et al.*, 1986). In addition, it is conceivable that CGRP may have trophic effects in the corneal epithelium and stroma, and a decrease in the number of such fibers may play a role in the pathogenesis of conditions, such as neuroparalytic keratitis.

V. Conclusions and Future Perspectives

The study of the biology and genetics of the calcium-regulating hormone, calcitonin, has led to the discovery not only of two unsuspected functional peptides, CGRP and amylin, but has also unraveled new systems of regulation. The next decade should see progress in at least three major areas: receptor cloning, post-receptor signal transduction mechanisms, and regulation of alternative splicing.

A. Strategies for Calcitonin Receptor Cloning

For several years, investigators have experienced major problems, despite sustained attempts to characterize calcitonin and CGRP receptors. The scarcity of the starting material and the difficulty in purifying the active form of the hydrophobic membrane protein have been the major impediments to any anticipated success. The alternative strategy to protein chemistry would, of course, be to clone the gene encoding the receptor molecule. Complementary DNA expression libraries could, in theory, be screened with CGRP, the true ligand. However, antiidiotypic immunological screening might be a more efficient method. Indeed, antibodies raised against "receptor-like" idiotypic determinants of antiligand antibodies or antiidiotypic monoclonals have previously been used to identify receptors. A more efficient means allowing the direct cloning of a full length cDNA containing all necessary expression sequences may be the cDNA screening system developed by Seed and colleagues (Seed and Aruffo, 1987; Seed, 1987). This would obviate multiple rounds of screening to identify full-length or overlapping clones. Briefly, it is a technique based on transient expression in *cos* cells and physical selection of expressing cells by adhesion to antibody coated dishes (so called "panning"). It allows a large number of cDNAs expressing surface molecules to be cloned quickly and allows monoclonal antibodies to be used effectively, unlike screening methods based on fusion protein expression (e.g., λ GTII) and also requires less antibody.

B. Post-Receptor Signaling

Studies on post-receptor signaling in osteoclasts are already underway in our and other laboratories. In order to establish any second messenger hypothesis, it is essential that time-resolved measurements are made. For this, inert photolabile precursors of second messengers (or "caged" second messengers) have proven ideal (Gurney and Lester, 1987; Walker *et al.,* 1987). The technique involves the introduction of these compounds into the cell cytoplasm by microinjection or permeabilization. The consequences of release of the active second messenger molecule by high energy flash photolysis on rapid changes in osteoclast activity or calcium transients can be accurately quantified. It appears likely that the next decade will unravel regulatory networks in osteoclasts and other hormone-responsive cells.

C. Factors Regulating Alternative Splicing of the Calcitonin–CGRP Gene

The factors regulating alternative splicing of the α-calcitonin–CGRP gene are, for practical purposes, unknown. Given that these factors act only on pre-mRNA, their elucidation appears to be formidable and progress is thus likely to be slow. On the other hand, attempts at elucidating promoter sequences and characterizing factors that regulate gene transcription are more likely to be successful, because techniques used to study the binding of factors to specific DNA sequences and to purify them are comparatively simple. The sequence elements in the promoter region of a gene that affects its transcription can be identified by their binding to specific regulatory factors. The method of analysis is simple: DNA sequences, which have bound a protein, are protected against DNAase digestion or retarded on gel electrophoresis. Once the recognition sequence has been identified, the transcription factor of interest can be purified by affinity chromatography using synthetic oligodeoxyribonucleotides of the DNA sequence, as binding elements. Indeed, a number of transcription factors have been purified using this approach; in one case (AP-1) the factor has been shown to be identical to an oncogene (c-*jun*) (Bohman *et al.,* 1987). These studies would become much easier if cell lines were to become easily available; these could used to study the expression of *in vitro* mutagenized promoters of genes, thus allowing genetic mapping of regions of interest.

REFERENCES

Abeyasekera, G., Datta, H. K., MacIntyre, I., Moonga, B. S., Patchell, A., and Zaidi, M. (1989). G proteins mediate the acute effects of calcitonin on isolated osteoclasts. *J. Physiol. (London)* **420,** 81P.

Aer, J. (1968). Effect of the thyrocalcitonin on urinary hydroxyproline and calcium in rats. *Endocrinology (Baltimore)* **83,** 379–380.

Agus, Z. S., Wasserstein, S., and Goldfarb, S. (1981). PTH, calcitonin cyclic nucleotides and the kidney. *Annu. Rev. Physiol.* **43,** 583.

Akisaka, T., and Gay, T. V. (1986). Ultracytochemical evidence for a proton pump adenosine triphosphate in chick osteoclasts. *Cell Tissue Res.* **245,** 507–512.

Alevizaki, M., Shiraishi, A., Rassool, F. V., Ferrier, G. J. M., MacIntyre, I., and Legon, S. (1986). The calcitonin-like sequence of the beta-CGRP gene. *FEBS Lett.* **206,** 47–52.

Alevizaki, M., Rassool, F. V., Collyear, K. L. S., MacIntyre, I., and Legon, S. (1987). A third calcitonin related sequence in the human genome. *Calcif. Tissue Int.* **41**(S2), 79.

Aliopoulious, M. A., Goldhaber, P., and Munson, P. L. (1965). Thyrocalcitonin inhibition of bone resorption induced by parathyroid hormone in tissue culture. *Science* **151,** 331.

Allan, E. (1983). Calcitonin in the treatment of intractible pain of malignancy. *Pharmacotherapeutica* **3,** 482–486.

Allison, J., Hall, L., MacIntyre, I., and Craig, R. K. (1981). The construction and partial characterization of plasmids containing complementary DNA sequences to human calcitonin precursor polyprotein. *Biochem. J.* **199,** 725–731.

Amara, S. G., David, D. N., Rosenfeld, M. G., Roos, B. A., and Evans, R. M. (1980). Characterization of rat calcitonin mRNA. *Proc. Natl. Acad. Sci. U.S.A.* **77,** 4444–4448.

Amara, S. G., Jonas, V., Rosenfeld, M. G., Ong, E. S., and Evans, R. M. (1982). Alternative RNA processing in calcitonin gene expression generates mRNAs encoding different polypeptide products. *Nature (London)* **298,** 240–244.

Amara, S. G., Arriza, J. L., Leff, S. E., Swanson, L. W., Evans, R. M., and Rosenfeld, M. G. (1985). Expression in brain of a messenger RNA encoding a novel neuropeptide homologous to calcitonin gene related peptide. *Science* **229,** 1094–1098.

Anand, P., Gibson, S. J., McGregor, G. P., Blank, M. A., Ghatei, M. A., Bacarese-Hamilton, A. J., and Polak, J. M. (1983). A VIP-containing system concentrated in the lumbosacral region of the human spinal cord. *Nature (London)* **305,** 143–144.

Anderson, R. E., Scharer, H., and Gay, C. V. (1982). Ultrastructural immunocytochemical localisation of carbonic anhydrase in normal and calcitonin-treated chick osteoclasts. *Anat. Rec.* **204,** 9.

Arnett, T. R., and Dempster, D. W. (1987). A comparative study of disaggregated chick and rat osteoclasts *in vitro:* effects of calcitonin and prostaglandins. *Endocrinology (Baltimore)* **120,** 602–608.

Avissar, S., Schreiber, G., Dannon, A., and Belmaker, R. H. (1988). Lithium inhibits adrenergic and cholinergic increase in GTP binding in rat cortex. *Nature (London)* **331,** 440–442.

Baghdiantz, A., Foster, G. V., Edwards, A., Kumar, M. A., Slack, E., Soliman, H. A., and MacIntyre, I. (1964). Extraction and purification of human calcitonin. *Nature (London)* **203,** 1027–1028.

Barga, P., Ferri, S., Santagostino, A., Oligiati, V. R., and Pecile, A. (1978). Lack of opiate receptor involvement in centrally induced calcitonin analgesia. *Life Sci.* **22,** 971–978.

Baron, R., and Vignery, A. (1981). Behavior of osteoclasts during a rapid change in their number induced by high doses of parathyroid hormone or calcitonin in intact rats. *Metab. Dis. Relat. Res.* **2,** 339–346.

Benjamin, N., Dollery, C. T., Fuller, R. W., Larkin, S., and McEwan, J. (1987). The effects of calcitonin gene-related peptide and substance P on resistance and capacitance vessels. *Br. J. Pharmacol.* **90,** Suppl., 43P.

Bevis, P. J. R., MacIntyre, I., Morris, H. R., and Zaidi, M. (1986a). On the presence of a potent vasodilator, calcitonin gene-related peptide (CGRP) in rat plasma. *J. Physiol. (London)* **376,** 24P.

Bevis, P. J. R., MacIntyre, I., and Zaidi, M. (1986b). Further evidence for the neural release of plasma calcitonin gene-related peptide. *Br. J. Pharmacol.* **88,** 314P.

Bevis, P. J. R., Zaidi, M., and MacIntyre, I. (1990). The dual effect of calcitonin gene-related peptide on plasma calcium levels in the chick. *Biochem. Biophys. Res. Commun.* **169,** 846–850.

Bohman, D., Bos, T. J., Adman, A., Nishimura, T., Vojt, P. K., and Tjian, R. (1987). Human proto-oncogene c-jun encode a DNA binding protein with structural and functional properties of transcriptor factor *AP-1. Science* **238,** 1386.

Bovenberg, R. A. L., van de Meerendonk, W. P. M., Bass, P. D., Steenbergh, P. H., Lips, C. J. M., and Jansz, H. S. (1986). Model for alternative RNA processing in human calcitonin gene expression. *Nucleic Acid Res.* **22,** 8785–8803.

Brain, S. D., and Williams, T. J. (1985). Inflammatory oedema induced by synergism between calcitonin gene-related peptide (CGRP) and mediators of increased vascular permeability. *Br. J. Pharmacol.* **86,** 855–860.

Brain, S. D., Williams, T. J., Tippins, J. R., Morris, H. R., and MacIntyre, I. (1985). Calcitonin gene-related peptide is a potent vasodilator. *Nature (London)* **313,** 54–56.

Brain, S. D., MacIntyre, I., and Williams, T. J. (1986). A second form of calcitonin gene-related peptide which is a potent vasodilator. *Eur. J. Pharmacol.* **124,** 349–352.

Breimer, L. H., MacIntyre, I., and Zaidi, M. (1988). Peptides from the calcitonin genes: molecular genetics, structure and function. *Biochem. J.* **255,** 377–390.

Brewer, H. B., and Ronan, R. (1969). Amino acid sequence of bovine thyrocalcitonin. *Proc. Natl. Sci. U.S.A.* **63,** 940.

Butler, J. M., Unger, W. G., and Hammond, B. R. (1979). Sensory mediation of the ocular response to neutral formaldehyde. *Exp. Eye Res.* **28,** 577–589.

Byfield, P. G. H., Clark, M. B., Turner, K., Foster, G. V., and MacIntyre, I. (1972). Immunochemical studies on human calcitonin M leading to information on the shape of the molecule. *Biochem. J.* **127,** 199–206.

Byfield, P. G. H., Matthews, E. W., Heersche, J. N. M., Boorman, G. A., Girgis, S. I., and MacIntyre, I. (1976a). Isolation of calcitonin from rat thyroid medullary thyroid carcinoma. *FEBS Lett.* **65,** 238.

Byfield, P. G. H., McLoughlin, J. L., Matthews, E. W., and MacIntyre, I. (1976b). A proposed structure for the rat calcitonin. *FEBS Lett.* **65,** 242.

Cao, H., and Gay, C. V. (1985). Effects of parathyroid hormone and calcitonin on carbonic anhydrase location in osteoclasts of cultured embryonic chick bone. *Experientia* **41,** 1472–1474.

Care, A. D. (1970). The effects of pancreozymin and secretin on calcitonin release. *Fed. Proc.* **29**, 253.

Carlsen, R. G. (1975). The possible role of cAMP in the neuro-trophic control of skeletal muscle. *J. Physiol. (London)* **247**, 343–361.

Caserani, R., Columbo, M., Oligiati, V. R., and Pecile, A. (1979). Calcitonin and prostaglandin system. *Life Sci.* **25**, 1851–1856.

Casey, P. J., and Gilman, A. F. (1988). G protein involvement in receptor-effector coupling. *J. Biol. Chem.* **263**, 2577–2580.

Chambers, T. J. (1982). Osteoblasts release osteoclasts from calcitonin-induced quiescence. *J. Cell Sci.* **57**, 247–253.

Chambers, T. J., and Ali, N. N. (1983). Inhibition of osteoclastic motility by prostaglandins I_2, E_1, E_2 and 6-oxo-E_1. *J. Pathol.* **139**, 383.

Chambers, T. J., and Magnus, C. J. (1982). Calcitonin alters behaviour of isolated osteoclasts. *J. Pathol.* **136**, 97–106.

Chambers, T. J., and Moore, C. J. (1983). The sensitivity of isolated osteoclasts to morphological transformation by calcitonin. *J. Clin. Endocrinol. Metab.* **57**, 819–824.

Chambers, T. J., Revell, P. A., Fuller, K., and Athanasou, N. A. (1984). Resorption of bone by isolated rabbit osteoclasts. *J. Cell Sci.* **66**, 383–399.

Chambers, T. J., McSheehy, P. M. J., Thomson, B. M., and Fuller, K. (1985a). The effect of calcium regulating hormones and prostaglandins on bone resorption by osteoclasts disaggregated from rabbit long bones. *Endocrinology (Baltimore)* **116**, 234–239.

Chambers, T. J., Fuller, K., McSheehy, P. M. J., and Pringle, J. A. S. (1985b). The effects of calcium regulating hormones on bone resorption by isolated human osteoclastoma cells. *J. Pathol.* **145**, 297–305.

Chambers, T. J., Chambers, J. C., Darby, J. A., and Fuller, K. (1986). The effect of human calcitonin on the cytoplasmic spreading of rat osteoclasts. *J. Clin. Endocrinol. Metab.* **63**, 1080–1085.

Chambers, T. J., Fuller, K., and Darby, J. A. (1987). Hormonal regulation of acid phosphatase release by osteoclasts disaggregated from neonatal rat bone. *J. Cell. Physiol.* **132**, 90–96.

Chausmer, A., Stevens, M. D., and Severn, C. (1982). Autoradiographic evidence for a calcitonin receptor on testicular Leidig cells. *Science* **216**, 735.

Chiba, T., Yanaguchi, A. Yamatani, T., Nakamura, A., Morishita, T., Inui, T., Fukase, M., Noda, T., and Fujita, T. (1989). Calcitonin gene-related peptide receptor antagonist human CGRP (8-37). *Am. J. Physiol.* **256**, E331–E335.

Clementi, G., Nicoletti, F., Patacchioli, F., Patti, F., Matera, M., and Scapagnini, U. (1983). Hypoprolactinaemic action of calcitonin and tuberoinfundibular dopaminergic system. *J. Neurochem.* **40**, 885.

Clementi, G., Prato, A., Conforto, G. and Scapagnini, U. (1984). Role of serotonin in the analgesic activity of calcitonin. *Eur. J. Pharmacol.* **98**, 449–451.

Clementi, G., Amico Roxus M., de Rapisarda, E., Caruso, A., Prato, A., Thrombadore, S., Priolo, G., and Scapagnini, U. (1985). The analgesic activity of calcitonin and the serotonergic system. *Eur. J. Pharmacol.* **108**, 71–75.

Cooper, C. W., Schwesinger, W. H., Mahgoub, A. M., and Ontjes, D. A. (1971). Thyrocalcitonin: stimulation of secretion by pentagastrin. *Science* **172**, 1238–1240.

Cooper, G. J. S., Willis, A. C., Clark, A., Turner, R. C., Sim, R. B., and Reid, K. B. M. (1987). Purification and characterization of a peptide from amyloid-rich pancreases of type-2 diabetic patients. *Proc. Natl. Acad. Sci. U.S.A.* **84**, 8628–8632.

Copp, D. H. and Cheney, B. A. (1962). Calcitonin—a hormone from the parathyroid that lowers the calcium level of the blood. *Nature (London)* **193**, 381–382.

Crawford A., Evans, D. B., Skjodt, H., Beresford, J. N., MacIntyre, I., and Russell, R. G.

G. (1991). The effect of calcitonin gene-related peptide on bone derived cells in culture. *Bone* (in press).

Datta, H. K., Zaidi, M., Wimalawansa, S. J., Ghatei, M. A., Beacham, J. L., Bloom, S. R., and MacIntyre, I. (1989a). *In vivo* and *in vitro* effects of amylin and amylin-amide on calcium metabolism in the rat and rabbit. *Biochem. Biophys. Res. Commun.* **162**, 876–881.

Datta, H. K., MacIntyre, I., and Zaidi, M. (1989b). The effect of ionised calcium on the morphology and function of isolated rat osteoclasts. *Biosci. Rep.* **9**, 247–251.

Datta, H. K., MacIntyre, I., and Zaidi, M. (1989c). Inhibition by elevated extracellular calcium of *in vitro* bone resorption by isolated rat osteoclasts. *J. Physiol. (London)* **413**, 98P.

Datta, H. K., MacIntyre, I., and Zaidi, M. (1990). Intracellular regulation of osteoclast function I: Lack of effects of voltage, nifedipine, BAYK8644 and diltaizem on calcium-activated calcium entry. *Biochem. Biophys. Res. Commun.* **167**, 183–188.

deLuise, M., Martin, T. J., and Melik, R. A. (1970). Inactivation and degradation of porcine calcitonin by rat liver and relative stability of salmon calcitonin. *J. Endocrinol.* **48**, 181–188.

Dempster, D. W., Murills, R. J., Horbert, W., and Arnett, T. R. (1987). Biological activity of chicken calcitonin: effects on neonatal rat and embryonic chick osteoclasts. *J. Bone Miner. Res.* **2**, 443–448.

de Vernejoul, M.-C., Horowitz, M., Demignon, J., Neff, L., and Baron, R. (1988). Bone resorption by isolated chick osteoclasts in culture is stimulated by murine spleen cell supernatant fluid (osteoclast activating factor) and inhibited by calcitonin and prostaglandin E2. *J. Bone Miner. Res.* **3**, 69–80.

Diez, Guerra, J., Zaidi, M., Bevis, P. J. R., MacIntyre, I., and Emson, P. C. (1987). Evidence for the release of calcitonin gene-related peptide and neurokinin A from sensory nerve terminals. *Neuroscience* **25**, 839–846.

D'Souza, S. M., MacIntyre, I., Girgis, S. I., and Mundy, G. R. (1989). Human synthetic calcitonin gene-related peptide inhibits bone resorption *in vitro*. *Endocrinology (Baltimore)* **119**, 58–62.

Dunn, G. A., and Brown, A. F. (1986). Alignment of fibroblasts on grooved surfaces described by a simple geometrical transformation. *J. Cell Sci.* **83**, 313–340.

Edbrooke, M. R., Parker, D., McVey, J. H., Riley, J. H., Sorensen, G. D., Pettengill, O. S., and Craig, R. K. (1985). Expression of the human calcitonin/CGRP gene in lung and thyroid carcinoma. *EMBO J.* **4**, 715–724.

Edvinsson, L., Fredholm, B. B., Hemel, E., Jansen, I., and Verrochia, C. (1985). Perivascular peptides relax cerebral arteries concomitant with stimulation of cyclic AMP accumulation or release of an endothelium derived relaxing factor in the cat. *Neurosci. Lett.* **58**, 213–217.

Elalouf, J. M., Roinel, N., and deRoffignac, C. (1985). Stimulation by human calcitonin of electrolyte transport in distal tubules of rat kidney. *Pfleugers Arch.* **399**, 111.

Emson, P. C., and Zaidi, M. (1989). Further evidence for the origin of calcitonin gene-related peptide in the rat. *J. Physiol.* **412**, 297–308.

Epand, R. M., Epand, R. F., Orlowski, R. C., Flanigan, E., and Stahl, G. L. (1985). A comparison of the interaction of glucagon, human parathyroid hormone (1–34)-peptide and calcitonin with dimyristoylphosphatidylglycerol and with dimyristoylphosphatidylcholine. *Biophys. Chem.* **23**, 39–48.

Epand, R. M., Epand, R. F., Orlowski, R. C., Seyler, J. K., and Collescott, R. L. (1986). Conformational flexibility and biological activity of salmon calcitonin. *Biochemistry* **25**, 1964–1968.

Findlay, D. M., deLuise, M., Michelangeli, V. P., Ellison, M., and Martin, T. J. (1980a).

Properties of calcitonin receptor and adenylate cyclase in BEN cells, a human cancer cell line. *Cancer Res.* **40**, 1311–1317.

Findlay, D. M., Michelangeli, V. P., Eisman, J. A., Frampton, R. J., Moseley, J. M., MacIntyre, I., Whitehead, R., and Martin, T. J. (1980b). Calcitonin and 1,25-dihydroxyvitamin D_3 receptors in human breast cancer cells. *Cancer Res.* **40**, 4764–4767.

Findlay, D. M., Michelangeli, V. P., Moseley, J. M., and Martin, T. J. (1981a). Calcitonin binding and degradation by two cultured human breast cancer cell lines (MCF7 and T47D). *Biochem. J.* **196**, 513–520.

Findlay, D. M., deLuise, M., Michelangeli, V. P., and Martin, T. J. (1981b). Independent downregulation of insulin and calcitonin receptors in human tumour cell lines. *Endocrinology (Baltimore)* **88**, 271–276.

Findlay, D. M., Ng, K. W., Niall, M., and Martin, T. J. (1982). Processing of calcitonin and epidermal growth factor after binding to receptors in human breast cancer cells (T47D). *Biochem. J.* **206**, 343–350.

Findlay, D. M., Michelangeli, V. P., Orlowski, R. C., and Martin, T. J. (1984). Relationship between internalisation and calcitonin-induced receptor loss in T47D cells. *Endocrinology (Baltimore)* **115**, 78–84.

Fischer, J. A., Tobler, P. H., Henke, H., and Tschopp, P. H. (1983). Salmon and human calcitonin-like peptides coexist in human thyroid and brain. *J. Clin. Endocrinol. Metab.* **57**, 1314–1316.

Fisher, D. A., Kikkawa, D. O., Rivier, J. E., Amara, S. G., Evans, R. M., and Rosenfeld, M. G. (1983). Stimulation of noradrenergic sympathetic outflow by calcitonin gene-related peptide. *Nature (London)* **305**, 534–536.

Fleming, N., Sliwinski-Lis, E., and Burke, D. N. (1989). G regulatory protein and muscarinic receptor signal transduction in mucous acini of rat submandibular gland. *Life Sci.* **44**, 1027–1033.

Foreman, J. C., Jordan, C. C., Oehme, P., and Renner, H. (1983). Structure activity relationship for some substance P-related peptide that causes wheel and flare reactions in human skin. *J. Physiol. (London)* **335**, 449.

Forrest, S. M., Ng, K. W., Findlay, D. M., Michelangeli, V. P., Livesey, S. A., Partridge, N. C., Zajac, J. D., and Martin, T. J. (1985). Characteristics of an osteoblast clonal cell line which responds to both parathyroid hormone and calcitonin. *Calcif. Tissue Int.* **37**, 51–56.

Foster, G. V., Baghdiantz, A., Kumar, M. A., Slack, E., Soliman, H. A., and MacIntyre, I. (1964). Thyroid origin of calcitonin. *Nature (London)* **202**, 1303–1305.

Foster, G. V., Joplin, G. F., MacIntyre, I., Melvin, K. E. W., and Slack, E. (1969). Effect of thyrocalcitonin in man. *Lancet* **i**, 107–109.

Fouchereau-Peron, M., Moukhtar, M. A., Benson, A. A., and Milhaud, G. (1981a). Demonstration of specific receptors for calcitonin in isolated trout gill cells. *Comp. Biochem. Physiol.* **68A**, 417–421.

Fouchereau-Peron, M., Moukhtar, M. A., Benson, A. A., and Milhaud, G. (1981b). Characterisation of specific receptors for calcitonin in porcine lung. *Proc. Natl. Acad. Sci. U.S.A.* **78**, 3973–3975.

Fraioli, F., Fabbri, A., Gnessi, L., Moretti, C., Santore, C., and Feleci, M. (1982). Subarachnoid injection of salmon calcitonin induces analgesia in man. *Eur. J. Pharmacol.* **78**, 381.

Freake, H. C., and MacIntyre, I. (1982). Specific binding sites of 1,25-dihydroxycholecalcitferol in human medullary thyroid carcinoma. *Biochem. J.* **206**, 181–184.

Fried, R. M., and Tashjian, A. H., Jr. (1986). Unusual sensitivity of cytosolic free calcium to changes in extracellular calcium in rat C-cells. *J. Biol. Chem.* **261**, 7669–7674.

Freidman, J., and Raisz, L. G. (1965). Thyrocalcitonin: inhibitor of bone resorption in tissue culture. *Science* **150,** 1465–1467.

Fritsch, H. A. R., van Noorden S., and Pearse, A. G. E. (1980). Calcitonin-like immunochemical staining in the alimentary tract of *Ciona Intestinalis. Cell Tissue Res.* **205,** 439–444.

Galante, L., Horton, R., Joplin, G. F., Woodhouse, N. J. F., and MacIntyre, I. (1971). Comparison of human, porcine and salmon synthetic calcitonins in man and the rat. *Clin. Sci.* **40,** 9–10.

Gamse, R., and Saria, A. (1985). Potentiation of tachykinin induced plasma protein extravasation by calcitonin gene-related peptide. *Eur. J. Pharmacol.* **114,** 61–66.

Gennari, C., and Fischer, J. A. (1985). Cardiovascular action of calcitonin gene-related peptide in humans. *Calcif. Tissue Int.* **37,** 581–584.

Ghatei, M. A., Gu, J., Mulderry, P. K., Allen, J. M., Morrison, J. F., Polak, J. M., and Bloom, S. R. (1984). Calcitonin gene-related peptide in the rat urogenital tract. *Peptides* **6,** 809–815.

Ghatei, M. A., Datta, H. K., Zaidi, M., Deborah-Watt, L., MacIntyre, I., and Bloom, S. R. (1989). Amylin and amylin-amide lack acute effect on plasma glucose and insulin. *J. Endocrinol.* **124,** R9–R11.

Gibson, S. J., Polak, J. M., Bloom, S. R., and Wall, P. D. (1981). The distribution of nine peptides in the rat spinal cord with special reference to substantia gelatinosa and on the area around the central canal (lamina X). *J. Comp. Neurol.* **201,** 65.

Gibson, S. J., Polak, J. M., Anand, P., Blank, M. A., Morrison, J. F. B., Kelly, J. S., and Bloom, S. R. (1984b). The distribution and origin of VIP in the spinal cord of six mammalian species. *Peptides* **5,** 201.

Gibson, S. J., Polak, J. M., Adrian, T. E., Allen, J. M., Kelly, J. S., and Bloom, S. R. (1984c). The distribution and origin of a novel brain peptide. neuropeptide Y in the spinal cord of several mammals. *J. Comp. Neurol.* **227,** 78.

Gilbey, S. G., & Ghatei, M. A., Bretherton-Watt, D., Zaidi, M., Jones, P. M., Perera, T., Beacham, J., Girgis, S. I., and Bloom, S. R. (1991). Islet amyloid peptide (IAPP): Production by osteoblast cell line and possible role as a paracrine regulator of osteoclast function in man. *Clin. Sci.* (in press).

Girgis, S. I. (1980). Immunochemical studies on calcitonin. *Ph.D. Thesis, Univ. of London.*

Glowacki, J., O'Sullivan, J., Miller, M., Wilke, D. W., and Deftos, L. J. (1985). Calcitonin produces hypercalcaemia in leopard sharks. *Endocrinology (Baltimore)* **116,** 827.

Goldring, S. R., Dayer, S. M., Ausiello, D. A., and Krane, S. M. (1978). A cell strain cultured from porcine kidney increases cyclic AMP content upon exposure to calcitonin and vasopressin. *Biochem. Biophys. Res. Commun.* **83,** 434–440.

Goltzman, D., and Mitchell, J. (1985). Interaction of calcitonin and calcitonin gene-related peptide at receptor sites in target tissues. *Science* **227,** 1343–1345.

Greenwald, S. E., Leuer, M. J., MacIntyre, I., Morris, H. R., and Tippins, J. G. (1986). Human calcitonin gene-related peptide is a potent dilator in the pig coronary circulation. *Br. J. Pharmacol.* **87,** 56P.

Gropp, C., Luster, W., and Havemann, K. (1985). Salmon and human calcitonin-like material in lung carcinoma. *Br. J. Cancer* **51,** 897–901.

Gu, J., Polak, J. M., Adrian, T. E., Allen, J. M., Tatemoto, K., and Bloom, S. R. (1983). Neuropeptide Y (NPY)-major cardiac neuropeptide. *Lancet* **i,** 1008–1009.

Gurney, A. M., and Lester, H. A. (1987). Light flash physiology with synthetic photosensitive compounds. *Physiol. Rev.* **67,** 583–617.

Gutierrez, G. E., Mundy, G. R., and Katz, M. S. (1984). Adenylate cyclase of osteoblast-like cells from rat osteosarcoma is stimulated by calcitonin as well as parathyroid hormone. *Endocrinology (Baltimore)* **115**, 2342–2346.

Habener, J. F., Singer, F. R., Deftos, L. J., Neer, R. M., and Potts, J. T., Jr. (1971). Explanation for the unusual potency of salmon calcitonin. *Nature (London)* **232**, 91–92.

Haller-Brem, S., Muff, R., Peterman, J. B., Born, W., Roos, B. A., and Fischer, J. A. (1987). Role of cytosolic free Ca^{2+} concentration in the secretion of CGRP and CT from medullary thyroid carcinoma cells. *Endocrinology (Baltimore)* **121**, 1272–1277.

Ham, J., Williams, J. C., and Ellison, M. I. (1979). Radioreceptor assay for the detection of biologically active forms of calcitonin. *J. Endocrinol.* **81**, 152.

Hanko, J., Hardebo, J. E., Kahlstrom, J. K., Owman, C., and Sundler, F. (1985). Calcitonin gene-related peptide is present in mammalian cardiovascular nerve fibres and dilates pial and peripheral arteries. *Neurosci. Lett.* **57**, 91–95.

Hass, H. G., Dambacher, M. A., Guncaga, J., and Lauffenberger, T. (1971). Renal effects of calcitonin and parathyroid extracts in man. Studies in hypoparathyroidism. *J. Clin. Invest.* **50**, 2689.

Heath, H., III, and Sizemore, G. W. (1983). Radioimmunoassay for calcitonin. *In* "Assay of Calcium Regulating Hormones (D. D. Bilke, ed.), pp. 229–244. Springer-Verlag, Berlin.

Heath, H., III, Body, J. J., and Fox, J. (1984). Radioimmunoassay of calcitonin in normal human plasma: problems, perspectives and prospects. *Biomed. Pharmacother.* **38**, 241–250.

Hedland, T., Hulth, A., and Johnell, O. (1983). Early effects of paratharmone and calcitonin on the number os osteoclasts and on serum calcium in rats. *Acta Orthop. Scand.* **54**, 802.

Heersche, J. N. M., Marcus, R., and Aurbach, G. D. (1974). Calcitonin and the formation of 3′-5′ AMP in the bone and kidney. *Endocrinology (Baltimore)* **94**, 241–247.

Heschler, J., Rosenthal, W., Trautwein, W., and Schultz, G. (1987). The GTP-binding protein, Go, regulates neuronal calcium channel. *Nature (London)* **325**, 445–447.

Hillyard, C. J., Myers, C., Abeyasekera, G., Stevenson, J. C., Craig, P. K., and MacIntyre, I. (1983). Katacalcin: a new plasma calcium lowering hormone. *Lancet* **I**, 846–848.

Hishikawa, R., Fukase, M., Yamatani, T., Kadowaki, S., and Fujita, T. (1985). Phorbol ester stimulates calcitonin secretion synergistically with A23187, and additively with dibutyryl cyclic AMP in a rat C cell line. *Biochem. Biophys. Res. Commun.* **132**, 424–429.

Holman, J. J., Craig, R. K., and Marshall, I. (1986). Human alpha- and beta-CGRP and rat alpha-CGRP are coronary vasodilators in the rat. *Peptides* **7**, 231–235.

Holtrop, N. E., Raisz, L. J., and Simmons, H. A. (1974). The effects of parathyroid hormone, colchicine and calcitonin on the ultrastructure and the activity of osteoclasts in organ culture. *J. Cell Biol.* **60**, 346–355.

Horiuchi, N., Takahashi, H., Matsumoto, T., Takahashi, N., Shimazawa, E., Suda, T., and Ogata, E. (1979). Salmon calcitonin-induced stimulation of 1,25, dihydroxyvitamin D_3 in rats involving a mechanism independent of adenosine 3′-5′-cyclic monophosphate. *Biochem. J.* **184**, 269.

Hughes, A., Thron, S., Martin, G., and Sever, P. (1985). Endothelial dependent relaxation of human arteries by peptide hormone. *Clin. Sci.* **13**, Suppl., 88P.

Hunt, N. H., Ellison, M., Underwood, J. C. E., and Martin, T. J. (1977). Properties of calcitonin receptor and adenylate cyclase in BEN cells, a human cancer cell line. *Br. J. Cancer* **35**, 777–784.

Inagaki, S., Shiotani, Y., Yamano, M., Shiosaka, S., Takagi, H., Tateishi, K., Hashimura, E., Hamoaka, T., and Tohyama, M. (1984). Distribution origin and fine structures of cholecsytokinin 8-like immunoreactive terminals in the nucleus ventromedialis hypothalami of the rat. *J. Neurosci.* **4,** 1289–1299.

Inagaki, S., Kito, S., Kubota, Y., Girgis, S., Hillyard, C. J., and MacIntyre, I. (1986). Autoradiographic localisation of calcitonin gene-related peptide binding sites in human and rat brains. *Brain Res.* **374,** 287–298.

Jacobs, J. W., Goodman, R. H., Chin, W. W., Dee, P. C., Habener, J. F., Bell, N. H., and Potts, J. T. (1981). Calcitonin messenger RNA encodes multiple polypeptides in a single precursor. *Science* **213,** 457–459.

Japmol, L. M., Axelrod, A., and Tessler, H. (1976). Pathways of the eye's response to tropical nitrogen mustard. *Invest. Ophthalmol. Visual Sci.* **15,** 486–489.

Jonas, V., Lin, C. R., Kawashima, E., Semon, D., Swanson, L. W., Mermod, J.-J., Evans, R. M., and Rosenfeld, M. G. (1985). Alternative mRNA processing events in human calcitonin/calcitonin gene related peptide gene expression. *Proc. Natl. Acad. Sci. U.S.A.* **82,** 1994–1998.

Kaiser, E. T., and Kezdi, F. J. (1984). Amphiphilic structure design of peptide hormones. *Science* **223,** 249–255.

Kallio, D. M., Ganat, P. R., and Minkin, C. (1972). Ultrastructural effects of calcitonin in osteoclasts in tissue culture. *J. Ultrastruct. Res.* **39,** 205.

Kawashima, H., Torikai, S., and Kurokawa, K. (1980). Localisation of 25-hydroxyvitamin D_3-1-alpha-hydroxylase and 24-hydroxylase along the rat nephron. *Proc. Natl. Acad. Sci. U.S.A.* **78,** 1199.

Kawashima, H., Torikas, S., and Kurokawa, K. (1981). Selective stimulation of 25-hydroxyvitamin D_1-hydroxylase by calcitonin in the proximal straight tubule of the rat kidney. *Nature (London)* **291,** 327–329.

Kawai, T., Takami, K., Shiosaka, S., Emson, P. C., Hillyard, C. J., MacIntyre, I., and Tohyama, M. (1985). Topographic localisation of calcitonin gene-related peptide in the rat brain: an immunohistochemical analysis. *Neuroscience* **15,** 747–763.

Kenney, A. D. (1971). Determination of calcitonin in plasma by bioassay. *Endocrinology (Baltimore)* **89,** 1005–1013.

Kimura, S., Sugita, Y., Kanazawa, I., Saito, A., and Goto, K. (1987). Isolation and amino acid sequence of calcitonin gene-related peptide from porcine spinal cord. *Neuropeptides* **9,** 75–82.

Kitajiri, M., Yamashita, T., Tohyama, Y., Kumazawa, T., Takeda, N., Kawasaki, Y., Matsunaga, T., Girgis, S., Hillyard, C. J., MacIntyre, I., Emson, P. C., Shiosaka, S., and Tohyama, M. (1985). Localisation of calcitonin gene-related peptide in the organ of Corti of the rat: an immunohistochemical study. *Brain Res.* **385,** 394–397.

Kiyama, H., Katayama, Y., Hillyard, C. J., Girgis, S., MacIntyre, I., Emson, P. C., and Tohyama, M. (1985). Occurrence of calcitonin gene-related peptide in the chicken amacrine cells. *Brain Res.* **327,** 367–369.

Kraenzlin, M. E., Ch'ng, J. L. C., Mulderry, P. K., Ghatei, M. A., and Bloom, S. R. (1985). Infusion of a novel peptide, calcitonin gene-related peptide (CGRP) in man. Pharmacokinetics and effects on gastric acid secretion and gastrointestinal hormones. *Regul. Pept.* **10,** 189–197.

Krahn, D. D., Gosnell, B. A., Levine, A. S., and Morley, J. E. R. (1984). The effects of calcitonin gene-related peptide on food intake. *Peptides* **5,** 861–864.

Krootila, K. (1988). Sensory nerves containing calcitonin gene-related peptide (CGRP) in relation to neurogenic inflammation in the eye. *Acad. Diss., Univ. of Helsinki.*

Krootila, K., Uusitalo, H., and Palkama, A. (1988). Effect of neurogenic irritation and calcitonin gene-related peptide (CGRP) on ocular blood flow in the rabbit. *Curr. Eye Res.* **7**, 695–703.

Kubota, M., Moseley, J. M., Butera, L., Dusting, G. J., MacDonald, P. S., and Martin, T. J. (1985). Calcitonin gene-related peptide stimulates cyclic AMP formation in rat aortic smooth muscle cells. *Biochem. Biophys. Res. Commun.* **138**, 88–94.

Kumar, M. A., Foster, G. V., and MacIntyre, I. (1963). A rapid-acting hormone which lowers plasma calcium. *Lancet* **ii**, 480–482.

Lamp, S. J., Findlay, D. M., Moseley, J. M., and Martin, T. J. (1981). Calcitonin induction of persistent activated state of adenylate cyclase in human breast cancer cells (T47D). *J. Biol. Chem.* **256**, 12269–12274.

Lasmoles, F., Julienne, A., Day, F., Minvielle, S., Milhaud, G., and Moukhtar, M. S. (1985a). Elucidation of the nucleotide sequence of chicken calcitonin mRNA: direct evidence for the expression of a lower verterbrae calcitonin like gene in man and rat. *EMBO J.* **4**, 2603–2607.

Lasmoles, F., Julienne, A., Desplan, C., Milhaud, G., and Moukhtar, M. S. (1985b). Structure of chicken calcitonin predicted by partial nucleotide sequence of its precursor. *FEBS Lett.* **180**, 113–116.

Lauffer, R., and Changeux, J. (1987). CGRP elevates cAMP levels in chick skeletal muscle: possible neurotropic role for a coexisting neuronal messenger. *EMBO J.* **6**, 901–906.

Leander, S., Brodin, E., Hakansou, R., Sundler, S., and Uddman, R. (1982). Neuronal substance P in oesophagus. Distribution and effects on motor activity. *Acta Physiol. Scand.* **115**, 427.

Lee, T., Takami, K., Kawai, Y., Girgis, S. I., Hillyard, C. J., MacIntyre, I., Emson, P. C., and Tohyama, M. (1985a). Distribution of calcitonin gene-related peptide in the rat peripheral nervous system with reference to its co-existence with substance P. *Neuroscience* **15**, 1227–1237.

Lee, Y., Kawai, Y., Shiosaka, S., Takami, K., Kiyama, H., Hillyard, C. J., Girgis, S., MacIntyre, I., Emson, P. C., and Tohyama, M. (1985b). Coexistence of calcitonin gene-related peptide and substance P-like peptide in single cells of the trigeminal ganglion of the rat: immunohistochemical analysis. *Brain Res.* **330**, 194–196.

Leff, S. E., Evans, R. M., and Rosenfeld, M. G. (1987). Splice commitment dictates neuron specific alternative RNA processing in calcitonin/CGRP gene expression. *Cell* **48**, 517–524.

Lehtosalo, J. I., Uusitalo, H., and Palkama, A. (1984). Sensory supply of the anterior uvea: a light and electron microscope study. *Exp. Brain Res.* **55**, 562–569.

Lembeck, F., and Gamse, R. (1982). Substance P in peripheral sensory processes. *In* "Substance P in the Nervous System" (R. Porter and M. O'Connor, eds.), pp. 35–54. Pitman, London.

Le Moullec, J. M., Julienne, A., Chenias, J., Lasmoles, F., Guliana, J. M., Milhaud, G., and Moukhtar, M. S. (1984). The complete sequence of human preprocalcitonin. *FEBS Lett.* **167**, 93–97.

Lenz, H. J., Mortrud, M. T., Rivier, J. E., and Brown, M. R. (1985). Central nervous system actions of calcitonin gene-related peptide on gastric acid secretion in the rat. *Gastroenterology* **88**, 539.

Luben, R. A., Wong, G. L., and Cohn, D. V. (1976). Biochemical characterization with parathormone and calcitonin of isolated bone cells: provisional identification of osteoclasts and osteoblasts. *Endocrinology (Baltimore)* **99**, 526–534.

Lundberg, J. A., Hua, X., Hokfelt, T., and Fischer, J. A. (1985). Co-existence of substance P and calcitonin gene-related peptide-like immunoreactivities in sensory nerves in relation to cardiovascular and bronchoconstrictor effects of capsaicin. *Eur. J. Pharmacol.* **108**, 315–319.

MacIntyre, I., and Zaidi, M. (1990). Calcitonin: some recent developments. *Proc. Steenbock Symp., Madison, Wis., 1989.* 233–240.

MacIntyre, I., Parsons, J. A., and Robinson, C. J. (1967). The effect of thyrocalcitonin on blood bone calcium equilibrium in the perfused tibiae of the cat. *J. Physiol. (London)* **191**, 393–405.

MacIntyre, I., Alevizaki, M., Bevis, P. J. R., and Zaidi, M. (1987a). Calcitonin and peptides from the calcitonin genes *Clin. Orthop. Relat. Res.* **21**, 45–54.

MacIntyre, I., Zaidi, M., Milet, C., and Bevis, P. J. R. (1987b). Hormonal regulation of extracellular calcium. *In* "Handbook of Experimental Pharmacology: Calcium in Drug Actions" (P. F. Baker, ed.), pp. 411–439. Springer-Verlag, Berlin.

MacIntyre, I., Kehley, A., Zaidi, M., and Seth, R. (1990). Biological activity of calcitonin and its assessment. *Exp. Gerontol.* **25**, 3–4.

Maier, R., Riniker, B., and Rittel, W. (1974). Analogues of human calcitonin I, Influence of modification of amino acid positions 29 and 31 and hypocalcaemia activities in the rat. *FEBS Lett.* **48**, 68–71.

Manning, M., Przybylski, A., Olma, A., Klis, W. A., Kruszynski, M., Wo, N. C., Pelton, G. H., and Sawyer, W. H. (1987). No requirement of cyclic conformation of antagonists in binding to vasopressin receptor. *Nature (London)* **329**, 839–840.

Martin, T. J., Robinson, C. J., and MacIntyre, I. (1966). The mode of action of thyrocalcitonin. *Lancet* **i**, 900–902.

Martin, T. J., Moseley, J. M., Findlay, D. M., and Michelangeli, V. P. (1980). Calcitonin production and calcitonin receptors in human cancers. *In* "Hormones in Normal and Abnormal Human Tissues" (K. Fotherby and S. B. Pal, eds.), pp. 429–457. de Gruyter, New York.

Marx, S. J., Woodward, C. J., and Aurbach, G. D. (1972). Calcitonin receptors of the kidney and bone. *Science* **178**, 998–1001.

Marx, S. J., Woodward, C. J., Aurbach, G. D., Glassman, H., and Keutmann, H. J. (1973). Renal receptors for calcitonin. Binding and degradation of hormone. *J. Biol. Chem.* **248**, 4797–4802.

Marx, S. J., Aurbach, G. D., Gavin, J. R., and Guell, J. W. (1974). Calcitonin receptors on cultured human lymphocytes. *J. Biol. Chem.* **249**, 6812–6816.

McCulloch, J., Uddman, R., Kingman, T., and Edvinsson, I. (1986). CGRP: functional role in cerebrovascular circulation. *Proc. Natl. Acad. Sci. U.S.A.* **83**, 5731–5735.

McEwan, J., Larkin, S., Davis, G., Chierchia, S., Brown, M., Stevenson, J., MacIntyre, I., and Masseri, A. (1986). Calcitonin gene-related peptide: a potent dilator of human epicardial coronary arteries. *Circulation* **74**, 1243–1247.

McEwan, J., Legon, S., Wimalawansa, S. J., Zaidi, M., Dollery, C. T., and MacIntyre, I. (1987). Calcitonin gene-related peptide: a review of its biology and its relevance to the cardiovascular system. *In* "Perspectives in Hypertension. Vol. II: The Endocrine Mechanisms in Hypertension" (J. H. Laragh, B. Brenner, and N. Kaplan, eds.), pp. 287–306. Raven, New York.

Michelangeli, V. P., Findlay, D. M., Moseley, J. M., and Martin, T. J. (1983). Mechanism of calcitonin induction of prolonged activation of adenylate cyclase in human cancer cells. *J. Cyclic Nucleotide Protein Phosphorylation Res.* **9**, 129–141.

Milhaud, G., Perault, A. M., and Moukhtar, M. S. (1965). Etude du mecanisme de l'action hypocalcemiante de la thyrocalcitonine. *C.R. Hebd. Seances Acad. Sci., Ser. D* **261**, 813.

Miller, A., Costa, M., Furness, J. B., and Chubb, I. W. (1981). Substance P immunoreactive sensory nerves in the rat iris and cornea. *Neurosci. Lett.* **23**, 243–247.

Minvielle, S., Cressent, M., Lasmoles, F., Julienne, A., Milhaud, G., and Moukhtar, M. S. (1986). Isolation and partial characterization of the calcitonin gene in a lower vertebrae. *FEBS Lett.* **203**, 7–10.

Minvielle, S., Cressent, M., Delehaye, M. C., Segond, N., Milhaud, G., Julienne, A., Moukhtar, M. S., and Lasmoles, F. (1987). Sequence and expression of the chicken calcitonin genes. *FEBS Lett.* **223**, 63–68.

Mitsuma, T., Nogimori, T., and Chaya, M. (1984). Peripheral administration of eel calcitonin inhibits thyrotropin secretion in the rat. *Eur. J. Pharmacol.* **102**, 123–128.

Moonga, B. S., Moss, D. W., Patchell, A., and Zaidi, M. (1990). Intracellular regulation of acid phosphatase secretion from isolated rat osteoclasts and further evidence for a functional role in bone resorption. *J. Physiol. (London)* **429**, 29–46.

Moran, J., Hunziker, W., and Fischer, J. A. (1978). Calcitonin and calcium ionophores: cyclic AMP responses in cells of a human lymphoid line. *Proc. Natl. Acad. Sci. U.S.A.* **8**, 3984.

Morikawa, T., Muniketa, E., Sakakibara, S., Noda, T., and Otani, M. (1976). *Experientia* **32**, 1104.

Morris, H. R., Panico, M., Etienne, T., Tippins, J., Girgis, S. I., and MacIntyre, I. (1984). Isolation and characterization of human calcitonin gene related peptide. *Nature (London)* **308**, 746–748.

Moseley, J. M., Findlay, D. M., Martin, T. J., and Gorman, J. J. (1982). Covalent cross-linking of a photoreactive derivative of calcitonin to human breast cancer cell receptors. *J. Biol. Chem.* **257**, 5846–5851.

Moseley, J. M., Findlay, D. M., Gorman, J. J., Michaelangeli, V. P., and Martin, T. J. (1983). The calcitonin receptor on T47D breast cancer cells. Evidence for glycosylation. *Biochem. J.* **212**, 609.

Mosselman, S., Hoppener, J. W., Zandberg, J., van Mansfeld, A. D. M., Geurts van Kessel, A. H. M., Lips, C. J. M., and Hansz, H. S. (1988). Islet amyloid polypeptide: identification and chromosomal localisation of the human gene. *FEBS Lett.* **239**, 227–232.

Muff, R., Nemeth, E. F., Haller-Brem, S., and Fischer, J. A. (1988). Regulation of hormone secretion and cytosolic calcium by extracellular calcium in PT cells and C-cells: role of voltage sensitive calcium channels. *Arch. Biochem. Biophys.* **265**, 128–135.

Mulderry, P. K., Ghatei, M. A., Rodrigo, K., Allen, J. M., Rosenfeld, M. G., Polak, J. M., and Bloom, S. R. (1985a). Calcitonin gene-related peptide in the cardiovascular tissues of the rat. *Neuroscience* **14**, 947–954.

Mulderry, P. K., Ghatei, M. A., Bishop, A. E., Allen, J. S., Polak, J. M., and Bloom, S. R. (1985b). Distribution and chromatographic characterisation of CGRP-like immunoreactivity in the brain and gut of the rat. *Regul. Pept.* **12**, 133–143.

Mulligan, G. (1988). Techniques used in the identification and analysis of function of pertussis toxin-sensitive guanine nucleotide binding proteins. *Biochem. J.* **255**, 1–13.

Murad, A., Brewer, H. B., Jr., and Vaugham, M. (1970). Effects of thyrocalcitonin on cyclic AMP formation by rat kidney and bone. *Proc. Natl. Acad. Sci. U.S.A.* **65**, 446.

Nakhla, A. M., and Majumdar, A. P. M. (1978). Calcitonin mediates changes in the plasma tryptophan and brain 5-hydroxy tryptamine and acetylcholinesterase activity in rats. *Biochem. J.* **170**, 445.

Neer, E. J., and Clapham, D. E. (1988). Roles of G protein subunits in transmembrane signalling. *Nature (London)* **333,** 129–134.

Neher, R., Riniker, B., Maier, R., Byfield, P. G. H., Gudmundsson, T. V., and MacIntyre, I. (1968). Human calcitonin. *Nature (London)* **220,** 984–986.

New, H. V., and Mudge, A. W. (1986). Calcitonin gene-related peptide regulates muscle acetylcholine receptors synthesis. *Nature (London)* **323,** 809–811.

Ng, K. W., Livesey, S. A., Larkins, R. J., and Martin, T. J. (1983). Calcitonin effects ongrowth and selective activation of type II isoenzyme of cyclic adenosine 3':5' monophosphate-dependent protein kinase in T47D human breast cancer cells. *Cancer Res.* **43,** 794.

Nguyen, K. Q., Sills, M. A., and Jacobawitz, D. M. (1986). Cardiovascular effects produced by microinjection of calcitonin gene-related peptide into the rat central amygdaloid nucleus. *Peptides* **7,** 337–339.

Niall, H. T., Keutmann, H. T., Copp, D. H., and Potts, J. T., Jr. (1969). The amino acid sequence of salmon ultimobranchial calcitonin. *Proc. Natl. Acad. Sci. U.S.A.* **64,** 771.

Nicholson, C. G., Moseley, J. M., Sexton, P. M., Mendelsohn, F. A. O., and Martin, T. J. (1986). Abundant calcitonin receptors in isolated rat osteoclasts. Biochemical and autoradiographic characterization. *J. Clin. Invest.* **78,** 355–360.

Nicoletti, F., Clementi, G., Patti, F., Canonico, P. L., diGiorgio, R. M., Matera, M., Pennsei, G., Angelussi, L., and Sapagnini, U. (1982). Effects of calcitonin on rat extrapyramidal motor system: behavioural and biochemical data. *Brain Res.* **250,** 381.

Norimatsu, H., Vander Weil, C. J., and Talmage, R. V. (1978). Electron microscope study of the effects of calcitonin on bone cells and extracellular milieu. *Clin. Orthop. Relat. Res.* **139,** 250–258.

O'Dor, R. K., Parkes, C. D., and Copp, D. H. (1969). The amino acid composition of salmon calcitonin. *Can. J. Biol.* **47,** 873.

Ohhashi, T., and Jacobowitz, D. M. (1985). Effects of calcitonin gene-related peptide in the neuroeffector mechanism of sympathetic nerve terminals in rat vas deferens. *Peptides* **4,** 989–991.

Oksala, O., Stjernschantz, J., Wahlestedt, C., and Hakanson, R. (1986). Calcitonin gene-related polypeptide: release in the eye. *Invest. Ophthalmol. Visual Sci.* **27,** Suppl., p. 356.

Oligiati, V. R., Guidobono, F., Lusisetto, G., Netti, C., Bianchi, C., and Pecile, A. (1981). Calcitonin inhibition of physiological and stimulated prolactin secretion in rat. *Life Sci.* **29,** 585.

Orlowski, R. C., Epand, R. M., and Stafford, A. R. (1987). Biological potent analogues of salmon CT which do not contain an N-terminal disulfide-bridge ring structure. *Eur. J. Biochem.* **162,** 399–402.

Otani, M., Yamauchi, H., Meguro, T., Kitazawa, S., Wanatabe, S., and Orimo, H. (1976). Isolation and characterisation of calcitonin from pericardium and oesophagus of the eel. *J. Biochem. (Tokyo)* **79,** 345.

Palkama, A., Uusitalo, H., and Lehtosalo, J. (1986). Innervation of the anterior segment of the eye featuring functional aspects. *In* "Neurohistochemistry Today" (P. Panula, H. Paivarinta, and S. Soinila, eds.), pp. 587–615. Alan R. Liss, New York.

Pecile, A., Ferri, S., Braga, P. C., and Olgiati, V. R. (1975). Effects of intracerebroventricular calcitonin in the conscious rabbit. *Experientia* **31,** 332–333.

Perez-Cano, R., Galan Galan, F., Girgis, S. I., Arnett, T. R., and MacIntyre, I. (1981). A human calcitonin-like molecule in the ultimobranchial body of the amphibian *(Rana pipiens). Experientia* **37**, 1116–1118.

Perez-Cano, R., Girgis, S. I., and MacIntyre, I. (1982a). Further evidence for calcitonin gene duplication: the identification of two different calcitonins in a fish, a reptile and two mammals. *Acta Endocrinol. (Copenhagen)* **100**, 256–261.

Perez-Cano, R., Girgis, S. I., Galan Galan, F., and MacIntyre, I. (1982b). Identification of both human and salmon calcitonin-like molecules in birds suggesting the existence of two calcitonin genes. *J. Endocrinol.* **92**, 351–355.

Perkins, E. S. (1957). Influence of the fifth cranial nerve on the intraocular pressure of the rabbit eye. *Br. J. Ophthalmol.* **41**, 257–300.

Poschl, E., Lindley, I., Hofer, E., Seifer, J.-M., Brunowsky, W., and Besemer, J. (1987). The structure of procalcitonin of the salmon as deduced from its cDNA sequence. *FEBS Lett.* **226**, 96–100.

Potts, J. T., Jr., Niall, H. D., Keutman, H. T., Brewer, H. B., and Deftos, L. J. (1968). The amino acid sequence of porcine calcitonin. *Proc. Natl. Acad. Sci. U.S.A.* **59**, 1321.

Potts, J. T., Jr., Niall, H. D., Keutman, H. T., Deftos, L. J., and Parsons, J. A. (1970). Calcitonin: recent chemical and immunological studies. *Calcitonin, Proc. Int. Symp. 2nd, London, 1969* pp. 56–73.

Przepiorka, D., Baylin, S. B., McBride, O. W., Testa, J. R., de Bustros, A., and Nelkin, B. D. (1984). The human calcitonin gene is located on the short arm of chromosome 11. *Biochem. Biophys. Res. Commun.* **120**, 493–499.

Rasmussen, H., Wong, M., Bolke, D., and Goodman, D. P. B. (1972). Hormonal control of the renal conversion of 25-hydroxycholecalciferol to 1,25 dihydroxycholecalciferol. *J. Clin. Invest.* **51**, 2502.

Raulias, D., Hagaman, J., Ontjes, D. A., Lundblad, R. L., and Kingdon, H. S. (1976). The complete amino acid sequence of rat thyrocalcitonin. *Eur. J. Biochem.* **64**, 607.

Reynolds, J. J., Dingle, J. T., Gudmundsson, T. V., and MacIntyre, I. (1968). Bone resorption in vitro and its inhibition by calcitonin. *Calcitonin, Proc. Int. Symp. Thyrocalcitonin C Cells, London, 1967* pp. 223–229.

Rifkin, B. R., Auszmann, J. M., Kleckner, A. P., Vernillo, A. T., and Fine, A. S. (1988). Calcitonin stimulates cAMP accumulation in chicken osteoclasts. *Life Sci.* **42**, 799–804.

Riley, J. H., Edbrooke, M. R., and Craig, R. K. (1986). Ectopic synthesis of high M_r calcitonin by the BEN lung carcinoma cell line reflects aberrant proteolytic processing. *FEBS Lett.* **198**, 71–79.

Riniker, B., Neher, R., Maier, R., Kahnt, F. W., Byfield, P. G. H., Gudmundsson, T. V., Galante, L., and MacIntyre, I. (1968). Menschliches calcitoni I. Isolierung und charakterisierung. *Helv. Chim. Acta* **51**, 1738–1742.

Rittel, W., Brugger, M., Kamber, B., Riniker, B., and Seiber, P. (1968). Thyrocalcitonin II. Die syntheses des alpha thyrocalcitonin. *Helv. Chim. Acta* **51**, 1378.

Rittel, W., Maier, R., Brugger, M., Kamber, B., Riniker, B., and Seiber, P. (1976). Structure–activity relationship of human calcitonin III. Biological activity of synthetic analogues with shortened or terminally modified peptide chains. *Experientia* **32**, 246–248.

Rizzo, A. J., and Goltzman, D. (1981). Calcitonin receptors in central nervous system of the rat. *Endocrinology (Baltimore)* **108**, 1672–1677.

Robinson, C. J., Martin, T. J., Matthews, E. W., and MacIntyre, I. (1967). Mode of action of thyrocalcitonin. *J. Endocrinol.* **39**, 71–79.

Robles Chillida, E. M., Rodrigo, J., Maya, I., Arnedo, A., and Comez, A. (1983). Ultrastructure of free nerve ending in the oesophagal epithelium. *J. Anat.* **133**, 237.

Rodrigo, J., Polak, J. M., Fernandez, L., Ghatei, M. A., Mulderry, P. K., and Bloom, S. R. (1985). Calcitonin gene-related peptide immunoreactivity sensory and motor nerves of the rat, cat and monkey oesophagus. *Gastroenterology* **88**, 444.

Roos, B. A., Fischer, J. A., Pignat, W., Allander, C. B., and Raisz, L. J. (1986). Evaluation of *in vivo* and *in vitro* calcium regulating actions of non calcitonin peptides produced via calcitonin gene expression. *Endocrinology (Baltimore)* **118**, 66–51.

Rosenfeld, M. G., Amara. S. G., Roos, B. A., Ong, E. S., and Evans, R. M. (1981). Altered expression of the calcitonin gene associated with RNA polymorphism. *Nature (London)* **290**, 63–65.

Rosenfeld, M. G., Mermod, J.-J., Amara, S. G., Swanson, L. W., Sawchenko, P. E., Rivier, J., Vale, W. W., and Evans, R. M. (1983). Production of a novel neuropeptide encoded by the calcitonin gene via tissue specific RNA processing. *Nature (London)* **304**, 129–135.

Sakanaka, M., Magari, S., Emson, P., Hillyard, C., Girgis, S. I., MacIntyre, I., and Tohyama, M. (1985). The calcitonin gene-related peptide containing fibre projections from the hypothalamus to the lateral septal area including its fine structures. *Brain Res.* **344**, 196–199.

Salmon, D. M., Azria, M., and Zanelli, J. M. (1983). Quantitative cytochemical responses to exogenously administered calcitonins in rat kidney and bone cells. *Mol. Cell. Endocrinol.* **33**, 293–304.

Seed, B. (1987). An LFA-3 cDNA encodes a phospholipid-linked membrane protein homologous to its receptor CD2. *Nature (London)* **329**, 840–842.

Seed, B., and Aruffo, A. (1987). Molecular cloning of the CD2 antigen, the T-cell erythrocyte receptor, by a rapid immunoselectric procedure. *Proc. Natl. Acad. Sci. U.S.A.* **84**, 3365–3369.

Seiber, P., Brugger, M., Kamber, P., Riniker, B., Rittel, W., Maier, R., and Staehelin, M. (1970). Synthesis and biological activity of peptide sequence related to porcine alpha-thyrocalcitonin. *Calcitonin, Proc. Int. Symp., 2nd, London, 1969* pp. 28–33.

Seifert, H., Sawchenko, P., Chestnut, J., Rivier, J., Vale, W., and Pandol, S. J. (1985). Receptor for calcitonin gene-related peptide: binding to exocrine pancreas mediates biological actions. *Am. J. Physiol.* **249**, G147–151.

Self, C. H. (1985). Enzyme amplification—a general method applied to provide an immuno-assisted assay for placental alkaline phosphatase. *J. Immunol. Methods* **76**, 389–393.

Seth, R., Zaidi, M., Fuller, J. Q., and Self, C. H. (1988). A highly specific and sensitive enzymeimmunometric assay for calcitonin gene-related peptide based on enzyme amplification. *J. Immunol. Methods* **111**, 11–16.

Seth, R., Motte, P., El Kholy, A., Datta, H. K., Zaidi, M., Kehley, A., Wimalawansa, S. J., Bohuon, C., and MacIntyre, I. (1989). Immunoreactive and biologically active calcitonin in medullary carcinoma of the thyroid. *J. Bone Miner. Res.* **4**, Suppl., p. 326.

Shimada, S., Shiosaka, S., Emson, P. C., Hillyard, C. J., Girgis, S. I., MacIntyre, I., and Tohyama, M. (1985a). Calcitonin gene-related peptidergic projection from the parabranchial area to the forebrain and diencephalon in the rat: an immunohistochemical analysis. *Neuroscience* **16**, 607–616.

Shimada, S., Shiosaka, S., Emson, P. C., Hillyard, C. J., Girgis, S. I., MacIntyre, I., and Tohyama, M. (1985b). Calcitonin gene-related peptide projection from the ventromedial thalamic nucleus to the insular cortex: a combination of retrograde transport and immunocytochemical study. *Brain Res.* **344**, 200–203.

Sigrist, S., Franco-Cereceda, A., Muff, R., Henke, H., Lundberg, J. M., and Fischer, J. A.

(1986). Specific receptor and cardiovascular effects of calcitonin gene-related peptide. *Endocrinology (Baltimore)* **119**, 381–387.

Sikri, K. L., Varndell, I. M., Hamid, Q. A., Wilson, B. S., Kameya, T., Ponder, B. A. J., Lloyd, R. V., Bloom, S. R., and Polak, J. M. (1985). Medullary carcinoma of the thyroid: an immunochemical and histochemical study of 25 cases using eight separate markers. *Cancer (Philadelphia)* **56**, 2481–2491.

Skofitsch, G., and Jacobowitz, D. M., (1985). Calcitonin gene-related peptide: detailed immunohistochemical distribution in the central nervous system. *Peptides* **6**, 747–752.

Steenbergh, P. H., Hoppener, J. W. M., Zandberg, J., Van de Ven, W. J. M., Jansz, H. S., and Lips, C. J. M. (1984). Calcitonin gene-related peptide-coding sequence is conserved in the human genome and is expressed in medullary thyroid carcinoma. *J. Clin. Endocrinol. Metab.* **59**, 358–360.

Steenbergh, P. H., Hoppener, J. W. M., Zandberg, J., Lips, C. J. M., and Jansz, H. S. (1985). A second human calcitonin/CGRP gene. *FEBS Lett.* **183**, 403–407.

Steenbergh, P. H., Hoppener, J. W. M., Zandberg, J., Visser, A., Lips, C. J. M., and Jansz, H. S. (1986). Structure and expression of the human calcitonin/CGRP genes. *FEBS Lett.* **209**, 97–103.

Sternweis, P. C., and Gilman, A. G. (1982). Aluminum: a requirement for activation of the regulatory component of adenylate cyclase by fluoride. *Proc. Natl. Acad. Sci. U.S.A.* **79**, 4888–4891.

Stevenson, J. C., Hillyard, C. J., MacIntyre, I., Cooper, H., and Whitehead, M. I. (1979). A physiological role for calcitonin: protection of maternal skeleton. *Lancet* **ii**, 769–770.

Stevenson, J. C., Abeyasekera, G., Hillyard, C. J., Phang, K. G., MacIntyre, I., Campbell, S., Lane, G., Townsend, P. T., Young, O., and Whitehead, M. I. (1983). Regulation of calcium regulating hormones by exogenous sex steroids in early post menopause. *Eur. J. Clin. Invest.* **13**, 481–487.

Stjernschantz, J., Sears, M., and Stjernschantz, L. (1981). Intraocular effect of substance P in the rabbit. *Invest. Ophthalmol. Visual Sci.* **20**, 53–60.

Stone, R. A., and McGlinn, A. M. (1988). Calcitonin gene-related peptide immunoreactive nerves in human and Rhesus monkey eyes. *Invest. Ophthalmol. Visual Sci.* **29**, 305–310.

Stone, R. A., Kuwayama, Y., Laties, A. M., and Schmidt, M. L. (1984). Guinea pig ocular nerves contain peptide of the cholecystokinin/gastrin family. *Exp. Eye Res.* **39**, 387–391.

Stone, R. A., Kuwayama, Y., Terenghi, G., and Polak, J. M. (1986). Calcitonin gene-related peptide: occurrence in corneal sensory nerves. *Exp. Eye Res.* **43**, 279–283.

Struthers, A., Brown, M. J., MacDonald, D. W., Beacham, J. L., Morris, H. R., and MacIntyre, I. (1986). Human CGRP: a potent endogenous vasodilator in man. *Clin. Sci.* **70**, 389–393.

Su, H. C., Wharton, J., Polak, J. M., Mulderry, P. K., Ghatei, M. A., Gibson, S. J., Terenghi, G., Morrison, J., Ballestra, J., and Bloom, S. R. (1986). Calcitonin gene-related peptide immunoreactivity in afferent neurones supplying the urinary tract: combined retrograde tracking and immunohistochemistry. *Neuroscience* **18**, 727.

Takami, K., Kawai, Y., Shiosaka, S., Lee, Y., Girgis, S. I., Hillyard, C. J., MacIntyre, I., Emson, P. C., and Tohyama, M. (1985a). Immunohistochemical evidence for the coexistence of calcitonin gene-related peptide and choline acetyltransferase-like immunoreactivity in neurones of the rat hypoglossal, facial and ambiguus nuclei. *Brain Res.* **328**, 386–389.

Takami, K., Kawai, Y., Uchida, S., Tohyama, M., Shiotani, Y., Yoshids, H., Emson, P. C.,

Girgis, S. L., Hillyard, C. J., and MacIntyre, I. (1985b). Effect of calcitonin gene-related peptide on contraction of striated muscle in the mouse. *Neurosci. Lett.* **60**, 227–230.

Tanuichi, H. (1984). The mechanism of protein folding. *In* "The Impact of Protein Chemistry on Biomedical Sciences" (A. N. Schechter, A. Dean, and R. F. Goldberger, eds.), pp. 67–81. Academic Press, Orlando, Florida.

Tashjian, A. H., Jr., Wright, D. R., Ivey, J. L., and Pont, A. (1978). Calcitonin binding sites in bone: relationship to biological responses and escape. *Recent Prog. in Horm. Res.* **34**, 285.

Terenghi, G., Polak, J. M., Ghatei, M. A., Mulderry, P. K., Butler, J. M., Unger, W., and Bloom, S. R. (1985). Distribution and origin of calcitonin gene-related peptide (CGRP) immunoreactivity in the sensory innervation of the mammalian eye. *J. Comp. Neurol.* **233**, 506–516.

Tippins, J. R., Morris, H. R., Panico, M., Etienne, T., Bevis, P., Girgis, S. MacIntyre, I., Azria, M., and Attinger, M. (1984). The myotropic and plasma calcium-modulating effects of calcitonin gene-related peptide (CGRP). *Neuropeptides* **4**, 425–434.

Tippins, J. R., Marzo, V. D., Panico, M., Morris, H. R., and MacIntyre, I. (1986). Investigation of the structure/activity relationship of human calcitonin gene-related peptide (CGRP). *Biochem. Biophys. Res. Commun.* **134**, 1306–1311.

Tschopp, F. A., Henke, H., Petermann, J. B., Tobler, P. H., Janzer, R., Hokfelt, T., Lundberg, J. M., Cuello, C., and Fischer, J. A. (1985). Calcitonin gene-related peptide and its binding sites in the human central nervous system and the pituitary. *Proc. Natl. Acad. Sci. U.S.A.* **82**, 248–252.

Twery, M. J., and Moss, R. L. (1985). Calcitonin and calcitonin gene-related peptide alter the excitability of neurones in the rat forebrain. *Peptides,* **6**, 373–378.

Unger, W. G., Terenghi, G., Ghatei, M. A., Polak, J. M., Ennis, K. W., Butler, J. M., Zhang, S. Q., Too, H. P., Polak, J. M., and Bllom, S. R. (1985). Calcitonin gene-related polypeptide as a mediator of the neurogenic ocular injury response. *J. Ocular Pharmacol.* **1**, 189–199.

Wahlestedt, C., Hakanson, R., Bedding, B., Bordin, E., Ekman, R., and Sundler, F. (1985). Intraocular effects of CGRP, a neuropeptide in sensory nerves. *In* "Tachykinin Antagonists" (R. Hakanson and F. Sundler, eds.), pp. 137–146. Elsevier, Amsterdam.

Wahlestedt, C., Bedding, B., Ekman, R., Oksala, O., Stjernschantz, J., and Hakanson, R. (1986). Calcitonin gene-related peptide in the eye: release by sensory nerve stimulation and effects associated with neurogenic inflammation. *Regul. Pep.* **16**, 107–115.

Walker, J. W., Somlyo, A. V., Goldman, Y. E., Somlyo, A. P., and Trentham, D. R. (1987). Kinetics of smooth and skeletal muscle activation by laser pulse photolysis of caged inositol 1,4,5-triphosphate. *Nature (London)* **327**, 249–252.

Wanaka, A., Matsuyama, T., Yoneda, S., Kamada, T., Emson, P. C., Hillyard, C. J., Girgis, S. I., MacIntyre, I., and Tohyama, M. (1987). Origins and distributions of calcitonin gene-related peptide-containing nerves in the wall of the cerebral arteries of the guinea pig, with special reference to co-existence with substance P. *Cell. Mol. Biol.* **33**, 201–209.

Warshawsky, F., Goltzman, D., Rouleau, M. F., and Bergeron, J. M. (1980). Direct *in vivo* demonstration by radioautography of specific binding sites for calcitonin in skeletal and renal tissues of rat. *J. Cell Biol.* **88**, 682–694.

Westermark, P., Wernstedt, C., Wilander, E., and Sletten, K. (1986). A novel peptide in the calcitonin gene-related peptide family as an amyloid fibril protein in the endocrine pancreas. *Biochem. Biophys. Res. Commun.* **140**, 827–831.

Westermark, P., Wernsted, C., Wilander, E., Hayden, D. W., O'Brien, T. D., and Johnson,

K. H. (1987a). Amyloid fibrils in human insulinoma and islets of Langerhans of the diabetic cat are derived from a neuropeptide-like protein also present in normal islet cells. *Proc. Natl. Acad. Sci. U.S.A.* **84**, 3881–3885.

Westermark, P., Wernstedt, C., O'Brien, T., Hayden, D. W., and Johnson, K. (1987b). Islet amyloid in type 2 human diabetes mellitus and adult diabetic cats contains a novel putative polypeptide hormone. *Am. J. Pathol.* **127**, 414–417.

Wharton, J., Polak, J. M., McGregor, G. P., Bishop, A. E., and Bloom, S. R. (1981). The distribution of substance P-like immunoreactive nerves in the guinea pig heart. *Neuroscience* **6**, 2193.

Williams, T. J. (1982). Vasoactive intestinal peptide is more potent than prostaglandin E_2 as a vasodilator and oedema potentiator in the rabbit skin. *Br. J. Pharmacol.* **77**, 505.

Wimalawansa, S. J., Emson, P. C., and MacIntyre, I. (1987). Regional distribution of calcitonin gene-related peptide and its specific binding sites in rat with particular reference to the nervous system. *Neuroendocrinology* **46**, 131–136.

Wohlwend, A., Malmstrom, K., Henke, H., Murer, H., Vassalli, J., and Fischer, J. A. (1985). Calcitonin and calcitonin gene-related peptide interact with the same receptor in cultured LLC-PK1 kidney cells. *Biochem. Biophys. Res. Commun.* **131**, 537–542.

Woodhouse, N. Y., Bordier, P., Fisher, M., Joplin, G. F., Reiner, M., Kalu, D. N., Foster, G. V., and MacIntyre, I. (1971). Human calcitonin in the treatment of Paget's bone disease. *Lancet* **i**, 1139–1143.

Wrann, M. M., and Fox, C. F. (1979). Identification of epidermal growth factor receptors in hyper-producing human epidermoid carcinoma line. *J. Biol. Chem.* **254**, 8083–8086.

Yamada, M., Matsumota, T., Su, K. W., and Ogata, E. (1985). Inhibition by prostaglandin E_2 of renal effects of calcitonin in rats. *Endocrinology (Baltimore)* **116**, 693–697.

Yatani, A., Codina, J., Imoto, Y., Reeves, J. P., Birnbaumer, L., and Brown, A. M. (1987). Direct regulation of mammalian cardiac calcium channels by a G protein. *Science* **238**, 1288–1292.

Zaidi, M., Bevis, P. J. R., Girgis, S. I., Lynch, C., Stevenson, J. C., and MacIntyre, I. (1985). Circulating CGRP comes from the perivascular nerves. *Eur. J. Pharmacol.* **117**, 283–284.

Zaidi, M., Bevis, P. J. R., Abeyasekera, G., Girgis, S. I., Wimalawansa, S. J., Morris, H. R., and MacIntyre, I. (1986a). The origin of circulating calcitonin gene-related peptide in the rat. *J. Endocrinol.* **110**, 185–190.

Zaidi, M., Chambers, T. J., Bevis, P. J. R., Passarella, E., Gaines Das, R. E., and MacIntyre, I. (1986b). Bone resorption by isolated osteoclasts—a new bioassay for calcitonin. *In* "Calcium Regulation and Bone Metabolism: Basic and Clinical Aspects" (D. V. Cohn, T. J. Martin, and P. J. Meunier, eds.), Int. Congr. Ser., No. 735, p. 892. Excerpta Med. Found., Amsterdam.

Zaidi, M., Breimer, L. H., and MacIntyre, I. (1987a). Biology of peptides from the calcitonin genes. *Q. J. Exp. Physiol.* **72**, 371–408.

Zaidi, M., Chambers, T. J., Gaines Das, R. E., Morris, H. R., and MacIntyre, I. (1987b). A direct effect of calcitonin gene-related peptide on isolated osteoclasts. *J. Endocrinol.* **115**, 511–518.

Zaidi, M., Fuller, K., Bevis, P. J. R., Gaines Das, R. E., Chambers, T. J., and MacIntyre, I. (1987c). Calcitonin gene-related peptide inhibits osteoclastic bone resorption: a comparative study. *Calcif. Tissues Int.* **40**, 149–154.

Zaidi, M., Wimalawansa, S. J., Lynch, C., and MacIntyre, I. (1987d). Characterisation of

CGRP-immunoreactivity and receptors, which co-exist on cloned cancer cells. *J. Endocrinol.* **112s,** 276.

Zaidi, M., Chambers, T. J., Bevis, P. J. R., Beacham, J. L., Gaines Das, R. E., and MacIntyre, I. (1988a). Effects of the peptides from the calcitonin genes on bone and bone cells. *Q. J. Exp. Physiol.* **73,** 471–485.

Zaidi, M., Girgis, S. I., and MacIntyre, I. (1988b). Development and assessment of a highly sensitive carboxyl-terminated-specific radioimmunoassay of calcitonin gene-related peptide. *Clin. Chem.* **34,** 655–660.

Zaidi, M., Chambers, T. J., Gaines Das, R. E., Passarella, E., and MacIntyre, I. (1988c). A novel ultrasensitive assay for biologically active calcitonin. *Ann. Clin. Biochem.* **24,** Suppl. p. 248.

Zaidi, M., Datta, H. K., Chambers, T. J., and MacIntyre, I. (1989a). Production and characterisation of immunoreactive CGRP from cloned CGRP receptor-positive rat osteogenic sarcoma cells (UMR 106.01). *Biochem. Biophys. Res. Commun.* **158,** 214–219.

Zaidi, M., Moonga, B., Moss, D. W., and MacIntyre, I. (1989b). Inhibition of osteoclastic acid phosphatase abolishes bone resorption. *Biochem. Biophys. Res. Commun.* **159,** 68–71.

Zaidi, M., Patchell, A., Datta, H. K., and MacIntyre, I. (1989d). Uncoupling of receptor-mediated cellular response by ionic lithium. *J. Endocrinol.* **123,** R 5–7.

Zaidi, M., Datta, H. K., Patchell, A., Abeyasekera, G., and MacIntyre, I. (1989e). High ambient calcium inhibits osteoclast function: a novel physiological mechanism. *Biochem. Biophys. Res. Commun.* **163,** 1461–1465.

Zaidi, M., Abeyasekera, G., and MacIntyre, I. (1989f). Endocrine distribution of calcitonin gene-related peptide and characterisation of its circulating forms. *J. Endocrinol. Invest.* **12,** 699–704.

Zaidi, M., Datta, H. K., and Bevis, P. J. R. (1990a). Kidney: a target organ for calcitonin gene-related peptide. *Exp. Physiol.* **75,** 27–32.

Zaidi, M., MacIntyre, I., and Datta, H. K. (1990b). Intracellular regulation of osteoclast function II: Unusual effects of verapamil. *Biochem. Biophys. Res. Commun.* **167,** 807–812.

Zaidi, M., Seth, R., Girgis, S. I., and Self, C. H. (1990c). An improved highly sensitive and specific amplified two-site enzymeimmunometric assay of calcitonin gene-related peptide. *Clin. Chem.* **36,** 1288–1294.

Zaidi, M., Chambers, T. J., Moonga, B. S., Oldoni, T., Passarella, E., Soncui, R., and MacIntyre, I. (1990d). A new approach for calcitonin determination based on target cell responsiveness. *J. Endocrinol. Invest.* **13** 119–126.

Zaidi, M., Datta, H. K., Moonga, B. S., and MacIntyre, I. (1990e). Evidence that the action of calcitonin on the osteoclast is mediated by two G proteins acting via separate post-receptor pathways. *J. Endocrinol.* **125,** 473–481.

Zaidi, M., Datta, H. K., Bevis, P. J. R., Wimalawansa, S. J., and MacIntyre, I. (1990f). Amylin-amide: a new bone-conserving peptide from the pancreas. *Exp. Physiol.* **75,** 529–536.

Zaidi, M., Brain, S. D., Tippins, J. R., DiMarzo, V., Moonga, B. S., Chambers, T. J., Morris, H. R., and MacIntyre, I. (1990g). Structure–activity relationship of human calcitonin gene-related peptide. *Biochem. J.* **269,** 775–780.

Zaidi, M., Patchell, A., Seth, R., Gaines, Das R. E., Chambers, T. J., and MacIntyre, I. (1990h). An ultrasensitive bioassay based on bone resorption by isolated osteoclasts used to measure biologically active calcitonin in plasma of patients with human medullary thyroid carcinoma. *J. Endocrinol.* (submitted).

Zaidi, M., Datta, H. K., Moonga, B. S., Huang, C. L. H., and MacIntyre, I. (1990i). Perchlorate is a powerful inhibitor of bone resorption. *Br. J. Rheumatol.* **24,** 106–107.

Zajac, J. D., Martin, T. J., Hudson, P., Niall, H., and Jacobs, J. W. (1985). Biosynthesis of calcitonin by human lung cancer cells. *Endocrinology (Baltimore)* **116,** 749–755.

Zalups, R. K., and Knox, P. G. (1983). Calcitonin decreases the renal tubular capacity for phosphate reabsorption. *Am. J. Physiol.* **245,** F345.

Pantothenic Acid in Health and Disease[1]

ARUN G. TAHILIANI[2] AND CATHY J. BEINLICH

Geisinger Clinic
Weis Center for Research
Danville, Pennsylvania 17822

I. INTRODUCTION

Pantothenic acid is an essential vitamin required for the biosynthesis of coenzyme A (CoA) in mammalian cells. Coenzyme A, an acyl group carrier, is a cofactor for a multitude of enzymatic reactions including the oxidation of fatty acids, carbohydrates, pyruvate, lactate, ketone bodies, and amino acids, as well as many synthetic reactions. Each tissue of the body appears to be capable of transporting

[1]Dedicated to the late Dr. James R. Neely.

[2]Present address: Department of Biomedical Sciences, University of South Alabama, Mobile, Alabama 36688.

pantothenic acid into the cell and synthesizing CoA from pantothenic acid, although the intracellular localization of these reactions remains uncertain. Although it has long been known that pantothenic acid is a precursor for CoA synthesis, the control of this pathway remains unclear. Besides being a component of CoA, pantothenic acid is also a structural component of acyl carrier protein (ACP), an essential component of the fatty acid synthetase complex, and is therefore required for fatty acid synthesis. Thus the importance of pantothenic acid in mammalian cells is dictated by the role of its metabolic products in cellular metabolism.

In this chapter, we have reviewed the literature with respect to the nutritional (sources, requirements, absorption, and elimination) as well as the biochemical aspects (cellular transport of pantothenic acid, synthesis, distribution and degradation of CoA) of pantothenic acid. We have also considered the implications of altered pantothenic acid metabolism in instances of hormonal imbalance or pathological conditions. In preparing this manuscript we have attempted to go beyond a review of the current literature to identify areas of discrepancy in experimental results, suggesting hypotheses to explain existing data, and identifying areas for future study.

II. PANTOTHENIC ACID

A. HISTORICAL OVERVIEW

Until the early 1900s, the components required for normal nutrition in humans were thought to include carbohydrates, proteins, minerals, water, and fats. During the period of 1906–1912, various experiments with rats suggested a requirement for small quantities of organic substances. The term *vitamin* was first suggested by Funk in 1912 to describe these vital factors (Funk, 1912). Pantothenic acid (from the Greek term "pantos" meaning everywhere) was discovered by Williams *et al.* (1933) and is one of the water soluble vitamins. The dietary requirement for pantothenic acid was recognized independently by Wooley *et al.* (1939) and by Jukes (1939, 1941). These two groups identified a factor present in tissue extracts that prevented a deficiency disease in fowls characterized by skin lesions. The "antidermatitis factor" and the "liver filtrate factor" from rats were subsequently identified as pantothenic acid. The vitamin has since been assigned the term vitamin B_5.

B. Dietary Sources and Requirements

Although pantothenic acid is found in virtually all plant and animal materials (Sauberlich, 1985), estimation of the dietary intake of pantothenic acid was complicated by the fact that it occurs as the free acid as well as in bound forms, i.e., in CoA and fatty acid synthetase. Thus, to estimate the intake of pantothenic acid accurately, it was necessary to convert bound pantothenic acid to the free form. A double enzyme system of intestinal alkaline phosphatase and pigeon liver extract was utilized by Zook *et al.* (1956) to release bound pantothenic acid before analyzing pantothenic acid content of various foods. Other groups also have used double enzyme hydrolysis methods to determine pantothenic acid content in foods (Orr, 1969; Walsh *et al.*, 1981b). Instability of the enzyme preparations and variations in hydrolytic procedures caused variability in the release of bound pantothenic acid and thus variability in the measurement of total pantothenic acid content. More recently, pantetheinase, an enzyme purified from pig kidney, has been used in conjunction with bovine intestinal alkaline phosphatase to liberate bound pantothenic acid in whole blood (Song *et al.*, 1985; Wittwer *et al.*, 1982, 1983). Free pantothenic acid thus released has been quantified by a variety of methods which are described in Section III,A. In addition to the variability attributable to pretreatment of foods to liberate bound pantothenic acid, another problem is the lack of a reference method for analysis of pantothenic acid.

Much of the information concerning pantothenic acid content of food was obtained using raw or unprocessed foods. Since this does not reflect the normal American diet, studies were undertaken to determine the pantothenic acid content of 75 processed and cooked foods (Walsh *et al.*, 1981b). Results from this study indicated that good sources of pantothenic acid included chicken, beef, potatoes, oat cereals, tomato products, and whole grains. Many highly processed foods including products from refined grains, fruit products, and meats and fish with added fat or cereal extenders were relatively low in pantothenic acid content. Schroeder (1971) found that the pantothenic acid content of vegetables decreased 37–57% and 46–78% during freezing and canning, respectively. Mean losses associated with canning of fish, meats, and dairy products were relatively lower (20, 26, and 35%, respectively). Processing and refining resulted in a 37–74% loss of pantothenic acid from whole grains.

Relatively little is known about the bioavailability of pantothenic acid in human beings. In one study (Tarr *et al.*, 1981), healthy male volunteers were fed two types of diet, both nutritionally equivalent to the average American diet. During period 1, the first 35 days, formula diet was supplemented with 8.2 mg of free pantothenic acid/day. Then a diet of natural food sources providing 11.5 mg pantothenic acid/day was given for 35 days, followed by the pantothenic acid-supplemented formula diet for the final 21-day period. Pantothenic acid intake and excretion were monitored by estimating pantothenic acid in the food and urine. The availability of pantothenic acid in the natural food diet was determined by comparing urinary pantothenic acid excretion while taking the natural diet to the average pantothenic acid excretion in the reference period (period 1) of pure pantothenic acid intake. Availability of the dietary pantothenic acid ranged from 40–60%, with a mean of 50%. Thus it appeared that determining pantothenic acid intake by assessing total dietary content overestimated pantothenic acid actually acquired.

Recommended dietary allowances (RDA) for pantothenic acid have not been established. However, it has been suggested that a safe and adequate intake for adults and adolescents is 4–7 mg/day (Food and Nutrition Board, 1980). These levels were recommended for a healthy population and did not consider special needs. Tarr et al. (1981) reported that the average American diet contained 5.8 mg/day of available pantothenic acid. Similarly, Bull and Buss (1982) and Katham and Kies (1984) estimated the pantothenic acid intake to be 5.1 and 5.5 mg/day, respectively. However, the latter studies did not estimate the bioavailability of pantothenic acid. Walsh et al. (1981a) analyzed the weekly dietary intake of pantothenic acid (excluding beverages) for nursing home residents to be 3.75 mg/day or 2.22 mg/1000 Kcal. An additional study found no difference in dietary pantothenic acid between institutionalized and noninstitutionalized elderly men and women (mean pantothenic acid intake of 5.9 mg/day or 2.9 mg/1000 Kcal) (Srinivasan et al., 1981). For adolescents, the mean dietary intake was calculated to be 6.25 mg/day for males and 4.14 mg/day for females. However, the nutrient density, i.e., milligrams pantothenic acid per 1000 kilocalories, was not different between the two sexes. Other studies that have investigated pantothenic acid intake in humans include that by Kathman and Kies (1984) in which the dietary intake in a group of 11 boys and girls was found to be 5.4 mg/day, and a study by Kerrey et al. (1968) that reported that the dietary intake of pantothenic acid in preschool children of a higher socioeconomic status was 3.8 mg/day, and that of children from a lower socioeconomic status was 5 mg/day. It is clear from these studies that the dietary intake of pantothenic acid in adults conforms to the recommended level of 4–7 mg/day. Intake appears to be somewhat lower in the elderly and in young children. If, however, the bioavailability of pantothenic acid from food supplies is less than 50%, as suggested by Tarr *et al.* (1981), then requirements for pantothenic acid may be more than currently accepted.

The nutritional status of pantothenic acid depends upon pantothenic acid intake and urinary excretion. In healthy young males, the relationship between pantothenate intake and urinary pantothenic acid excretion appeared to be parabolic over an intake range of 0–10 mg pantothenic acid/day (Fry *et al.*, 1976). The urinary excretion of pantothenic acid decreased from 3.05 to 0.79 mg/day in subjects fed a pantothenic acid deficient diet, and increased from 3.95 to 5.84 mg/day in subjects supplemented with 10 mg pantothenic acid/day. After 9 weeks of taking controlled diets, the deficient and supplemented groups were each given a bolus dose of 100 mg pantothenic acid/day for 7 days and the excretion of pantothenic acid was monitored. On day 1 after the bolus, the deprived group retained 63% of the test dose while the group which had received a pantothenic acid supplement retained 48% of the dose. However, by day 7, both the groups retained 40% of the bolus. A significant positive correlation between the pantothenic acid intake and urinary excretion in adults has also been reported by several other groups (Song *et al.*, 1985; Kathman and Kies, 1984; Fox and Linkswiler, 1961; Cohenour and Calloway, 1972; Srinivasan *et al.*, 1981; Eissenstat *et al.*, 1986). In contrast to the results from adults, Kathman and Kies (1984) did not find a positive correlation between pantothenic acid intake and excretion in adolescents.

The effect of pregnancy and lactation on the nutritional status of pantothenic acid has been studied. Song *et al.* (1985) found that the dietary intake of pantothenic acid in pregnant or lactating women (2.75 mg/1000 Kcal) was no different from a group of nonpregnant women. Similarly, Cohenour and Calloway (1972) reported that the pantothenic acid intake of pregnant teenagers was no different from that of nonpregnant teenagers, although the intakes in both groups were near or below the lower level of the suggested safe and adequate intake. Although the average blood content of pantothenate in either the pregnant or lactating group was lower than in the control group, no difference in fasting concentration in plasma or in urinary excretion between the two groups could be detected (Song *et al.*, 1985; Cohenour and Calloway, 1972). This may indicate an increased need for this vitamin during pregnancy, as observed in animal studies (Hurley, 1967). No differences were found in pantothenic acid levels of blood collected at different times of gestation or within 3 months postpartum

(Cohenour and Calloway, 1972; Song *et al.*, 1985). With regard to human milk, it was found that pantothenic acid levels in term milk were significantly correlated with maternal dietary intake and urinary excretion as well as with pantothenic acid levels in maternal circulation (Song *et al.*, 1984; Johnston *et al.*, 1981). Oral contraceptives did appear to cause a significant change in pantothenic acid status (Lewis and King, 1980).

C. DEFICIENCIES

Perhaps due to the ubiquitous nature of pantothenic acid, spontaneous deficiency of pantothenic acid in humans has not been reported. Pantothenic acid deficiency was produced experimentally in humans fed a diet deficient in pantothenic acid along with a pantothenic acid antagonist, ω-methylpantothenic acid (Bean and Hodges, 1954; Hodges *et al.*, 1958). The most common symptoms associated with pantothenic acid deficiency were headache, fatigue, and a sensation of weakness. Other symptoms included personality changes, sleep disturbances, impaired motor coordination, and gastrointestinal disturbances. Metabolic alterations included a loss of eosinopenic response to adrenocorticotropin (ACTH), and increased sensitivity to insulin. Although early results suggested impaired adrenal cortical function (Bean and Hodges, 1954), this did not appear to be consistent (Hodges *et al.*, 1958), since pantothenic acid-deficient humans showed normal urinary excretion of 17-keto steroids, normal glucose tolerance, and normal blood and urine sodium. In a more recent study, human volunteers fed a semisynthetic, pantothenic acid-free diet for 9 weeks did not develop clinical signs of pantothenic acid deficiency. However, the pantothenic acid-restricted group appeared listless and complained of fatigue (Fry *et al.*, 1976). Low serum pantothenic acid has also been suggested to be associated with an increased incidence of hypertension (Koyanagi *et al.*, 1966).

The effects of pantothenic acid deficiency have been studied in a variety of animal models. In guinea pigs, there was a sharp increase in bound pantothenic acid and in CoA in the perinatal period (Hurley, 1967). In addition, 1 week of pantothenic acid deficiency reduced the number of young born alive. The effect of pantothenic acid restriction was especially severe during the ninth week of gestation (total gestation is 10 weeks). Restriction of pantothenic acid in the tenth week of gestation produced an increase in liver fat of the newborn (Hurley and Volkert, 1965). Pantothenic acid deficiency during the prenatal and neonatal periods also caused altered growth and maturation of the small intestine in the rat (Ramakrishnan and Subramaniam, 1978). The brain lipids in neonates from maternal rats fed pantothenic acid-deficient diets were reduced in comparison to neonates from maternal rats receiving a normal diet. However, food consumption by the group fed a pantothenic acid-deficient diet was reduced. Pair-fed rats receiving control diet in amounts matching consumption by the pantothenic acid-deficient group also exhibited similar decreases in brain lipids (Rajalakshmi and Nakhasi, 1975), suggesting that the observed effects in the pantothenic acid-deficient group were due to decreased food intake rather than pantothenate deficiency.

In the adult male, pantothenic acid deficiency causes a variety of effects, including altered intestinal transport in swine (Nelson, 1968), depressed heme synthesis resulting in anemia in monkeys (McCall et al., 1946), and a decreased need for vitamin B_6 (pyridoxine) in mice and rats (Huang and Kies, 1981). In addition, pantothenic acid deficiency may have contributed to hypertension in rats after unilateral adrenonephrectomy (Schwabedel et al., 1985), altered the immune response in rats (Axelrod, 1981), and altered the incorporation of amino acids in serum albumin (Roy and Axelrod, 1971).

An extensive study by Smith et al. (1987) indicated that mice maintained on a pantothenic acid-deficient diet for 65–105 days show decreased pantothenate content in all tissues studied as compared to animals on a pantothenic acid-supplemented diet. The total CoA was reduced in all tissues except the brain and epididymal fat pads. After a 48-hour fast, the total CoA level increased in the heart and liver of both groups; it remained lower, however, in the pantothenic acid deficient group. Liver glycogen levels were decreased and liver ketone levels were increased in the fasted, deficient mice. Pantothenic acid-deficient animals subjected to exercise showed lower stamina and lower glycogen levels in liver and muscle. Liver ketone bodies were elevated in the deficient group at rest and after exercise. This indicated an inability to maintain glycogen levels in the pantothenic acid-deficient group, but a normal ketogenic response to exercise and fast in spite of reduced liver total CoA. Reduced liver fructose 1,6-diphosphate 1-phosphohydrolase, increased glucose 6-phosphatase, and decreased liver glycogen, suggestive of impaired gluconeogenesis have been observed in pantothenic acid deficient rats (Srinivasan and Belavady, 1976). Liver total CoA was reduced in chicks fed a pantothenic acid-deficient diet (Cupo and Donaldson, 1986). Although the rate of lipid accumulation in vivo was reduced in chicks, lipogenesis in vitro (as determined by specific activities of acetyl CoA carboxylase and fatty acid synthetase) was unchanged. In a study by Reibel et al.

(1982), rats fed a pantothenic acid-deficient diet for 4–8 weeks had a reduced pantothenic acid content in the heart, kidney, gastrocnemius, testes, and liver, as well as a reduced growth rate. However, CoA levels in these tissues were maintained at normal levels. A 48-hour fast resulted in increased liver and heart CoA content in both the pantothenic acid-deficient and control animals. Similar effects on tissue CoA content have been observed in experimental diabetes and are discussed at length in Section V. The reason for the differences observed in CoA content of tissues from pantothenic acid-deficient animals is unclear and may reflect species differences in response to decreased pantothenic acid intake.

III. PANTOTHENIC ACID IN BIOLOGICAL SYSTEMS

A. ASSAY

Pantothenic acid can be quantitated by microbiological assay or by radioimmunoassay. Although various microbiological procedures, utilizing *Saccharomyces carlsbergenesis* (Tsuji, 1966), *Pediococcus acidilactici* NC1B 6990 (Solberg and Hegna, 1979), and *Lactobacillus and arabinosus* (Skeggs and Wright, 1944) have been described, the most widely used microbiological assay, described by Skeggs and Wright (1944) was based on the growth requirement of *Lactobacillus* for pantothenic acid. *L. plantarum* were grown in a pantothenate-containing medium after which they were washed with and resuspended in a pantothenate-free medium. Tubes containing either known amounts of pantothenate or neutralized biological samples were seeded with bacteria and grown for 24 hours, after which bacterial density was determined spectrophotometrically. The standard curve was typically in the range of 2–40 nM pantothenate. Fatty acids stimulate the growth of bacteria in media containing suboptimal concentrations of pantothenic acid, but interference from other compounds appears minimal. Recovery of pantothenate from various samples is close to 100%, interassay coefficient of variation is ~17%, and results obtained with this method agree with those obtained using other pantothenate-requiring bacteria.

A radioimmunoassay has also been used to determine pantothenic acid in biological samples (Wyse *et al.*, 1979). Pantothenic acid was conjugated with denatured, reduced albumin and an immune response was elicited in rabbits. Antiserum was collected and a competitive binding assay was carried out with increasing amounts of unlabeled pantothenic acid. The method was sensitive enough to allow determinations of pantothenic acid in the nanomole range and the results obtained with the assay were consistent with those obtained using the microbiological assay. The reproducibility of the radioimmunoassay was better than that of the microbiological assay with an intra-assay coefficient of variation of 2.9% and an interassay coefficient of variation of 3.3%. Although the immunoassay was time consuming initially, i.e., for preparing the ligand and obtaining antiserum, the actual assay was completed within a short time. On the other hand, the microbiological assay was a 2–3 day procedure, i.e., from growing the inoculum to seeding the standards and samples to determining the turbidity. A plot of results for pantothenic acid in blood using the radioimmunoassay versus microbiological assay gave a line described by y (radioimmunoassay) = 0.72 x (microbiological assay) + 280, r = 0.8 (Wyse et al., 1979). Similarly good correlations were found with pantothenic acid assays on extracts of hearts from control and diabetic rats by the two assays: y (radioimmunoassay) = 1.22 x microbiological assay − 46, r = 0.85. Interestingly, the pantothenic acid content of hearts from 48-hour streptozotocin diabetic rats was reduced by about 50% as compared to control when measured by radioimmunoassay (Reibel et al., 1981b; Beinlich et al., 1990). When pantothenic acid content of these tissue extracts was measured using the microbiological assay, it was unchanged from control (Beinlich et al., 1990). After 4 days of diabetes, the pantothenic acid content was 83 and 88% of control levels using radioimmunoassay and microbiological assay, respectively (Beinlich et al., 1990). This suggested that acute diabetes resulted in the generation of some metabolite capable of interfering with one of these assays.

Attempts have also been made to assay pantothenic acid using chromatographic methods, but these methods were unsuitable as outlined in the next paragraph. Hence, chromatography has been used only to separate pantothenic acid from the intermediates of the CoA biosynthetic pathway and thus to study flux through various enzymes (Nakamura et al., 1972; Smith, 1978). The procedure using paper chromatography involved spotting samples on diethylaminoethyl (DEAE)-cellulose paper and developing the chromatogram with double-distilled formic acid by ascending chromatography. Using this method, the positions of standard 4'-phosphopantetheine (4'-PP), dephospho-CoA, and CoA were established after spraying with cyanide and nitroprusside (for sulfhydryl groups) (Waldi, 1965). The position of pantothenic acid was located with the aid of commercially available radiolabeled pantothenic acid, while the intermediates between pantothenic acid and

4'-PP (see Fig. 2) were located by radioactive standards prepared in the laboratory.

High pressure liquid chromatography (HPLC) systems have been developed to separate the intermediates of the CoA biosynthetic pathway (Robishaw et al., 1982). Separation was carried out using a C_{18} reverse phase column with 20 mM phosphate and acetonitrile as the solvent system. The column was equilibrated with phosphate and after injection of sample, a gradient of 0–8% acetonitrile was established over 35 minutes. The system was maintained at 8% acetonitrile for an additional 15 minutes to elute all the intermediates. Another solvent system used successfully in our laboratory for separating CoA intermediates is a modification of the method described by Corkey et al. (1981) for separating acyl esters of CoA. A higher concentration of phosphate (100 mM) and methanol were used. The C_{18} column was equilibrated with 8% methanol and a gradient of 8–20% methanol over 80 minutes was used. This method was similar to that reported by Halvorsen and Skrede (1980) to separate the intermediates of CoA biosynthesis and the disulfides of CoA and dephospho-CoA. The advantage of HPLC was that it simultaneously provided quantitation of CoA and its esters (by optical absorbance at 254 nm) and separation of pantothenate and the intermediates of the CoA biosynthetic pathway (using radioactive precursors). This was particularly useful in studying the effects of elevated levels of acyl CoAs on pantothenate incorporation or monitoring changes in concentrations of acyl esters under various conditions of incubation. Pantothenate could not be assayed simultaneously since it absorbed at 205 nm, a wavelength at which a large number of compounds in biological samples also absorb.

B. ABSORPTION, DISTRIBUTION, AND ELIMINATION

Investigation of the absorption of dietary pantothenic acid poses several questions, including (1) are both free and bound forms of pantothenic acid absorbed; (2) what is the mechanism of absorption; and (3) is pantothenic acid metabolized or altered during absorption. Turner and Hughes (1962) suggested that CoA was converted to either pantothenic acid or pantetheine (PaSH) by the intestinal mucosa in everted sacs of rat intestine. Since transport of pantothenic acid against a concentration gradient in the preparation was not observed, it was concluded that the compound was absorbed by passive diffusion. Additional studies using isolated rat intestine indicated that orally administered CoA was hydrolyzed to pantothenic acid in the intestinal lumen via the formation of dephospho-CoA, phosphopantetheine and

PaSH (Shibata *et al.*, 1983). Intestinal tissue absorbed pantothenic acid and PaSH but not CoA, dephospho-CoA, or phosphopantetheine. The intestinal tissue PaSH was hydrolyzed to pantothenic acid for transport to the blood. Ono *et al.* (1974) suggested that pantethine was more readily absorbed than calcium pantothenate when administered orally to rats. Pantethine was found to be partially hydrolyzed to pantothenic acid during absorption. Pantetheinase, an enzyme that hydrolyzes either pantethine or PaSH is found in intestinal cells (Ono *et al.*, 1974; Shibata *et al.*, 1983). Absorption of pantothenic acid by passive diffusion (Shibata *et al.*, 1983) was suggested, since saturation was not observed over a wide concentration range. Also, no significant difference in the rate of pantothenic acid transport was found in the upper, middle, or lower segments of the intestine. In contrast to the results obtained by Shibata *et al.* (1983), Fenstermacher and Rose (1986) reported data indicating a specific transport mechanism for pantothenic acid in the rat and chicken intestine. They compared brush border transport in various segments of isolated rat intestine and found that the jejunum exhibited the greatest rate of pantothenic acid transport. This absorption was shown to be unidirectional, sodium-dependent, and to demonstrate saturation kinetics ($K_m = 17 \mu M$; $V_{max} = 972$ pmol/cm^2/hour at Na = 145 meq/liter). The process appeared to be energy-dependent without substrate conversion. Similar results were obtained using chick enterocytes. Perhaps earlier studies did not find saturation for pantothenic acid transport because higher concentrations of pantothenic acid were used. Fenstermacher and Rose (1986) suggested a model of intestinal transport whereby uptake from the intestinal lumen was mediated by a sodium-dependent transporter with a 1 : 1 coupling ratio that utilized the electrochemical gradient as the energy source. The electrochemical gradient, maintained by the Na$^+$,K$^+$-ATPase on the basolateral membrane, favored the entry of sodium and thus pantothenic acid into the cell from the lumen. The importance of bacterial production of pantothenic acid in mammalian intestine in preventing pantothenate deficiency is not known. The adult ruminant appears to be independent of dietary pantothenic acid, since sufficient quantities of pantothenic acid are obtained via rumen microorganisms (Finlayson and Seeley, 1983). In adult sheep fitted with duodenal and ileal reentry cannulae, there was an increase in total pantothenic acid and CoA before the small intestine. A positive correlation was observed between the total pantothenic acid reaching the duodenum and the microbial dry matter synthesized in the rumen (Finlayson and Seeley, 1983). In the latter study it appeared that CoA-bound pantothenic acid, upon entering the small intestine, was hydrolyzed to release free pantothenic acid and that free pantothenic acid was absorbed by a passive mechanism. The increase in total pantothenic acid before the small intestine suggested that *de novo* synthesis of pantothenic acid occurred within the rumen.

Following intestinal absorption, pantothenic acid is transported to various tissues by blood. Pantothenic acid in blood was primarily represented by the bound forms in erythrocytes (Eissenstat *et al.*, 1986). Plasma levels of pantothenic acid were low and correlated poorly with pantothenic acid in whole blood (Cohenour and Calloway, 1972) or with dietary intake (Song *et al.*, 1985). The correlation between blood pantothenic acid levels and dietary pantothenic acid intake has been described as low (Song *et al.*, 1985) to moderate (Srinivasan *et al.*, 1981). Baker *et al.* (1969) reported a large increase in red cell but not plasma pantothenic acid after an intravenous load of pantothenic acid. The plasma level reached a peak in 10 minutes and decreased gradually thereafter. These data suggested that pantothenic acid was taken up rapidly by red cells and/or tissues.

Tissue distribution of pantothenic acid has been studied by determining tissue distribution of radioactivity after oral administration of radioactive pantothenic acid. In rats, similar distribution of radioactivity was obtained with [^{14}C] CoA or [^{14}C]pantothenic acid. Five hours after oral administration, trace amounts of radioactivity were found in blood, while approximately 40% of the dose was present in muscle. Liver and intestinal tissue each contained about 10% of the total dose (Shibata *et al.*, 1983). In dogs, plasma pantothenic acid peaked 2–2.5 hours after an oral dose of [^{14}C]pantothenic acid followed by declining concentrations ($t_{1/2}$ = 2.8 hour). In contrast, intravenous injection of [^{14}C]pantothenic acid resulted in rapidly falling plasma ([^{14}C]pantothenic acid during the first 2 hours after administration and a $t_{1/2}$ of 2.5 hours thereafter (Taylor *et al.*, 1974). The apparent volume of distribution for pantothenic acid was calculated and approached the value for total extracellular fluid. The maximal concentration of blood total pantothenic acid was observed 2–4.5 hours after oral ingestion of either PaSH or calcium pantothenate in rats (Ono *et al.*, 1974).

Investigation of the pantothenic acid content of various organs from rats indicated relatively high concentrations (284 and 245 nmol/g dry tissue weight, respectively) (Reibel *et al.*, 1981b) in the heart and kidney. Further, the pantothenic acid content of tissues appears to be under hormonal control since pantothenic acid concentrations are influenced by diabetes or starvation (Reibel *et al.*, 1981b).

Pantothenic acid is eliminated via urinary excretion. As previously discussed, there was a positive correlation between urinary excretion and dietary intake of pantothenic acid in adults (Song *et al.*, 1985; Eissenstat *et al.*, 1986; Kathman and Kies, 1984). Karnitz *et al.* (1984), using isolated perfused kidney, observed that pantothenic acid was largely reabsorbed at physiological concentrations, while at higher concentrations there was tubular secretion of pantothenic acid. The tubular secretion of pantothenic acid was inhibited by penicillin, suggesting a secretory mechanism common to weak organic acids. Transport of pantothenic acid by brush border membrane vesicles from kidney indicated that transport of [^{14}C]pantothenic acid was a sodium-dependent process with a K_m of 7.3 μM or 16 μM and V_{max} of 23.8 pmol/mg/minute or 6.7 pmol/mg/10 seconds (Karnitz *et al.*, 1984; Barbarat and Podevin, 1986, respectively). Barbarat and Podevin (1986) suggested that pantothenic acid transport occurred by an electrogenic sodium/pantothenate cotransport system specific for pantothenic acid. Mechanisms for active reabsorption and secretion of pantothenic acid in the kidney, along with the positive correlation between dietary intake and urinary excretion, suggested that this organ may be involved in regulation of body stores of pantothenic acid.

Although blood concentrations of pantothenic acid in human diabetics was unchanged from nondiabetics, urinary excretion of pantothenic acid was increased in diabetics and was further elevated with induction of diabetic ketosis (Hatano *et al.*, 1967). In animal studies, however, Reibel *et al.* (1981b) found decreased urinary excretion of pantothenic acid in diabetic rats, even though serum pantothenic acid was elevated as compared to controls. A review of studies investigating pantothenic acid status in alcoholics indicated reduced urinary excretion and blood levels (Bonjour, 1980). Malnutrition, often associated with alcoholism, may cause decreased intake of pantothenic acid. Tao and Fox (1976) suggested that alteration of urinary excretion in alcoholics indicated an inability to efficiently utilize dietary pantothenic acid. This speculation was based upon the observation that in chronic alcoholics, excretion approximated intake at the beginning of a rehabilitation program but was decreased at the end of rehabilitation. This hypothesis was supported by animal studies indicating that chronic ethanol ingestion decreased pantothenic acid content in rat heart and possibly in liver (Israel and Smith, 1987). Ethanol administration to rats *in vivo* or added to cultured hepatocytes *in vitro* inhibited conversion of [^{14}C]pantothenic acid to [^{14}C]CoA by inhibition of pantothenate kinase (Iannucci *et al.*, 1982; Israel and Smith, 1987). This inhibition appeared to be the result of metabolism of ethanol to acetyl CoA (Smith *et al.*, 1987).

Although no urinary metabolite of pantothenic acid has been described in humans, Taylor *et al.* (1972) have reported a urinary metabolite of pantothenic acid in dogs. After oral administration of [^{14}C]pantothenic acid, 80–90% of the oral dose was absorbed. Urinary excretion was slow, with 0.5% of the oral dose excreted unchanged in urine within 24 hours and 40% of the dose excreted as the β-glucoronide ester in 7 days. The renal clearance of unchanged vitamin in dogs was consistent with tubular reabsorption, whereas clearance of the β-glucoronide ester was higher (Taylor *et al.*, 1972). More recent studies using HPLC analysis of dog urine and feces after oral administration of [^{3}H]pantothenic acid indicated that 30% of the radioactivity was recovered in feces within 4 days, and an additional 25% was recovered in urine within 9 days. Analysis of the radioactivity recovered from urine indicated that in addition to [^{3}H]pantothenic acid, a metabolite identical to that identified by Taylor *et al.* (1972) was found; only [^{3}H]pantothenic acid was detected in extracts of fecal material. Structural identification by enzymatic analysis, and gas-chromatography/mass spectroscopy (GC/MS) and nuclear magnetic resonance (NMR) analysis indicated the metabolite to be the vitamin β-glucoside, rather than the β-glucoronide (Nakano *et al.*, 1986). Species differences in renal clearance may exist since analysis of rat urine indicated unchanged pantothenic acid with no vitamin ester detected (Taylor *et al.*, 1972).

C. CELLULAR TRANSPORT

The first step in the metabolism of pantothenic acid is transport into cells. Pantothenic acid appeared to be cotransported with sodium, using the sodium electrochemical gradient for uphill movement in heart (Lopaschuk *et al.*, 1987; C. J. Beinlich, unpublished observations), liver (Smith and Milner, 1985), kidney (Karnitz *et al.*, 1984; Barbarat and Podevin, 1986), intestinal cells (Fenstermacher and Rose, 1986), and perhaps isolated rat adipocytes (Sugarman and Monro, 1980). In rat liver parenchymal cells (Smith and Milner, 1985) and chick intestinal cells (Fenstermacher and Rose, 1986), pantothenate and sodium were transported in a 1 : 1 ratio, while in rabbit brush border membrane vesicles, evidence indicated an electrogenic transport with a 1 : 2 pantothenate : sodium ratio (Barbarat and Podevin, 1986). In the heart (Robishaw *et al.*, 1982), liver (Smith and Milner, 1985), kidney (Karnitz *et al.*, 1984), and intestinal cells (Fenstermacher and Rose, 1986), there was uptake of vitamin without apparent conversion of pantothenic acid, while in brain slices, transport was accompanied by rapid phosphorylation (Spector, 1986).

The kinetics of pantothenic acid transport were shown to be similar in several tissues with the K_m reported to be 11 μM in heart (Beinlich *et al.*, 1989; Lopaschuk *et al.*, 1987), and liver (Smith and Milner, 1985), 7–16 μM in renal brush border membrane vesicles (Karnitz *et al.*, 1984; Barbarat and Podevin, 1986), and 17 μM for intestine (Fenstermacher and Rose, 1986). The V_{max} for pantothenic acid transport was reported to be 228 nmol/g dry heart/30 minutes (Lopaschuk *et al.*, 1987), and 630 nmol/g dry heart/hour in the isolated perfused heart (Beinlich *et al.*, 1989), 28.8 pmol/mg/minute (Karnitz *et al.*, 1984), or 6.7 pmol/mg/10 seconds (Barbarat and Podevin, 1986) in kidney, 350 nmol/mg/minute in the liver (Smith and Milner, 1985), and 972 pmol/cm^2/hour in rat intestine (Fenstermacher and Rose, 1986). Recalculation of these data to express transport in nanomoles per milligram of protein per hour (assuming 750 mg protein/g dry heart tissue) gives similar V_{max} values for the heart (1.1 nmol/mg/hour, 0.84 nmol/mg/hour), liver (2.1 nmol/mg/hour) and kidney (1.4 nmol/mg/hour, 2.4 nmol/mg/hour).

The transport system for pantothenic acid appears to be quite specific, since analogs of pantothenic acid and various carboxylic acids did not inhibit transport in brush border membrane vesicles (Barbarat and Podevin, 1986) or in cultured liver cells (Smith and Milner, 1985). In the perfused working heart a group of seven amino acids inhibited pantothenic acid transport at perfusate concentrations of 0.7 mM with no further inhibition at 1.2 mM (Lopaschuk *et al.*, 1987). Using the Langendorf preparation for perfusing hearts, we have not, however, been able to confirm these results (Beinlich *et al.*, 1990). The apparent discrepancy may reflect different experimental models, since cardiac work was shown to stimulate pantothenic acid transport (Lopaschuk *et al.*, 1987). Pantethine, unlike most analogs of pantothenic acid, appeared to inhibit pantothenic acid uptake by the isolated perfused heart. Further investigation, however, suggested that this was due to conversion of pantethine to pantothenic acid (Beinlich *et al.*, 1990). High concentrations of medium chain length saturated fatty acids inhibited pantothenic acid transport in the isolated perfused heart (Beinlich *et al.*, 1990), and in brain slices (Spector, 1986). Probenecid, an inhibitor of epithelial transport of weak organic acids, and biotin, a water soluble B vitamin, also inhibited pantothenic acid transport in these two preparations. In the isolated perfused heart, both probenicid and biotin were competitive inhibitors of pantothenic acid transport with K_i values of 85 μM and 31 μM, respectively (Beinlich *et al.*, 1990). Although biotin and pantothenic acid may share some transport characteristics (Beinlich *et al.*, 1990; Said and Redha, 1987), it is unlikely that inhibition of pantothenic acid transport by biotin is physiologically important, since the plasma concentration of biotin (20 nM, Ikeda *et al.*, 1979) is far below the K_i for pantothenic acid transport. Further conformational and structural requirements for transport are unknown at this time.

The transport of pantothenic acid across the blood–brain barrier appeared to be saturable with a K_m of 19 μM and a V_{max} of 0.21 nmol/g/minute. In contrast to other tissues, transport across the blood–brain barrier did not appear to be dependent on the sodium gradient. This was indicated by the lack of effect of poly-L-lysine, an inhibitor of sodium transport (Spector, 1986). Experiments using rabbit brain slices indicated transport of pantothenic acid by a saturable system which was inhibited by probenicid and medium chain fatty acids but insensitive to extracellular sodium concentration (Spector, 1986). In contrast, pantothenic acid transport in the isolated choroid plexus appeared to be a sodium-dependent active uptake process that was sensitive to inhibition by probenecid, *N*-ethylmaleimide and poly-L-lysine (Spector and Boose, 1984). Characteristics of pantothenic acid transport in various tissues are summarized in Table I. The similarity of pantothenic acid transport in tissues other than the brain suggested the possibility of a common transport mechanism. The lack of sodium dependence for pantothenic acid transport across the blood–brain barrier may indicate a separate mechanism for pantothenic acid transport in that organ.

The factors regulating pantothenic acid transport are undefined and may vary from tissue to tissue. *In vivo* studies with rats indicated that fasting or diabetes cause increased [^{14}C]pantothenic acid uptake, higher pantothenic acid levels, increased incorporation of [^{14}C]pantothenic acid into CoA, and elevated CoA levels in the liver (Reibel *et al.*, 1981b). In the heart, however, fasting and diabetes led to increased [^{14}C]pantothenic acid incorporation into CoA and increased CoA levels, while [^{14}C]pantothenic acid uptake and tissue pantothenic acid levels were reduced. Uptake of [^{14}C]pantothenic acid was reduced slightly in skeletal muscle and diaphragm, but not in kidney of diabetic rats (Reibel *et al.*, 1981b). Cardiac CoA levels increased as early as 6 hours following induction of diabetes with high doses of alloxan (60 mg/kg) (Neely *et al.*, 1982), remained elevated for several days, and returned to control levels by 9 days (Beinlich *et al.*, 1989a). In rats subjected to lower doses of alloxan (37.5 mg/kg), myocardial CoA levels

TABLE I
CHARACTERISTICS OF PANTOTHENATE TRANSPORT IN DIVERSE TISSUES

Tissue	Sodium dependent	K_m (μM)	V_{max}[a]	V_{max}[b] (nmol/ mg/hr)	Reference
Heart	Yes	10.7	417 nmol/g/30 min	1.1	Lopaschuk et al. (1987)[c]
	Yes	11	630 nmol/g/hr	0.84	Beinlich et al. (1989)[d]
Liver	Yes	11	350 nmol/mg protein/min	2.1	Smith and Milner (1985)[e]
Kidney	Yes	7.3	23.8 pmol/mg protein/min	1.4	Karnitz et al. (1984)
	Yes	16	6.7 pmol/mg protein/10 sec	2.4	Barbarat and Podevin et al. (1986)
Intestine	Yes	17	972 pmol/cm²/hr		Fenstermacher and Rose (1986)
Brain	No	19	0.21 nmol/g/min		Spector (1986)[f]

[a] V_{max} as reported by authors.

[b] V_{max} recalculated in nmol/mg protein/hour. In the heart, 1 g dry tissues contains 750 mg protein.

[c] Transport inhibited by a mixture of seven amino acids at 0.7 mM.

[d] Transport inhibited by biotin, probenecid, octanoic acid, and nonanoic acid.

[e] Transport weakly inhibited by 3-hydroxybutyrate, 2-oxovalerate, and panthenol.

[f] Transport inhibited by probenecid, nonanoic acid, and biotin.

were elevated within 24 hours and remained elevated for at least 21 days (Neely et al., 1982). In contrast to the in vivo studies, in vitro synthesis of CoA was reduced in hearts from alloxan diabetic rats, and after 9 days of diabetes, synthesis was 26% that of hearts from control rats. Reduced synthesis was accompanied by decreased pantothenic acid transport and phosphorylation (Beinlich et al., 1989). Myocardial pantothenic acid transport, as measured in vitro, was reduced by 70% after 48 hours of streptozotocin diabetes and remained reduced during 10 weeks of diabetes (Beinlich et al., 1990). Concurrently, pantothenic acid content decreased and, after 10 weeks of diabetes, intracellular pantothenic acid was 67 μM. Although this was considerably lower than intracellular pantothenic acid levels from control hearts (180 μM), it was significantly higher than the K_m of pantothenate kinase for pantothenic acid (18 μM) (Fisher et al., 1985). CoA levels increased within 24 hours of streptozotocin injection and remained elevated during 10 weeks of diabetes. From these studies it appeared that pantothenic acid transport was not rate limiting for CoA synthesis in chronic streptozotocin diabetic rats. The binding affinity (K_m) for pantothenic acid transport was not changed in hearts from diabetic animals, while the V_{max} was reduced to 26% of control, indicating a reduced number of effective transporters (Beinlich *et al.*, 1989).

The defect in myocardial pantothenic acid transport was corrected by *in vivo* insulin treatment (Beinlich *et al.*, 1990; Lopaschuk *et al.*, 1987). Treatment of rats with thyroxine or triiodothyroxine, hormones that also are altered in diabetes, did not affect *in vitro* transport of pantothenic acid. Lopaschuk (1988), using the isolated working heart preparation, reported that perfusion with buffer containing insulin, 1.2 mM palmitate, and 11 mM glucose restored pantothenic acid transport in hearts from untreated diabetic BB Wistar rats (spontaneously diabetic rats), and improved pantothenic acid uptake in hearts from 48-hour streptozotocin diabetic rats. In contrast, using the Langendorf preparation, Beinlich *et al.* (1990) did not observe any improvement of pantothenic acid transport in hearts from streptozotocin diabetic rats when perfused with insulin, palmitate, and glucose. These differences may reflect differences in experimental models, since cardiac work has been shown to increase pantothenic acid transport (Lopaschuk *et al.*, 1987).

It is clear that pantothenic acid is transported into cells, apparently by a sodium-dependent mechanism. Furthermore, the process appears to be subject to hormonal perturbations, the mechanisms involved being unclear. Controversy exists whether the effects of hormonal alterations are direct or secondary effects of hormonal deficiency. Available studies, which are mostly short term, do not indicate that altered pantothenate transport significantly affects CoA homeostasis. However, this does not mean that pantothenate transport will not be a significant factor in CoA homeostasis over long-term alterations in pantothenate transport. One approach that might answer some of these questions is to isolate the pantothenate transporter and study it as a separate entity in reconstituted vesicles. This approach may also help understand the alterations of pantothenate transport in disease conditions at the molecular level.

D. MICROBIAL METABOLISM

Although pantothenic acid cannot be synthesized by animals, most microorganisms are capable of producing pantothenic acid from its precursors, pantoic acid and β-alanine (Brown and Williamson, 1982). Pantoate is synthesized from α-ketovalerate via a two-step reaction requiring tetrahydrofolate and NADPH (Fig. 1). The suggestion that

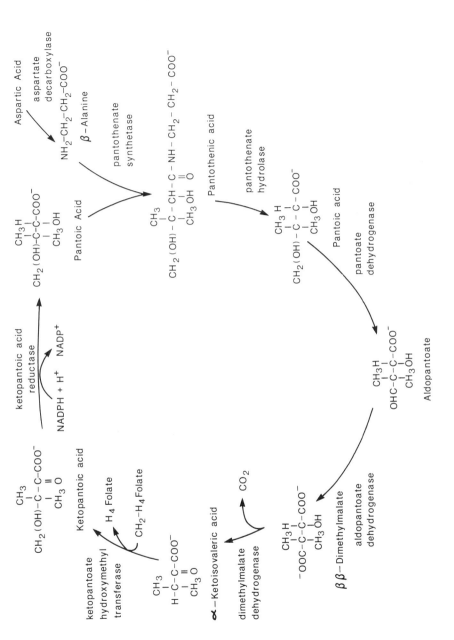

FIG. 1. Schematic diagram representing the synthetic and degradative pathway for pantothenic acid in bacteria (Vallari and Rock, 1985; Brown and Williamson, 1982; Magee and Snell, 1966).

one of the intermediates in this reaction was ketopantoic acid was confirmed by identification of a class of *Escherichia coli* mutants that utilized ketopantoate instead of pantoate. Evidence that whole cells of a strain of *E. coli* synthesized ketopantoate and pantoate from α-ketoisovaleric acid while certain pantoate-requiring mutants could not, suggested that α-ketoisovaleric acid was the precursor for ketopantoic acid (Brown and Williamson, 1982). Teller *et al.* (1976) identified the tetrahydrofolate-dependent enzyme, ketopantoate hydroxymethyltransferase, as the enzyme catalyzing the conversion of α-ketoisovalerate to ketopantoate. Ketopantoic acid reductase, an enzyme that catalyzes the formation of D-pantoic acid from ketopantoic acid has been characterized (Shimuzu *et al.*, 1988). The β-alanine required for biosynthesis of pantothenic acid is produced by α-decarboxylation of aspartic acid. This decarboxylase exists in the wild-type strain but not in a mutant of *E. coli* (M99-2) that required either β-alanine or pantothenate (Brown and Williamson, 1982).

Snell and colleagues described bacterial degradation of pantothenic acid by *Pseudomonas* P-2, an organism that can grow aerobically with pantothenate as a sole source of carbon and nitrogen (Goodhue and Snell, 1966; Nurmikko *et al.*, 1966; Magee and Snell, 1966). Their data indicated that in *Pseudomonas* P-2, pantothenic acid was hydrolyzed to pantoic acid and β-alanine by an inducible enzyme, pantothenate hydrolase (Nurmikko *et al.*, 1966). Pantoate was oxidized by pantoate dehydrogenase to a previously unknown compound, aldopantoic acid (Goodhue and Snell, 1966). Two enzymes, D-adlopantoate dehydrogenase and dimethyl malate dehydrogenase completed the enzymatic conversion of aldopantoate to α-ketoisovalerate (Magee and Snell, 1966). Thus, the biosynthetic and degradative pathways for pantothenic acid appear to be distinct even though α-ketoisovalerate is a common intermediate.

Bacteria can synthesize pantothenic acid and several strains also transport it (Germinario and Waller, 1977; Mantsala, 1973; Vallari and Rock, 1985; Nakamura and Tamura, 1973). The active transport systems in gram-negative bacteria were classified as osmotic shock-sensitive or shock-resistant systems. The osmotic shock-sensitive systems showed a requirement for phosphate bond energy and were associated with a periplasmic substrate binding protein, while shock-resistant transport was coupled to the membrane electrochemical gradient and involved membrane-bound permeases (Vallari and Rock, 1985). Nakamura and Tamura (1973) described a pantothenic acid transport system in *E. coli* K-12 having characteristics of an active transport process. The pantothenic acid uptake was energy-, temperature-, and pH-dependent. Transport was markedly inhibited by sulfhydryl reagents and 2,4-dinitrophenol. The apparent K_m for transport was 300 nM. Additional studies (Vallari and Rock, 1985) found pantothenic acid transport in *E. coli* K-12 to be specific for pantothenate with a K_m of 400 nM and a V_{max} of 1.6 pmol/minute/10^8 cells. Pantothenic acid uptake was not reduced in osmotically shocked cells or by ATP depletion with arsenate. Transport was reduced, however, by dissipation of the membrane electrochemical gradient. Pantothenate transport into *E. coli* K-12 cells did not require phosphorylation (Vallari and Rock, 1985; Nakamura and Tamura, 1973). These results were consistent with a transport system that concentrates pantothenic acid by sodium cotransport. In contrast, studies with *E. coli* V-5/41 showed transport activity for pantothenic acid that was reduced by osmotic shock (Mantsala, 1973). Other characteristics of this transport included inhibition by 2,4-dinitrophenol and sodium azide, a K_m of 25 μM, and sensitivity to pH and temperature. This investigation did not report the effect of osmotic shock on cell viability or on established transport systems. An energy-dependent transport system for pantothenic acid in *Lactobacillus plantarum* exhibited pH and temperature sensitivity, substrate saturation, and competitive inhibition by panthenol and pantoyltaurine (Germinario and Waller, 1977).

IV. COENZYME A IN BIOLOGICAL SYSTEMS

A. ASSAY

A number of assays are available for determining the CoA content of biological samples. An enzymatic assay described by Garland *et al.* (1965) is based on the conversion of NAD to NADH in the presence of α-ketoglutarate, CoA, and α-ketoglutarate dehydrogenase, i.e.,

$$\text{CoA} + \alpha\text{-ketoglutarate} + \text{NAD}^+ \xrightarrow{\ \ \ \ \ \ \ \ \ \ \ \ \ \ } \text{succinyl CoA} + \text{CO}_2 + \text{H}^+ + \text{NADH}$$
$$\text{α-ketoglutarate dehydrogenase} \tag{1}$$

Production of NADH is monitored flurometrically resulting in assay sensitivity in the nanomolar range. Although some cross-reactivity is caused by dephospho-CoA (the K_m value for dephospho-CoA is about 600 times that of CoA), acyl esters of CoA do not interfere with the assay. Acyl esters can be assayed by hydrolyzing prior to assay. Acetyl CoA can be assayed by converting it to free CoA either by alkaline hydrolysis or by enzymatic hydrolysis using phosphotransacetylase plus arsenate, i.e.,

$$acetyl\ CoA \xrightarrow[\text{arsenate, phosphotransacetylase}]{\text{alkaline hydrolysis OR}} acetate + CoA \qquad (2)$$

Another enzymatic assay for CoA entails the sequential use of phosphotransacetylase, citrate synthase, and L-glutamate-oxaloacetate transaminase. Coenzyme A is first converted to acetyl CoA which then reacts with radiolabeled oxaloacetate to form radiolabeled citrate. The excess radiolabeled oxaloacetate is converted to radiolabeled aspartate, which is removed from the reaction mixture by addition of a cation exchanger. Radiolabeled citrate in the supernatant is determined and this correlates with the acetyl CoA present in the sample. Sensitivity of this assay is in the picomolar range. Knights and Drew (1988) described a radioisotopic CoA assay in which conversion of CoA to radiolabeled palmitoyl CoA in the presence of radiolabeled palmitate and acyl CoA synthetase was determined. The assay was linear over a wide range of CoA concentrations (1 pmol–2 nmol). Acetyl CoA, dephospho-CoA, or oxidized CoA did not interfere with the assay, making the assay suitable for CoA determinations in pathological states where concentrations of acyl esters of CoA may be altered. The assay is relatively simple to set up and has the advantage of rapid CoA determination in a large number of samples.

Paper chromatography (Nakamura *et al.*, 1972; Smith, 1978) and HPLC also have been used to determine CoA in tissue samples. These methods were described in Section III,A and as previously mentioned, the HPLC method has the added advantage of simultaneous determinations of acyl CoAs.

B. Biosynthesis

After uptake into cells, pantothenic acid is converted to CoA via a number of enzymatic reactions as depicted in Fig. 2. The following sections describe each of these steps in some detail.

It should be pointed out at the outset that although a significant amount of literature is available on pantothenate kinase, its *in vivo* regulation remains obscure. By the end of this section, it will become clear that if CoA derivatives were the only means of regulation for pantothenate kinase, it would be difficult to explain the biosynthesis of CoA. Thus, there must be other factors that stimulate or otherwise regulate its activity and identification of these factors will be pivotal in elucidating the regulation of CoA biosynthesis.

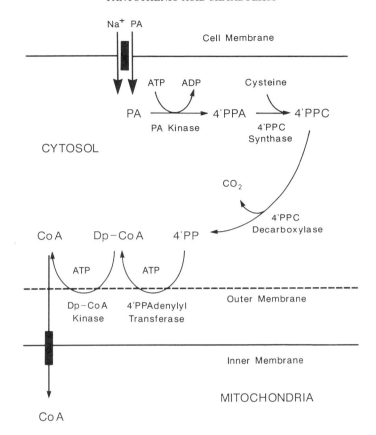

FIG. 2. Schematic representation of CoA metabolism. Pantothenic acid (PA) is taken up by an Na$^+$-dependent uptake process and is converted to 4'-phosphopantothenic acid (4'-PPA) by pantothenate kinase (PA kinase), the rate-limiting enzyme in the biosynthesis of CoA. 4'-Phosphopantothenic acid then condenses with cysteine to form 4'-phosphopantothenoyl cysteine (4'-PPC) which is subsequently decarboxylated to 4'-phosphopantotheine (4'-PP). In the final steps of the synthetic pathway, an adenine moeity from ATP is transferred to 4'-PP to form dephospho-CoA (Dp-CoA) which is subsequently phosphorylated to CoA. Synthesis of CoA, which is cytosolic in cardiac cells is followed by its transport into mitochondria apparently by a specific transport process.

1. *Pantothenate Kinase: The Rate Limiting Step*

The first step in the biosynthetic pathway of CoA is the phosphorylation of pantothenic acid catalyzed by the enzyme pantothenate kinase (EC 2.7.1.33). The 4'-OH position of pantothenic acid reacts via Mg^{2+} and ATP to produce 4'-phosphopantothenic acid (4'-PPA). Partial purification of the rat liver enzyme using ammonium sulfate fractionation (Brown, 1959) and protamine precipitation (Abiko, 1967a) revealed that a 1 : 1 ATP–Mg^{2+} complex was an active substrate for the enzyme. The apparent K_m values for pantothenate and the ATP–Mg complex were 0.011 mM and 1 mM, respectively, and the pH optimum was 6.1 (Abiko *et al.*, 1972). In more recent studies, pantothenate kinase from the rat heart showed a pH optimum between 6 and 9, used ATP–Mg as the nucleotide substrate and displayed apparent K_m values for pantothenate and ATP–Mg of 0.018 mM and 0.6 mM, respectively (Fisher *et al.*, 1985). The enzyme was located in the cytosol in mammalian systems studied (Smith *et al.*, 1978; Skrede and Halvorsen, 1979). Pantothenate kinase was also capable of phosphorylating pantothenate-related substrates such as PaSH, pantothenoyl cysteine, and pantothenyl alcohol (Abiko, 1975).

A large number of studies suggested that pantothenate kinase is an important regulatory step in the overall synthesis of CoA. Abiko *et al.* (1972) reported that rat liver pantothenate kinase was inhibited to varying extents by intermediates of the CoA synthetic pathway, the most significant inhibition observed in the presence of 4′-PP or CoA (about 50% inhibition with 250 μM of either compound). These findings, along with reports that estimated the concentrations of 4′-PP and CoA in rat liver to be approximately 220 and 360 μM, respectively (Nakamura *et al.*, 1970; Kuwagata, 1971), suggested that the kinase was not fully active in liver cells and that regulation by these compounds may be relevant physiologically. Similar results were obtained in another study on rat liver pantothenate kinase (Halvorsen and Skrede, 1982). However, the K_i for CoA (47 μM) was considerably lower than that reported in the previous study. In addition, the acetyl, propionyl, and malonyl esters of CoA were found to be strong inhibitors of pantothenate kinase, with K_i values in the range of 1–3 μM. Inhibition of pantothenate kinase by CoA and its derivates has also been studied in rat kidney (Karasawa *et al.*, 1972), and rat heart (Fisher and Neely, 1985; Fisher *et al.*, 1985). In the kidney, CoA, dephospho-CoA, and 4′-PP were found to be inhibitory, the K_i value for CoA was 72 μM (Karasawa *et al.*, 1972). However, in the rat heart, the K_i value of 0.2 μM for CoA was much lower than that in either liver or kidney (Fisher *et al.*, 1985). In contrast to the results in liver (Halvorsen and Skrede, 1982), acetyl CoA was only slightly more potent than free CoA at inhibiting pantothenate kinase (Fisher *et al.*, 1985). Since the reported concentration of total CoA (free and esterified) in the cytosol of myocardial cells was approximately 14 μM (Idell-Wenger *et al.*, 1978), pantothenate kinase would be expected to be completely inhibited at all times. Thus, for the CoA biosynthetic pathway to operate *in vivo*, other mechanisms of control must exist. One potential regulator of pantothenate kinase is carnitine, since this compound reversed the inhibitory effects of CoA on pantothenate kinase in rat hearts (K_a of 270 μM for deinhibition). While the inhibition of pantothenate kinase by CoA was noncompetitive with respect to pantothenate, deinhibition by carnitine was competitive with respect to CoA, suggesting that carnitine and CoA compete for the same site and that this site is distinct from that occupied by pantothenate (Fisher et al., 1985). Due to its high cytosolic concentration (2.6 mM, Idell-Wenger et al., 1978) carnitine would be expected to counteract at least some of the inhibitory effects of CoA and its esters. However, as predicted in the study by Fisher et al. (1985), the activity of pantothenate kinase would be only 13% of its maximal activity even at the highest physiological concentration of carnitine. Myocardial biosynthesis of CoA in vivo, as determined from pantothenate incorporation into CoA, is estimated to be in the range of 0.15–0.37 nmol/minute/g dry. This rate is 12- to 30-fold lower than maximal rates of myocardial CoA biosynthesis obtained in vitro (Robishaw and Neely, 1984). The results of these studies indicate that the CoA biosynthetic pathway must operate far below its maximal capacity under normal conditions, or that other factors act to deinhibit pantothenate kinase and provide a physiological means of regulation.

The effects of various in vivo and in vitro conditions on cellular CoA levels appear to be mediated by altering the activity of pantothenate kinase. Starvation and diabetes are two conditions that have been studied with respect to pantothenate metabolism. Hepatic CoA levels were significantly elevated in fasted or diabetic rats (Smith et al., 1978). Although the mechanism of this elevation has not been determined, the following explanations have been suggested. Starvation and diabetes cause mobilization of fatty acids, resulting in an increase in the ratio of acylated to unacylated CoA (Randle et al., 1966). By virtue of their hydrophobicity, the long chain derivatives of CoA may bind to membranes and thereby reduce the effective concentrations of inhibitory CoAs. This would result in deinhibition of pantothenate kinase. This theory, however, is not supported by data from the isolated perfused rat heart, since inhibition of pantothenate phosphorylation (indicative of pantothenate kinase inhibition) was observed in the presence of palmitate (Reibel et al., 1981b), a condition known to elevate the long chain acyl CoA pool (Oram et al., 1973). The increase in CoA content in livers of fasted and diabetic animals develops despite an increase in acetyl CoA. This finding is unexpected in view of the observations of Halvorsen and Skrede (1982) that acetyl CoA is a potent inhibitor of CoA synthesis. The authors explained their findings on the basis that the increase in acetyl CoA was probably mainly mitochondrial, since acetyl CoA levels are reported to be 10–30 times higher in mitochondria than in the cytosol (Williamson and Corkey, 1979). Although the increase in acetyl CoA may be mitochondrial, cytosolic acetyl CoA levels may not differ between liver cells of diabetic rats as compared to controls; thus, acetyl CoA may not be a factor. Also, this hypothesis does not satisfactorily explain the elevation of *myocardial* CoA in diabetic or fasted animals, since acetyl CoA and CoA are almost equipotent at inhibiting myocardial pantothenate kinase (Fisher *et al.*, 1985).

A significant increase in the CoA content of liver, skeletal muscle, heart, and kidney of clofibrate-treated rats has been reported (Voltti *et al.*, 1979). The increase in CoA was accompanied by increased incorporation of labeled pantothenic acid into CoA, as well as a decrease in the disappearance of labeled CoA from the respective tissues, suggesting that both the synthetic and the degradative pathways were affected. (Voltti *et al.*, 1979). However, subsequent studies demonstrated that clofibrate treatment significantly increased the activity of pantothenate kinase, indicating that stimulation of the synthetic pathway (rather than inhibition of the degradative pathway) was primarily responsible for the observed increase in CoA levels (Skrede and Halvorsen, 1979; Halvorsen and Skrede, 1982). In addition, the potency of CoA and its derivatives for inhibiting pantothenate kinase was reduced in clofibrate-treated rats (Halvorsen and Skrede, 1982), which may have also contributed to the increased levels of CoA in these rats. The decreased potency of the inhibitors may be a significant determinant of CoA biosynthesis in the clofibrate-treated rats, since CoA levels increased despite elevated levels of acetyl CoA in clofibrate-treated rat livers (Voltti *et al.*, 1979). It is not known, however, whether the increase was in the cytosolic or mitochondrial compartments. An increase in the mitochondrial compartment alone would be irrelevant to the regulation of pantothenate kinase, an exclusively cytosolic enzyme.

Data from *in vitro* studies also suggest pantothenate kinase is the rate-limiting step of the CoA biosynthetic pathway. In isolated rat hearts perfused with palmitate, pyruvate, or β-hydroxybutyrate, i.e., conditions that increase acetyl CoA and decrease free CoA (Garland and Randle, 1964; Oram *et al.*, 1973; Whitmer *et al.*, 1978), the incorporation of pantothenate into CoA was significantly reduced (Reibel *et al.*, 1981a). On the other hand, conditions that decreased acetyl CoA, such as perfusion without substrate or with only glucose, increased the incorporation of pantothenate into CoA (Reibel *et al.*, 1981a), suggesting that acetyl CoA (rather than free CoA) regulates CoA synthesis. This suggestion is intriguing since both acetyl CoA and CoA are equipotent inhibitors of the myocardial pantothenate kinase (Fisher *et al.*, 1985). The contention that CoA synthesis was controlled by acetyl CoA exclusively was not supported by results obtained in hearts perfused with insulin. With insulin added to the perfusate, myocardial acetyl CoA levels increased and free CoA levels decreased. Although the insulin-induced elevation of acetyl CoA was much smaller than that caused by pyruvate, insulin-induced inhibition of pantothenate phosphorylation was much greater than that induced by pyruvate (Reibel *et al.*, 1981a). These data suggest that direct hormonal regulation of pantothenate kinase exists in myocardial cells. Robishaw and Neely (1984) measured the flux of intermediates through each step of the CoA synthetic pathway and found that perfusion with energy substrates decreased pantothenate phosphorylation in the heart. However, without substrate, phosphorylation was stimulated and control of CoA synthesis was shifted from pantothenate kinase to the next step in the pathway, i.e., 4'-phosphopantothenate cysteine synthetase. This suggested that pantothenate kinase was the rate-limiting step in the overall biosynthesis of CoA (Robishaw and Neely, 1984).

Control of CoA synthesis also has been studied in bacterial preparations. Unlike mammalian systems, which lack the ability to synthesize pantothenic acid, *E. coli* and other microorganisms are capable of synthesizing pantothenic acid from β-alanine and pantoic acid (Fig. 1) (Maas, 1952; Brown, 1959). There are, however, mutants of *E. coli* and *S. typhimurium* that cannot synthesize pantothenate (Demerec *et al.*, 1959; Ortega *et al.*, 1975). In a study of an *E. coli* β-alanine auxotroph, strain SJ16, it was observed that CoA synthesis was a direct function of the β-alanine concentration up to 8 μM external β-alanine (Jackowski and Rock, 1981). Beyond that concentration, pantothenate was excreted into the medium, suggesting that utilization, rather than production of pantothenate, was rate limiting. Relatively small amounts of other intermediates of the CoA synthetic pathway were detected in the external medium, further supporting the concept that pantothenate kinase was the rate-limiting step in CoA synthesis. However, in another study, an increase in CoA was observed when the bacterial growth medium was supplemented with 100 μM pantothenate, or with 100 μM β-alanine (Cronan *et al.*, 1982). These findings are not easily reconciled with those from the previous report, and suggest that pantothenate kinase may not be the absolute rate-limiting step in bacterial CoA biosynthesis. It is interesting to note that bacteria can grow apparently normally over a 10-fold range of CoA concentrations, suggesting that strict control of the CoA synthetic pathway is not essential for growth (Alberts and Vagelos, 1966; Polacco and Cronan, 1981; Cronan *et al.,* 1982). On the other hand, there may be other alterations, still undetected, in the metabolic profile produced by the altered CoA content.

2. *Synthesis of 4'-Phosphopantotheine from 4'-Phosphopantothenate*

After phosphorylation of pantothenate, the next step in the biosynthetic pathway of CoA is the condensation of 4'-phosphopantothenate with cysteine to form 4'-phosphopantothenoyl cysteine. The reaction is catalyzed by the enzyme 4'-phosphopantothenoyl cysteine synthetase (EC 6.3.2.5). This enzyme has not been studied to the same extent as pantothenate kinase. The isolated enzyme displays a molecular weight around 37,000. At pH 7.5 (optimal for the enzyme), the K_m value for 4'-phosphopantothenate was 71–83 μM (Abiko, 1967a). The synthetase was found to be specific for 4'-phosphopantothenate and did not catalyze the condensation of pantothenate with cysteine; a CoA synthetic pathway that was originally suggested by Hoaglund and Novelli (1954). The requirement for a phosphorylated substrate appears to be absolute, since the enzyme was competitively inhibited by phosphopantothenyl alcohol, whereas pantothenyl alcohol was without effect (Abiko, 1967a). While the mammalian enzyme appeared to be specific for cysteine (Hoaglund and Novelli, 1954), the bacterial enzyme also utilized β-mercaptoethylamine, the disulfide of β-mercaptoethylamine, or α-methylcysteine, instead of cysteine (Brown, 1959). The condensation step is probably not a rate-controlling reaction since in the isolated perfused rat heart 4'-phosphopantothenate disappeared rapidly when cysteine was added to the perfusion buffer (Robishaw and Neely, 1984). However, in the absence of cysteine, 4'-phosphopantothenate accumulated, suggesting that the availability of substrate was limiting.

4'-Phosphopantetheine is formed by the action of 4'-phosphopantothenoyl cysteine decarboxylase (EC 4.1.1.36) on 4'-phosphopantothenoyl cysteine. Abiko (1967b) demonstrated that the enzyme decarboxylated only the phosphorylated compound and was inhibited by the product. The pH optimum was 8 and the apparent K_m for 4'-phosphopantothenyl cysteine was between 0.15 and 1.5 mM. While pantothenate kinase and 4'-phosphopantothenyl cysteine synthetase required ATP, the decarboxylase was inhibited by ATP. Analogs of ATP, including ADP or AMP, however, did not affect the enzyme. The reaction rate was increased by sulfhydryl (SH) compounds such as dithiotheritol, cysteine, and β-mercaptoethanol, and was inhibited by sulfhydryl reagents, suggesting that the protein—SH groups may be important for activity (Scandurra *et al.*, 1974). The decarboxylation does not appear to be a rate-controlling step in the overall synthetic pathway, since the substrate 4'-phosphopantothenyl cysteine could not be detected in the isolated perfused heart under conditions which caused maximal stimulation of CoA synthesis (Robishaw and Neely, 1984).

3. *Synthesis of CoA from 4'-Phosphopantotheine*

The final two steps of the CoA synthetic pathway involve the conversion of 4'-PP to CoA via dephospho-CoA. The first step, catalyzed by 4'-phosphopantetheine adenyltransferase (EC 2.7.7.3) (dephospho-CoA pyrophosphorylase), involves the addition of an 5'-AMP group from ATP to the phosphopantetheine moiety. This enzyme was reported to have a pH optimum of 8; apparent K_ms were 0.14 mM for 4'-phosphopantetheine, and 1 mM for ATP. Mg^{2+} was required for activity. On the other hand, dephospho-CoA kinase (EC 2.7.1.24), which phosphorylates dephospho-CoA at the 3'-OH position of the ribose, showed a pH optimum of 10, and the K_ms for dephospho-CoA and ATP were 0.12 mM and 0.36 mM, respectively (Abiko, 1975). Attempts to isolate the two enzymes as separate proteins have been unsuccessful. In one study, protamine sulfate treatment plus ammonium sulfate fractionation and purification by cellulose chromatography gave a 250-fold purified preparation (Suzuki *et al.*, 1967). In another study, 18,000-fold purification using sodium dodecyl sulfate-polyacrylamide gel electrophoresis (SDS/PAGE) yielded an enzyme preparation with a molecular weight around 57,000 (the native enzyme obtained by Sephadex G-150 had a molecular weight of about 115,000) (Worrall and Tubbs, 1983). In neither study was it possible to separate the two enzymes, suggesting that they exist as a bifunctional complex. The reaction catalyzed by pyrophosphorylase is the only reversible step in the entire CoA biosynthetic pathway. While dephospho-CoA inhibited the pyrophosphorylase (K_i = 0.02 mM), the kinase did not appear to be inhibited by CoA (Skrede and Halvorsen, 1983).

4. *Localization of CoA Biosynthetic Enzymes*

Localization of CoA biosynthetic enzymes has been studied in some detail. All the participating enzymes have been isolated from the soluble fraction of rat liver (Abiko, 1975), suggesting a cytosolic localization. The first three enzymes (responsible for the conversion of pantothenic acid to 4'-PP) have not been found in mitochondria; mitochondrial preparations do not detectably convert pantothenic acid, 4'-PPA or 4'-phosphopantothenoyl cysteine to their respective products. On the other hand, mitochondria can convert 4'-PP and de-

phospho-CoA to CoA, suggesting that dephospho-CoA pyrophosphorylase and dephospho-CoA kinase exist in the mitochondrial
fraction of liver cells (Skrede and Halvorsen, 1979). Further fractionation of the mitochondria revealed that these enzymes exist in the inner
membrane fraction of mitochondria (Skrede and Halvorsen, 1979). A
later study from the same laboratory demonstrated that these enzymes were localized within the mitochondrial matrix, rather than the
inner membrane (Skrede and Halvorsen, 1983). Although Skrede and
Halvorsen (1983) demonstrated the enzymes within the mitochondrial
matrix, there was no indication that synthesis of CoA occurred within
the matrix. Studies from our laboratory have suggested that CoA synthesis from 4'-PP in mitochondria isolated from rat heart was extra-
mitochondrial (Tahiliani and Neely, 1987a). This suggested that the
CoA synthetic enzymes associated with mitochondria are on the mitochondrial membrane, but that their conformation is outwardly facing,
such that the substrates and products are extramitochondrial, i.e.,
cytosolic.

As mentioned, it has been suggested that dephospho-CoA
pyrophosphorylase and dephospho-CoA kinase exist as a bifunctional
complex, since attempts to separate the activities of the two enzymes
were unsuccessful (Suzuki *et al.,* 1967; Worrall and Tubbs, 1983). In
view of the latter, it is interesting to note that Skrede and Halvorsen
(1983) reported that within the mitochondrial pool of these enzymes,
the dephospho-CoA kinase was not as readily released by disruption
techniques as the 4'-phosphopantetheine adenylyltransferase. It was
suggested that the kinase might be located more superficially (in the
membrane) than the transferase (which might be within the matrix).
This, however, remains to be demonstrated. Whatever the intra-
organelle localization, there is little argument that there are two pools
of 4'-phosphopantetheine adenylyltransferase and dephospho-CoA
kinase. The teleological significance of this finding is presently unclear. Coenzyme A pools are relatively stable under physiological conditions and turnover of the factor appears to be slow. Under varied
pathological conditions, however, CoA content of tissues can change
rapidly (Smith, 1978). It is thus tempting to speculate that physiologically, the cytosolic pool of CoA-synthesizing enzymes maintains CoA
concentrations, and that under pathological conditions, the mitochondrial pool of 4'-phosphopantetheine adenylyltransferase and dephospho-CoA kinase is activated to elevate CoA levels.

In *Saccharomyces cerevisiae* (Baker's yeast), the biosynthetic pathway is apparently not as structured as the bacterial or mammalian
systems. In this organism, a multienzyme complex [CoA-synthesizing

protein complex (CoA-SPC)] may exist, since all the CoA synthesizing activity was found in one large (MW > 200,000) lysate-insoluble protein (Bucovaz *et al.*, 1980).

C. Cellular Distribution

The CoA concentrations vary among all tissues studied. The heart contains approximately 100 nmol/g tissue (Reibel *et al.*, 1982). The contents of kidney, testes, diaphragm, adrenal, and gastrocnemius muscle decrease in that order (Reibel *et al.*, 1982). The reported amounts of total hepatic CoA vary considerably, ranging from 136 to 434 nmol/g tissue (Table II). Perhaps this reflects the various assay methods used since a standard acid extraction procedure was used by most of these groups. The discrepancy in liver CoA levels makes it difficult to estimate the intracellular distribution of CoA. For instance, using the values for total hepatic CoA reported by Garland *et al.* (1965), approximately 80% is mitochondrial (assuming that 1 g of

TABLE II

Hepatic CoA Content as Reported by Several Laboratories

Total tissue CoA (nmol/g wet)				
Free	Acid-soluble	Acid-insoluble	Total	Reference
368[a]	17[b]	53	434	Tubbs and Garland (1964)
77[c]	64[c]	20[c]	160	Garland *et al.* (1965)
			170	Nakamura *et al.* (1972)
			388	Smith *et al.* (1978)
			397	Skrede and Halvorsen (1979)
78	58[b]	30	166	Voltti *et al.* (1979)
119	30[b]	18	167	Voltti and Hassinen (1980)
110	96	27	245	Pacanis *et al.* (1981)
			155[d]	Reibel *et al.* (1981b)
			136[d]	Reibel *et al.* (1982)
226	103	58	387	Swartzentruber and Harris (1987)
127	104[e]			Corkey *et al.* (1988)

[a]Calculated as the difference between total acid soluble CoA and acetyl CoA.

[b]Acetyl CoA levels.

[c]Calculated as sum of cytosolic and mitochondrial CoA (assuming 65 mg mitochondria/g liver).

[d]Calculated from reported values in nmol/g dry (assuming a wet:dry ratio of 3:5).

[e]Calculated as difference between total acid-soluble CoA and free CoA.

liver contains 65.5 mg mitochondria) (Beggs and Randle, 1988) and 20% cytosolic. On the other hand, approximately 65% and 50% of the tissue CoA is mitochondrial if calculations are based on the values reported by Smith *et al.* (1978) and Voltti and Hassinen (1980), respectively. Williamson and Corkey (1979) suggested that 75% of the total hepatic CoA was mitochondrial. Thus, although it is clear that a significant proportion of hepatic CoA is in the mitochondrial compartment, the actual distribution is debatable. Of the total myocardial CoA, nearly 95% was reported to be mitochondrial and the remainder cytosolic (see below) (Idell-Wenger *et al.*, 1978).

It has been generally accepted that the inner mitochondrial membrane is impermeable to CoA. (Yates and Garland, 1966; Ciman and Siliprandi, 1968). However, swelling-induced leakage of CoA from mitochondria has been demonstrated by various groups (Brenner-Holzach and Raaflaub, 1954; Bremer *et al.*, 1972) and more recently, a mitochondrial transport system for CoA was discovered in our laboratory (Tahiliani and Neely, 1987b). It was observed that mitochondria accumulated radiolabeled CoA in two distinct phases. The first was an energy-independent, temperature-independent, nonsaturable process which probably reflected nonspecific binding of CoA to CoA and adenine-recognizing sites in mitochondrial membranes. This was followed by a slower energy- and temperature-dependent, saturable process which probably represents specific CoA transport into mitochondria (Tahiliani and Neely, 1987b). Further work on the transport system suggested that the slower, delayed phase (transport) was driven by the membrane electrical gradient (Tahiliani, 1989). Absolute pH also modulated transport, probably via alteration of the absolute intramitochondrial pH rather than the proton gradient or the absolute medium pH (Fig. 3). In this respect, transport of CoA appeared to be similar to the mitochondrial exchange of aspartate and glutamate which, although electrogenic, was modulated by matrix pH. The transport operates within the physiological range of cytosolic CoA. The proximity of the K_m for CoA (17 μM in heart mitochondria) to the concentration of cytosolic CoA in myocardial cells (14 μM) (Idell-Wenger *et al.*, 1978), suggests that transport regulates distribution of CoA in myocardial cells. More recently, transport has been observed in rat liver mitochondria as well, and results with respect to driving forces were identical to those obtained in rat heart mitochondria (A. G. Tahiliani, unpublished observations).

The existence of a mitochondrial transport system helps reconcile some previously reported data with respect to CoA metabolism. The first of these is the differential distribution of CoA between the mito-

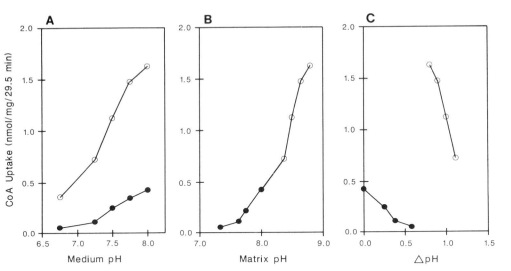

Fig. 3. Dependence of mitochondrial CoA uptake on various pH-related parameters. (A) Coenzyme A uptake increases as medium pH increases such that maximal uptake is seen at pH$_{(ext)}$ 8 in the presence (○) or absence (●) or nigericin. (B) On the other hand, a single curve is obtained when uptake is plotted against matrix pH either in the presence or absence of nigericin. (C) No correlation between the membrane proton gradient and CoA uptake is observed. (Modified from Tahiliani, 1989.)

chondrial and cytosolic fractions. In rat heart, the measured cytosolic CoA was 14 μM, and the mitochondrial content was reported to be about 2.25 mM (Idell-Wenger et al., 1978). Since the mitochondrial content of myocardial tissue was about 53 mg/g wet weight (Idell-Wenger et al., 1978), the total CoA in the mitochondrial compartment was 120 nmol/g of wet tissue, while the cytosolic content was 12 nmol/g of wet tissue weight. Thus, in the myocardium, mitochondria contained about 95% of the total cellular CoA, while the cytosol contains the remainder. The figures reported for heart mitochondria may be overestimated, since mitochondria have a significant capacity for binding CoA (Tahiliani and Neely, 1987b) that was not accounted for in the Idell-Wenger study. Nonetheless, it is clear that the distribution of CoA between mitochondria and cytosol is uneven and that in the heart, mitochondria contain a larger proportion of the total CoA. In rat liver, based on values reported by Garland et al. (1965), the concentration of total CoA in the cytosol was approximately 43 μM (34.4 nmol/g tissue and assuming that 80% of the tissue is water) and the mitochondrial content of CoA was reported to be approximately 2.2 mM (assuming a water volume of 1 μl/mg protein). These figures translate to a distribution of 20% cytosolic and 80% mitochondrial. These results, along with the finding that synthesis of CoA may be extra-mitochondrial (Tahiliani and Neely, 1987a), suggested a transfer system for CoA from the cytosol into the mitochondria. Second, as stated earlier, the CoA content of certain tissues such as heart and liver increases in pathological conditions such as diabetes and starvation (Reibel et al., 1981a,b). Since pantothenate kinase (and, by implication, CoA synthesis) is subject to feedback inhibition by CoA, the transport system could be viewed as a means of removing CoA from the cytosolic compartment and thereby regulating pantothenate kinase and thus overall CoA biosynthesis. The third concept that can be explained on the basis of a CoA transporter is CoA degradation; this is discussed in Section IV,D.

In addition to CoA, carnitine also plays a major role in fatty acid metabolism. It is pertinent in the context of this article to point out that the ratio of carnitine to CoA may relate to the metabolic function of the tissue. For instance, in cardiac tissue, the ratio of cytosolic carnitine to CoA is higher than that in hepatic tissue. Since cytosolic CoA determines the formation of acyl CoA, and cytosolic carnitine directs acyl groups into mitochondria, the higher carnitine : CoA ratio in cardiac tissue may relate to the higher oxidative capacity of this tissue; the lower carnitine : CoA ratio in liver may relate to the higher capacity of this tissue to synthesize triglycerides (for review see Opie, 1979).

D. BIODEGRADATION

Relatively little is known about the regulation of CoA degradation. Degradation is the exact reverse of the biosynthetic pathway until the formation of 4'-PP (Fig. 4). Thus, the first step in the degradation pathway is dephosphorylation of CoA at the 3' position of the ribose to dephospho-CoA. Mitochondria isolated from diverse tissues were capable of degrading CoA to dephospho-CoA; the degradation, however, appeared to be due to lysosomal contamination of mitochondrial preparations (Bremer et al., 1972). This conclusion was based on the finding that the lysosomal fraction degrades CoA to dephospho-CoA and that lysosome-free mitochondria were not capable of degrading CoA. A specific enzyme responsible for the degradation of CoA has not been identified. Instead, dephosphorylation of CoA appeared to be mediated via a nonspecific phosphate-sensitive lysosomal phosphatase. Moreover, CoA was converted to dephospho-CoA in isolated liver mitochondria

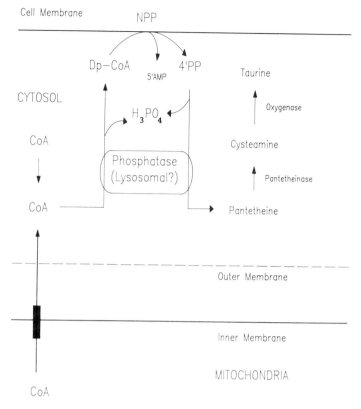

FIG. 4. Schematic representation of CoA degradation. CoA (mitochondrial and/or cyto-solic) appears to be degraded by acid phosphatases, which may be lysosomal in origin, to dephospho-CoA ((Dp-CoA). The latter is degraded to 4′-phosphopantetheine (4′-PP) by a plasma membrane nucleotide pyrophosphatase (NPP). 4′-Phosphopantetheine in turn is dephosphorylated, apparently by lysosomal phosphatase, to pantetheine. Pantetheinase then degrades pantetheine to cysteamine, which is finally converted to taurine.

only when CoA leaked out of mitochondria (the leakage was induced by such means as calcium, oleate, or sonication), suggesting that the conversion occurred outside the mitochondrial matrix (Bremer *et al.*, 1972). The degradation was prevented by P_i or by ATP. This has been explained on the basis of direct inhibition of the enzyme by P_i and rephosphorylation of dephospho-CoA to CoA with ATP.

Dephospho-CoA was degraded to 4′-PP and 5′-AMP by a pyrophosphatase located in the plasma membrane fraction of the liver (Franklin and Trams, 1971; Skrede, 1973). Although the enzyme also degraded CoA, the reaction rate with CoA was less than 10% of the rate with dephospho-CoA (K_m = 300 μM for free CoA). However, the best substrate for the enzyme appeared to be acyl CoA (K_m for acyl CoA was 9 μM) (Trams et al., 1968; Franklin and Trams, 1971). Microsomal and nuclear fractions of the liver were also capable of degrading dephospho-CoA; this, however, appeared to be due to contamination of these fractions by the plasma membrane (Bremer et al., 1972; Skrede, 1973). The K_m for dephospho-CoA was 20 μM, pH optimum was 7.8, and the enzyme was competitively inhibited by nucleotides with a pyrophosphate bond (Skrede, 1973). Activity of the enzyme was also dependent on divalent cations. On the basis of these characteristics, which are similar to those of a nucleotide pyrophosphatase isolated from the plasma membrane of rat liver (Bischoff et al., 1975), it was suggested that dephospho-CoA pyrophosphatase is identical to nucleotide pyrophosphatase. In a study by Lopaschuk and Neely (1987a), the effect of fatty acids on CoA degradation was studied in isolated perfused rat hearts. Coenzyme A levels were elevated by perfusing hearts with cysteine in the absence of any exogenous substrate. Palmitate was then added and tissue CoA content was determined at intervals. It was found that upon addition of palmitate, acyl CoA levels increased. While total CoA levels remained constant in hearts perfused with glucose and pyruvate, a significant decrease in total CoA was observed in hearts perfused with palmitate (Lopaschuk and Neely, 1987a). Furthermore, it was observed that degradation of CoA was restricted to the cytosolic compartment, supporting previous findings that the degrading enzymes were extramitochondrial. This study implied that the loss of total CoA from hearts perfused with palmitate was a result of elevated acyl CoA which would be recognized as a substrate by the nucleotide pyrophosphatase. Since the K_m of the liver enzyme for acyl CoA (8–9 μM) was reported to be much lower than that for free CoA (300 μM), (Franklin and Trams, 1971), the acyl CoA would be degraded more readily than free CoA.

The next step of the degradative pathway is the breakdown of 4'-PP to PaSH by the action of a phosphatase. The source of this phosphatase is not known, but it may be lysosomal since degradation of 4'-PP was inhibited by fluoride (Cavallini et al., 1966; Dupre et al., 1970). Pantetheine thus formed was degraded by pantetheinase to pantothenic acid and cysteamine (Dupre et al., 1970). The pantetheinase from horse kidney exhibited a low pH optimum (4.5–5), had an apparent K_m for PaSH of 5 mM and was inhibited by pantothenic acid (Cavallini et al., 1966). In the rat liver and kidney, the enzyme was found distributed between the microsomal and lysosomal fractions. The reported K_ms were much lower than in horse kidney: 95 μM and 36 μM for liver and kidney, respectively (Abiko, 1975). The pH optimum for the enzyme from rat liver and kidney was between 6 and 7, which was higher than that for the horse kidney.

The final step in the degradative pathway of CoA in mammals is the metabolism of cysteamine to hypotaurine by the action of oxygenase (Cavallini *et al.*, 1966). Bacteria, however, can metabolize pantothenate further to β-alanine and pantoic acid, the reaction being catalyzed by pantothenase (EC 3.1.5.22) (Arias, 1978).

The scattered localization of CoA-degrading enzymes makes it difficult to envision operation of the CoA degradative system *in vivo*. Since the phosphatase responsible for degrading CoA to dephospho-CoA is localized in the lysosomes, CoA would have to be transported into this subcellular compartment (in the case of mitochondrial CoA, an additional step, i.e., efflux from mitochondria would be involved). Dephospho-CoA thus formed would have to exit the lysosomes and be transferred to the plasma membrane where the nucleotide pyrophosphatase is located and the resulting 4'-PP would then have to be transferred back to the lysosomes, where it would undergo further degradation. Alternatively, if one were to assume that the degradation of CoA occurs via breakdown of acyl CoA rather than free CoA, although some of the previously outlined transfer processes would be circumvented, the process would still involve transfer of substrates back and forth between various compartments. Another apparent problem with the latter theory is that it does not provide for degradation of mitochondrial CoA, which makes up a large proportion of cellular CoA. In order to accommodate mitochondrial CoA into this scheme, one would have to speculate that upon efflux from mitochondria, CoA is converted to acyl CoA (the machinery for which is available) and then degraded. In either case, it would appear that the cell is geared to minimize the breakdown of CoA. In view of the slow turnover of CoA, and the fact that CoA acts only as a nonconsumable substrate in reactions requiring it, this may well be the case.

The phosphatase and the nucleotide pyrophosphatase enzymes are apparently not very specific and display high K_ms for the nonacylated substrates; hence, they probably do not provide a fine-tuned control for CoA degradation. Were it assumed that the mitochondrial CoA transport system described by Tahiliani and Neely (1987b) operates in reverse, i.e., mediates efflux of CoA from mitochondria, one could propose that the transport system serves as a mechanism of fine control not only for the distribution of CoA in cell compartments, but also for maintenance of total CoA in the cell via control of degradation. The data of Lopaschuk and Neely (1987a) indicating that the stimulated degradation of CoA caused by addition of fatty acids to the perfusate was restricted to the cytosolic compartment can be reconciled with such a hypothesis.

V. ALTERED PANTOTHENATE METABOLISM

A. HORMONE-INDUCED ALTERATIONS

The effects of hormones on pantothenate metabolism have been studied directly, such as in tissue culture, or indirectly by observing changes induced by conditions in which hormonal control is altered, as in diabetes or food deprivation. Conclusions that effects seen in diabetic or fasted animals are a direct consequence of insulin lack or glucagon excess, however, should be viewed with reservation, since these conditions produce a wide variety of secondary effects. Experimental diabetes significantly increased the CoA content in various tissues. A 2-fold increase in the CoA content of liver was observed as early as 48 hours after induction of diabetes or fasting (Reibel *et al.*, 1981b; Smith *et al.*, 1978). Although myocardial CoA levels were not elevated in the study by Smith *et al.* (1978), Reibel *et al.* (1981b) observed a significant elevation of cardiac content of CoA. A similar increase was also reported by Neely *et al.* (1982) within 6 hours of induction of diabetes. Diabetes and fasting were each associated with little change in the pantothenic acid content of the liver. In the myocardium, no change (in fasted animals), or a large decrease (in diabetic animals) in pantothenic acid content was observed. In rats maintained on a pantothenate-deficient diet, myocardial pantothenate concentrations decreased to approximately 10% of control animals. Despite this massive decrease in pantothenate, diabetes and fasting elevated CoA levels to the same extent observed in pantothenate-sufficient rats (Reibel *et al.*, 1982), suggesting that the effect of these states was on the biosynthetic/degradative pathways rather than on the availability of pantothenate. This hypothesis was further supported by more recent work from this laboratory in which elevation of CoA levels accompanied by decreased pantothenate transport was observed within 24 hours of streptozotocin diabetes (Beinlich *et al.*, 1990). Although the pantothenate transport remained depressed over 10 weeks of diabetes, and pantothenate levels in the myocardium were decreased to approximately 40% of control level, total tissue CoA levels did not decrease over that time period. Within the CoA pool, the diabetes- or fasting-induced increase appears mainly in the acyl rather than free CoA fraction (Smith *et al.*, 1978; Beinlich *et al.*, 1990). It is not known whether this is the cause (see Section IV,B), or a result of the observed increase. The changes in CoA levels are supported by studies in which incorporation of radiolabeled pantothenate into CoA was monitored. Fasting increased incorporation of pantothenate into CoA in rat liver (Smith, 1978) and in heart (Reibel *et al.*, 1981b) *in vivo*. Surprisingly, however, pantothenate incorporation into CoA in hearts isolated from diabetic rats and perfused *in vitro* was significantly depressed (Reibel *et al.*, 1981a; Beinlich *et al.*, 1989). Insulin was found to inhibit pantothenate incorporation into CoA in perfused hearts isolated from normal rats. It was thus suggested that high concentrations of CoA in diabetic or fasted rats could be due to the deinhibition of pantothenate kinase, a result of insulin lack.

The maintenance of high CoA content despite very low pantothenate levels raises some interesting possibilities regarding the homeostasis of CoA. One possibility that has been considered relates to the biosynthetic pathway of CoA. The K_m of pantothenate kinase (the rate-limiting step in CoA biosynthesis) appears to be much lower than the lowest reported levels of pantothenic acid (67 μM, Beinlich *et al.*, 1990) in pantothenate sufficient diabetic rats. However, in pantothenate-deficient diabetic rats, myocardial pantothenate levels decreased to approximately 9 μM (calculated from Reibel *et al.*, 1982), which is about one-half the K_m. The fact that CoA content did not decrease suggests that either the biosynthetic pathway is stimulated in diabetes (i.e., by a decrease in K_m of pantothenate kinase) as was suggested by increased incorporation of [^{14}C]pantothenate into CoA *in vivo*, or that the degradation pathway is affected. There are no available reports on the kinetic characteristics of pantothenate kinase from diabetic tissues. The other aspect is that of CoA degradation. Diabetes might completely inhibit CoA degradation and thereby maintain elevated CoA content despite low pantothenate. Alternatively, CoA degradation products could be shuttled back into the biosynthetic pathway such that very little CoA is completely degraded. Such a system has been proposed for CoA homeostasis in bacteria whereby CoA supplies 4′-PP to the acyl carrier protein, which in turn supplies 4′-PP to the CoA biosynthetic pathway (Fig. 5) (Jackowski and Rock, 1984). However, until the degradative scheme for CoA in mammalian systems is proved beyond mere speculation, these alternatives cannot be confirmed. A third possibility regarding the elevated CoA levels involves the CoA transport system. We have observed that the mitochondrial CoA transport system was significantly inhibited in hearts from 24- and 48-hour

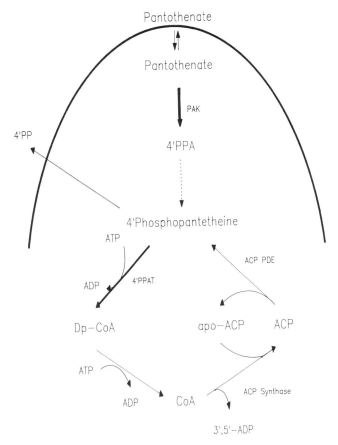

FIG. 5. Recycling of 4'-phosphopantetheine (4'-PP) in *E. coli*. The 4'-PP prosthetic group is transferred from CoA to apo-acyl carrier protein (ACP) to form holo-ACP, a reaction catalyzed by ACP synthase. Holo-ACP is degraded by ACP phosphodiesterase (ACP PDE) to 4'-PP and apo-ACP. The latter can accept 4'-PP from CoA. It is suggested that 4'-PP adenylyl transferase (4'-PPAT) is the other rate-limiting step (the first being pantothenate kinase, PAK), at least in bacteria, since 4'-PP is the only other intermediate which can be detected in the extracellular space. (After Jackowski and Rock, 1984.)

diabetic rats (A. G. Tahiliani, unpublished observations). If, like most other mitochondrial transport systems, the CoA transport system mediates both efflux and influx (particularly if CoA degradation is mitochondrial), decreased efflux may well prevent CoA degradation in diabetic animals. It should also be pointed out that there are significant elevations in the cytosolic compartment (from 37 μm to 93 μM) even though the increase is found mainly in the mitochondrial compartment (from 2.0 to 2.6 nmol/mg protein). The preceding possibility remains to be investigated.

The effect of glucocorticoids on CoA content has also been studied. Nakamura *et al.* (1970) reported decreased CoA content in livers from adrenalectomized rats. More direct evidence of the effects of glucocorticoid and other hormones has been presented by Smith and Savage (1980) by studying the effects of hormones on cultured hepatocytes. Glucagon or dibutyryl cyclic AMP (cAMP) increased, while insulin decreased the incorporation of pantothenate into CoA. While dexamethasone alone did not affect pantothenate incorporation, it potentiated the effects of glucagon or dibutyryl cAMP (Smith and Savage, 1980). These changes in pantothenate incorporation were not accompanied by increased tissue content of pantothenate or by increased uptake of pantothenate, suggesting that the effects of the hormones were on the enzymes of the biosynthetic or degradative pathways, rather than on the availability of pantothenate. The mechanism by which these changes are brought about is not clear. In the study by Smith and Savage (1980), cycloheximide inhibited the basal rate of pantothenate incorporation into CoA and also abolished the stimulatory effect of glucagon and dibutyryl cAMP. This finding suggested that turnover of one (or more) of the enzymes was rapid enough that inhibition of its synthesis could be rate limiting for CoA synthesis. However, the hypothesis that hormonal effects are mediated via protein synthesis does not explain the inhibitory effect of insulin, since insulin stimulates protein synthesis. Neither is the effect of insulin explained on the basis of elevated acetyl CoA levels (see Section IV,B). It could be hypothesized that the effect of insulin is mediated via stimulation of CoA degradation. Lopaschuk and Neely (1987b) have demonstrated, on the contrary, that insulin inhibits the degradation of CoA. Thus the mechanism of the effect of diabetes and insulin on CoA synthesis remains open for investigation.

Hyperthyroidism increases CoA content in rat liver (Tabachanick and Bonnycastle, 1954), and cold exposure increases the uptake of pantothenic acid and the levels of CoA in the liver (Tsujikawa and Kimura, 1981). Since cold exposure increases thyroid activity (Itoh and Kuroshima, 1970), it was suggested that the cold-induced increases in CoA may be related to hyperthyroidism (Tsujikawa and Kimura, 1981). However, the details of the mechanism by which thyroid hormone stimulates CoA synthesis, which may well be mediated via stimulation of protein synthesis, remains to be demonstrated.

B. Pathological Conditions

Beyond diseases reflecting hormonal perturbations, a variety of other pathological conditions also affect pantothenate metabolism. Alcoholism has been studied in some detail. A significant decrease in pantothenate-containing compounds was reported in livers of alcoholics with fatty or cirrhotic livers (Leevy *et al.*, 1960, 1965; Leevy and Baker, 1963; Baker *et al.*, 1964). In alcoholics who did not have an accompanying vitamin deficiency, the decrease in hepatic pantothenate was accompanied by increased circulating pantothenate, suggesting that intestinal absorption and availability of pantothenate were not affected by alcohol. In malnourished alcoholics, however, circulating pantothenate levels also decreased (Tao and Fox, 1976).

Animal studies have reported decreased uptake of pantothenate into the heart (58% of control) and liver (75% of control) of rats treated with ethanol (Israel and Smith, 1987). Despite decreased pantothenate, however, CoA was not decreased in tissues from ethanol-treated animals; a situation somewhat reminiscent of pantothenate metabolism in diabetes. Kondrup and Grunnet (1973) reported similar hepatic CoA content in control rats and those given alcohol for 4 weeks. Similarly, Bode *et al.* (1978) observed only a small increase in hepatic CoA content of rats treated with ethanol for 4 months. In contrast, a more recent study by Smith and co-workers (Israel and Smith, 1987) demonstrated a small (10–22%) *decrease* in myocardial CoA content after approximately 4 weeks of alcoholic treatment. In contrast with the results from *in vivo* studies, acute treatment of hepatocytes with alcohol did not affect pantothenate content (Iannucci *et al.*, 1982). *In vitro* incorporation of pantothenate into CoA, however, was significantly inhibited by alcohol, the effect apparently being mediated by acetaldehyde (Iannucci *et al.*, 1982). Acetaldehyde-induced inhibition in turn, it has been suggested, may be mediated via acetyl CoA (Smith *et al.*, 1987). The magnitude of the decrease in CoA content *in vivo* following chronic alcohol treatment (10–22%) was much smaller than the reported *in vitro* inhibition of pantothenate incorporation into CoA (~20–50% of control in liver), suggesting that other regulatory factors are probably involved *in vivo*. The *in vitro* effects do agree closely with the acute effects of alcohol on pantothenate incorporation into CoA *in vivo,* suggesting that there may be adaptation in response to chronic alcohol use returning CoA levels to normal. The questions that obviously arise are (1) what are the *in vivo* factors responsible for the adaptation; and (2) how long is it before the systems adapt to ethanol. It would be important to carry out systematic studies to determine tissue CoA content at stages of alcohol treatment and determine whether they parallel the ability of tissues *in vivo* (such as the isolated perfused rat heart or hepatocytes) to synthesize CoA from pantothenate. Known regulators of CoA biosynthesis such as acetyl CoA and carnitine would also have to be examined and other regulators identified.

A few studies have investigated pantothenate or CoA metabolism in other pathological conditions. Studies on tumor-bearing mice have reported significantly reduced CoA levels in livers of mice bearing TLX-5 lymphoma or C_3H mammary tumors (McAllister *et al.*, 1982, 1988). Other tumors, such as sarcoma 180 and fibrosarcoma were also associated with decreased hepatic CoA levels, although the decrease was not as dramatic as that in TLX-5 lymphoma or C_3H-bearing mice (McAllister *et al.*, 1988). Similarly, Rapp (1973) reported decreased CoA levels in various organs of animals subjected to various tumors. In parallel with the decrease in hepatic CoA, pantothenate and 4'-phosphopantothenate levels were increased 7- to 10-fold in livers from mice bearing the TLX-5 lymphoma (McAllister *et al.*, 1988). Although the hepatic pantothenate levels were almost similar to those in controls, hepatic 4'-phosphopantothenate levels were significantly elevated in mice bearing sarcoma 180 or fibrosarcoma. The mechanism of these changes is unknown. It was suggested that the increase in pantothenate was the result of CoA degradation in livers from these animals. However, there was no evidence for this speculation. Alternatively, elevated pantothenate could reflect stimulated pantothenate transport. The mechanism of increased pantothenate content could be easily resolved by studying tissue radioactivity after injection of radioactive pantothenate (Smith, 1978; Reibel *et al.*, 1981b). Such a study would also give some idea of the effect of tumors on the rate of incorporation of pantothenate into CoA.

The decrease in acetyl CoA in parallel with decreased "total" CoA provides further support to the hypothesis that acetyl CoA may not be a predominant regulator of CoA biosynthesis as discussed in Section IV,B, since a decrease in acetyl CoA would be expected to elevate CoA levels. Elevation of 4'-phosphopantothenate content suggested stimulation (or deinhibition) of pantothenate kinase. The fact that CoA content was reduced despite a stimulation of pantothenate kinase suggests that, at least under these conditions, some other step(s) in the biosynthetic or degradative pathways determines CoA content. From the limited data available it is not possible to speculate what this step(s) may be.

Other conditions known to affect CoA metabolism are vitamin B_{12}

deficiency (Brass *et al.*, 1990) and Reye syndrome (RS) (Corkey *et al.*, 1988). Total hepatic CoA content was increased as a result of chronic B_{12} deficiency in rats (320 nmol/g wet versus 166 nmol/g wet in controls). The increase was found mainly in the acid-soluble forms of CoA. This condition was associated with decreased methylmalonyl-CoA mutase activity, increased levels of circulating methylmalonic acid and increased propionyl- and methylmalonyl-CoA. The authors suggested that the increase in CoA reflected mitochondrial sequestration of CoA by these acids. Moreover, incubation of isolated hepatocytes with propionic acid caused significant stimulation of pantothenate incorporation into CoA (Brass *et al.*, 1990). In contrast to vitamin B_{12} deficiency, Corkey *et al.* (1988) reported a decrease in the total acid-soluble CoA in livers of patients suffering from RS and medium chain acyl CoA dehydrogenase deficiency (MCAD) (89 nmol/g tissue in RS, 185 nmol/g wet in MCAD versus 261 nmol/g wet in controls). The decrease probably did not reflect a redistribution from the acid-soluble to the acid-insoluble pool of CoA, since long-chain acyl CoA concentrations were not altered in RS (Kang *et al.*, 1982). Within the acid-soluble pool, there was a large shift of CoA from the free form to other short-chain acyl esters (some of which are not normally found) such that free CoA was reduced to less than 10% of control values (154 nmol/g wet in control versus 11 nmol/g wet in RS). The reason for this large decrease in CoA is unclear; one possibility, however is the altered state of mitochondria in RS patients (Partin *et al.*, 1971). Leakage of CoA from damaged mitochondria could lead to its degradation in lysosomes and the plasma membrane. Alternatively, it could be hypothesized that the decrease in CoA was mediated by a 9-fold increase in the acetyl CoA : CoA ratio (0.25 in controls versus 2.2 in RS) which would inhibit pantothenate kinase, and thereby CoA biosynthesis. For that matter, any of the unusual CoA esters which were elevated in RS could exert an inhibitory effect on CoA biosynthesis and thereby decrease CoA levels. The increase in unusual acyl CoA esters was suggested to be due to a primary defect in mitochondrial β-oxidation at the level of various acyl CoA dehydrogenases, since such a defect would prevent medium- and short-chain acyl CoA esters from being metabolized.

C. Implications of Altered CoA Metabolism

It should be obvious by now that the major biological significance of pantothenate relates to its function as a precursor of CoA. Moreover, tissue CoA content does not appear to relate to tissue pantothenate levels. Although this does not necessarily mean abnormal pantothenate homeostasis will not produce dire consequences (as actually suggested by the clinical deficiency studies), we will limit this discussion to the implications of altered CoA metabolism. By virtue of its essential role in acylation reactions, altered CoA metabolism can produce significant effects on biological systems. Diverse enzyme systems are affected by altered CoA metabolism. Most of these effects relate to shifts within the CoA pool, i.e., between free, acid-soluble and acid-insoluble pools, rather than alterations of the entire tissue CoA pool.

Normally, most cellular CoA is in the unacylated form, i.e., as CoASH. However, as demonstrated by *in vitro* experiments in isolated perfused rat hearts, acylated CoA increases dramatically in hearts perfused with fatty acids or other substrates (Oram *et al.*, 1973; Olson *et al.*, 1978). The ratio of acyl CoA to free CoA has been shown to be an important determinant of the activity of a number of enzymes. Pyruvate dehydrogenase was regulated by the acetyl CoA : CoA ratio (Kerbey *et al.*, 1979) while α-ketoglutarate dehydrogenase was regulated by the succinyl CoA : CoA ratio (LaNoue *et al.*, 1972). The ratio of succinyl CoA : acetyl CoA determines the activity of citrate synthase (LeNoue *et al.*, 1972), while pyruvate carboxylase is stimulated by acetyl and other esters of CoA (Scrutton and Utter, 1967; Cooper and Benedict, 1968). Long-chain acyl esters of CoA are known to affect multiple systems, including carnitine acetyltransferase (Chase, 1967), mitochondrial tricarboxylate transport (Shug and Shrago, 1973), adenine nucleotide translocation (Pande and Blanchaer, 1971; Shug and Shrago, 1973; Ho and Pande, 1974), oxidative phosphorylation (Pande and Blanchaer, 1971; Borutaite *et al.*, 1989), fatty acyl CoA synthetase (Oram *et al.*, 1975), glutamate and malate dehydrogenases (Kawaguchi and Bloch, 1976), and the cardiac sodium pump (Wood *et al.*, 1977; Kakar *et al.*, 1987). Hence, abnormal CoA metabolism can adversely affect a number of systems including those of energy metabolism.

The effect of altered total CoA content is perhaps best exemplified by the effects of maleate on biological systems. Maleate is the *cis* isomer of fumarate which can accept CoA from succinyl CoA, a reaction mediated by succinyl CoA : 3-oxoacid CoA transferase (Fenselau and Wallis, 1974; White and Jencks, 1976). In this process, CoA is converted to a stable thioether which is metabolically inert (Pacanis and Rogulski, 1981; Pacanis *et al.*, 1981). Upon incubation of isolated mitochondria with maleate, a rapid and dramatic decrease in total CoA content is observed (Pacanis *et al.*, 1981). Similarly, CoA in kidneys from rats treated with maleate is significantly reduced in amount (Pacanis *et al.*, 1981). The effect is most prominent in kidney and not observed in liver; this is consistent with the high activity of enzyme in kidney and lack of the enzyme in liver (Williamson *et al.*, 1971; Tildon and Sevdalian, 1972). The most prominent effects of maleate *in vitro* include inhibition of oxidation of CoA-dependent substrates, i.e., α-keto-glutarate, pyruvate, palmitoyl carnitine, and acetoacetate, and inhibition of oxygen uptake and oxidative phosphorylation (Rogulski *et al.*, 1974). In addition, in rats treated with maleate, renal ATP levels fall to about 20% of normal, the cytosolic NAD : NADH ratio increases, and renal gluconeogenesis is inhibited (Rogulski *et al.*, 1975). The effects of maleate are manifested as Fanconi syndrome, with marked diuresis, phosphaturia, glycosuria, and aminoaciduria (Angielski and Rogulski, 1975). Impairment of renal function by maleate has been reported in dogs (Berliner *et al.*, 1950), rabbits (Angielski and Rogulski, 1962), and rats (Harrison and Harrison, 154; Worthen, 1963). Although the effects of maleate are restricted to the kidney (probably, as mentioned, due to abundance of the transferase in that organ), these studies with maleate underscore the importance of CoA for proper functioning of biological systems.

VI. OTHER ROLES OF PANTOTHENIC ACID

A. ACYL CARRIER PROTEIN OF FATTY ACID SYNTHETASE

Although CoA accounts for a large proportion of cellular pantothenic acid, other cellular molecules also contain the pantothenic acid moeity. One such form of bound pantothenic acid is the acyl carrier protein (ACP). Although evidence suggests that ACP may be associated with a number of proteins or protein complexes, ACP associated with fatty acid synthetase is perhaps best studied. Fatty acid synthetase is an ubiquitous complex of seven soluble enzymes, well characterized in bacteria and plants (Perkins *et al.*, 1962; Volpe and Vagelos, 1973). The components of the complex appear to be less organized in mammalian species and individual components of the mammalian complex have yet to be separated. Initial studies in bacterial cells showed that the ACP contains residues of β-alanine and taurine (which is an oxidation product of cysteamine), and these findings established a link between ACP and CoA, since CoA also contained these components (Sauer *et al.*, 1964; Majerus *et al.*, 1965a). Further studies demonstrated that the ACP contained 1 mole of pantoic acid and 1 mole of phosphate per mole of protein (Majerus *et al.*, 1965b). The absence of adenine and ribose units suggested that ACP contained the 4'-PP part of CoA. This was confirmed by isolating the prosthetic group of ACP following alkaline hydrolysis and incubating it with ATP, dephospho-CoA pyrophosphorylase, and dephospho-CoA kinase, and identifying the product as CoA. Further studies revealed that the 4'-PP moeity was attached to ACP by a phosphate ester bond through the serine hydroxyl group of the ACP protein (Majerus *et al.*, 1965a,b). Subsequently, mammalian (Volpe and Vagelos, 1973) and avian ACP (Williamson and Wakil, 1966) were also found to contain 4'-PP as the prosthetic group. Acyl carrier protein of *E. coli* was isolated and the sequence was found to contain 77 residues with two serines at positions 27 and 36. 4'-Phosphopantetheine was found to be bound covalently to the serine at the 36 position. Mammalian ACP was also covalently attached to 4'-PP by the same type of bond utilizing serine at position 36 of the rabbit fatty acid synthetase (Smith and Libertini, 1979) and at position 231 of the rat fatty acid synthetase, which corresponds to serine 36 of rabbit and *E. coli* (Witkowski *et al.*, 1987). Further, mammalian ACP exhibited about 25% sequence homology with the monofunctional acyl carrier proteins of *E. coli,* spinach, and barley (Witkowski *et al.*, 1987). Similarly, chicken and *E. coli* ACPs were found to be approximately 28% homologous, whereas chicken and rat ACPs were 65% homologous (Huang *et al.*, 1989). Thus it appeared that ACP from mammalian and avian sources were more similar to each other than ACPs from bacteria and plants, which are more closely related to each other. Investigation of the three-dimensional structure of *E. coli* and chicken ACP suggested that there are four α helices, three of which line a hydrophobic cavity (which may be involved in the binding and transport of acyl groups) (Mayo and Prestegard, 1985; Holak *et al.*, 1988; Huang *et al.*, 1989).

The biologically active holo-ACP was synthesized from apo-ACP and CoA; the reaction was catalyzed by holo-ACP synthetase with 3',5'-ADP as the reaction product (Vagelos and Larrabee, 1967; Elovson and Vagelos, 1968). The enzyme had apparent K_ms of 0.4 μM and 150 μM for apo-ACP and CoA respectively. Although holo-ACP synthetase represented only 0.01% of the total soluble protein in *E. coli,* the total activity of 10 nmol holo-ACP formed/min was sufficient to account for all the synthesis of ACP in exponentially growing cells, since *E. coli* contain only 50 nM ACP (Alberts and Vagelos, 1966). Release of apo-ACP (inactive ACP) and 4'-PP from holo-ACP is brought about by ACP hydrolase. The enzyme is very specific for intact ACP, since peptides of the ACP were not hydrolyzed by ACP hydrolase (Vagelos and Larrabee, 1967). Cross-reactivity between ACP from at least two different bacterial strains has been observed (Vagelos and Larrabee, 1967).

Since 4'-PP is an intermediate in both the biosynthesis and degradation of CoA, either of these pathways could supply 4'-PP for synthesis of holo-ACP. When pantothenate auxotrophs were transferred from a pantothenate-supplemented medium to a pantothenate-deficient medium, the prosthetic group of ACP was obtained from CoA, suggesting a precursor–product relationship between CoA and ACP (Powell *et al.*, 1969). In these organisms, it was also found that at low concentrations of pantothenate, about 94% of the pantothenate was in the ACP pool and only at higher concentrations of pantothenate was CoA synthesized. Also, the levels of ACP remained constant beyond 0.5 μM pantothenate while the levels of CoA increased with increasing concentrations of pantothenate. When these bacteria were transferred to a pantothenate-deficient medium, ACP content remained constant, while the level of CoA decreased significantly. These results suggested that ACP was maintained at the expense of CoA in bacteria (Vagelos *et al.*, 1966). The reverse was observed in another study where pantothenate auxotrophs were incubated with a limited amount of labeled pantothenate. Almost all the radioactivity was found in the ACP pool of cells which had stopped growing due to lack of pantothenate (Alberts and Vagelos, 1966). When these cells were transferred to a medium containing unlabeled pantothenate, the radioactivity was shifted to the CoA pool. These results suggest that ACP also acted as a precursor for CoA. It is interesting to note that the turnover rate for 4'-PP was much faster than that for the entire ACP (Alberts and Vagelos, 1966). It was thus suggested that a small part of the fatty acid synthetase complex (containing the prosthetic group) was periodically removed and replaced. Because of the absolute dependence of the synthetase activity on the prosthetic group, this turnover could provide a fine control of fatty acid synthesis.

The role of the ACP : apo-ACP ratio in regulating lipid biosynthesis was studied by Jackowski and Rock (1983). These studies demonstrated that in normally growing *E. coli,* apo-ACP concentrations are very low and remain so even when the concentration of CoA, the presursor for ACP, is severely depressed (i.e., a condition where the supply of the prosthetic group was absent) confirming previous observations that ACP levels are maintained at the expense of CoA. Also, in one strain of *E. coli* (MP4) which is conditionally defective in ACP synthetase, normal growth (suggesting normal lipid synthesis) was observed despite a large pool (70% of total ACP) of apo-ACP. It was suggested that normal cells contain all the ACP in the active form and that the ACP : apo-ACP ratio may not be important in lipid biosynthesis. In another study (Jackowski and Rock, 1984), metabolism of 4'-PP in *E. coli* was studied using double-label experiments, in which the intracellular pool of pantothenate-containing compounds (ACP and CoA) was labeled first with β-[3-^{3}H]alanine and then with β-[1-^{14}C]alanine. Since the precursor in the latter part of the experiment was β-[1-^{14}C]alanine, excreted metabolites of the biosynthetic pathway would contain only ^{14}C, whereas if they originated from the degradative pathway, they would contain ^{14}C and ^{3}H. The ratio of ^{3}H : ^{14}C 4'-PP in the extracellular medium was identical to that of intracellular ACP, suggesting that the excreted 4'-PP was derived from the degradation of ACP and not from the biosynthetic pathway leading to CoA (Jackowski and Rock, 1984). Pantothenate and 4'-PP were the only two intermediates of the pathway that accumulated in the medium of cells that were incubated with β-alanine, suggesting that the enzymes responsible for the consumption of these two compounds are probably the rate-controlling steps (Jackowski and Rock, 1984) (Fig. 5). The results of this study suggest that 4'-PP adenyl transferase may be an additional rate-controlling step in the metabolism of pantothenate-containing compounds. The finding that 4'-PP excreted into the extracellular compartment could not be utilized by the cells has important implications (at least in bacteria) with respect to the control of CoA and ACP concentrations, since it provided a mechanism by which an irreversible decrease in the content of pantothenate-containing compounds may be achieved.

As previously mentioned, fatty acid synthetase is less structured in mammalian systems and consequently has not yet been resolved into its constituent enzymes. Early studies demonstrated that while the fatty acid synthetase complex from mammalian tissues existed as a multifunctional complex (Majerus et al., 1965a), it contained a protein-bound 4'-PP moiety, identified using methods used previously to identify the protein-bound 4'-PP molecule in E. coli (Larrabee et al., 1965). The pigeon fatty acid synthetase complex can be reversibly dissociated into two separate subunits by limited elastase proteolysis (Kumar et al., 1970; Kumar and Porter, 1972; Lornitzo et al., 1974; Puri and Porter, 1981, 1982). Elastase digestion of rabbit mammary gland fatty acid synthetase released a 4'-PP containing protein similar in size and homologous to the ACP of E. coli; this suggested that the multifunctional complex of mammals may have arisen from gene fusion of monofunctional ancestors (McCarthy et al., 1983).

The turnover rate of 4'-PP has been studied in diverse mammalian tissues. In the rat liver, the half-life for fatty acid synthetase was 71–108 hours, while maximal incorporation of 4'-PP into fatty acid synthetase was found within 14 hours. This suggested that while the enzyme complex may be synthesized in toto, the prosthetic group may be removed and replaced many times before the entire complex is catabolized (Tweto *et al.*, 1971). Further studies on liver, adipose tissue, and brain also demonstrated that 4'-PP of ACP was replaced in hours, while the fatty acid synthetase had a half-life in days (Volpe and Vagelos, 1973). The turnover was the slowest in brain and the fastest in rat liver. Moreover, the time course of the incorporation of labeled 4'-PP into CoA or ACP revealed that incorporation into CoA always preceded that into ACP, which supports the previous suggestion that the prosthetic group of ACP may be obtained from CoA. Earlier studies showed no evidence for ACP hydrolase in mammalian tissues despite clear demonstrations of turnover of the prosthetic group of ACP (Volpe and Vagelos, 1973), raising the question of the mode of regulation of fatty acid synthetase. One suggestion was that since acetyl CoA carboxylase (the first enzyme in the fatty acid biosynthetic pathway) was altered *in vitro* by phosphorylation–dephosphorylation, fatty acid synthesis in mammalian systems may be controlled by ATP or AMP (Carlson and Kim, 1973). More recent studies, however, found ACP hydrolase in rat liver (Roncari, 1974) and a subsequent study reported its partial purification (Sobhy, 1979). All of these studies used 3-day fasted rats; activity was not detectable in fed or 2-day fasted animals. Evidence for the existence of an enzyme capable of converting apo-fatty acid synthetase into the holoenzyme, the other factor involved in the turnover of 4'-PP, has been presented in mammalian systems (Yu and Burton, 1974; Craig *et al.*, 1972).

The effect of altered nutritional status on turnover of the prosthetic group of ACP has been studied. Decreased exchange of 4'-PP between CoA and fatty acid synthetase in livers from starved rats was followed by increased exchange during fat-free feeding (Volpe and Vagelos, 1973). This is compatible with findings noted above; ACP hydrolase was detected only in 3-day starved animals (Sobhy, 1979). Since starvation causes profound increases in fatty acid liberation, fatty acid synthesis would be expected to minimized and this could account for the observed increase in activity of the hydrolase, and thereby decreased activity of fatty acid synthetase. On the other hand, the reverse would be true during fat-free feeding.

B. ACYL CARRIER PROTEIN OF OTHER PROTEIN COMPLEXES

From the previous account, it is obvious that ACP (and thus 4'-PP) is an essential part of the fatty acid synthetase complex and thus fatty acid synthesis. There is evidence in the literature suggesting that 4'-PP may also be an essential part of other proteins (or protein complexes). One study reported the isolation of two proteins containing 4′-PP moieties from monkey brain (Reichelt, 1971). Although the function of these proteins was not known, one of them could be acylated, suggesting that it may be an acyl carrier group in some brain enzyme. Citrate lyase, which catalyzes the cleavage of citrate to acetate and oxaloacetate, from *Klebsiella aerogenes* contains 3 mol of phosphopantothenate/mol of enzyme (Srere *et al.*, 1972). This was later confirmed in a pantothenate auxotroph of *Klebsiella pneumoniae,* which incorporated [^{14}C]pantothenate solely into the ACP of citrate lyase (Singh *et al.,* 1975). Activity of the enzyme was dependent on the *S*-acetyl moeity of the cysteamine residue of 4′-PP (Dimroth *et al.,* 1973; Basu *et al.,* 1983). In *E. coli,* the synthesis of membrane-derived oligosaccharides was catalyzed by a system that was composed of a membrane enzyme and a soluble factor (Weissborn and Kennedy, 1984). The soluble factor has been isolated and is identical to ACP of fatty acid synthetase (Therisod *et al.,* 1986). It is interesting to note that the prosthetic group of ACP (4′-PP) is not required for the synthesis of membrane-derived oligosaccharides, showing that the function of ACP in lipid synthesis is different from its function in oligosaccharide synthesis (Therisod and Kennedy, 1987). Other studies on *Neurospora crassa* have demonstrated that one subunit of cytochrome *c* oxidase and two subunits of ATPase/ATP synthetase bear a covalent derivative of pantothenic acid (Plesofsky-Vig and Brambl, 1984; Brambl and Plesofsky-Vig, 1986). An additional study showed that the pantothenate derivative was 4′-PP, and also presented evidence for the existence of at least three other cytoplasmic proteins derived from pantothenic acid, one of which was fatty acid synthetase (Lakin-Thomas and Brody, 1985). Thus there seem to be a number of proteins besides fatty acid synthetase that contain 4′-PP as an essential part. The prosthetic group may act as either a regulatory unit of these proteins or may serve as a carrier group in an enzymatic reaction (as with fatty acid synthetase).

VII. SUMMARY

In summary, the vitamin pantothenic acid is an integral part of the acylation carriers, CoA and acyl carrier protein (ACP). The vitamin is readily available from diverse dietary sources, a fact which is underscored by the difficulty encountered in attempting to induce pantothenate deficiency. Although pantothenic acid deficiency has not been linked with any particular disease, deficiency of the vitamin results in generalized malaise clinically. In view of the fact that pantothenate is required for the synthesis of CoA, it is surprising that tissue CoA levels are not altered in pantothenate deficiency. This suggests that the cell is equipped to conserve its pantothenate content, possibly by a recycling mechanism for utilizing pantothenate obtained from degradation of pantothenate-containing molecules.

Although the steps involved in the conversion of pantothenate to CoA have been characterized, much remains to be done to understand the regulation of CoA synthesis. In particular, in view of what is known about the *in vitro* regulation of pantothenate kinase, it is surprising that the enzyme is active *in vivo,* since factors that are known to inhibit the enzyme are present in excess of the concentrations known to inhibit the enzyme. Thus, other physiological regulatory factors (which are largely unknown) must counteract the effects of these inhibitors, since the pantothenate-to-CoA conversion is operative *in vivo.* Another step in the biosynthetic pathway that may be rate limiting is the conversion of 4′-phosphopantetheine (4′-PP) to dephospho-CoA, a step catalyzed by 4′-phosphopantetheine adenylyltransferase. In mammalian systems, this step may occur in the mitochondria or in the cytosol. The teleological significance of these two pathways remains to be established, particularly since mitochondria are capable of transporting CoA from the cytosol.

Altered homeostasis of CoA has been observed in diverse disease states including starvation, diabetes, alcoholism, Reye syndrome (RS), medium-chain acyl CoA dehydrogenase deficiency, vitamin B_{12} deficiency, and certain tumors. Hormones, such as glucocorticoids, insulin, and glucagon, as well as drugs, such as clofibrate, also affect tissue CoA levels. It is not known whether the abnormal metabolism observed in these conditions is the result of altered CoA metabolism or whether CoA levels change in response to hormonal or nonhormonal perturbations brought about in these conditions. In other words, a cause–effect relation remains to be elucidated. It is also not known whether the altered CoA metabolism (be it cause or result of abnormal metabolism) can be implicated in the manifestations of a disease.

Besides CoA, pantothenic acid is also an integral part of the ACP molecule. Thus, altered pantothenic acid homeostasis would be expected to affect not only the fatty acid catabolism pathways (by the involvement of CoA in fatty acid activation, β-oxidation pathway, and the Krebs cycle) but also in the fatty acid synthetic pathway (by virtue of the involvement of ACP in fatty acid synthase). More recent studies have approached these problems at a molecular level and such studies may well provide some of the answers being sought currently. For instance, now that the structure of ACP is known, it will be of significant interest to determine how the protein functions and how it is regulated. It will also be of interest to determine whether the structure is altered in disease states and how these alterations, if any, relate to the manifestations of disease. It is hoped that this chapter will stimulate interest in the field of pantothenic acid, CoA, and ACPs not only at the molecular level, but also at the tissue and whole body level.

ACKNOWLEDGMENT

Work was supported by Grant HL37937 from the National Institutes of Health and the Weis Center for Research.

REFERENCES

Abiko, Y. (1967a). Investigations of pantothenic acid and its related compounds. IX. Biochemical studies. 4. Separation and substrate specificity of pantothenate kinase and phosphopantothenoylcysteine synthetase. *J. Biochem. (Tokyo)* **61**, 290–299.

Abiko, Y. (1967b). Investigations on pantothenic acid and its related compounds. X. Biochemical studies. 5. Purification and substrate specificity of pantothenoylcysteine decarboxylase from rat liver. *J. Biochem. (Tokyo)* **61**, 300–308.

Abiko, Y. (1975). Metabolism of coenzyme A. *In* "Metabolic Pathways" (D. Greenburg, ed.), Vol. 7, pp. 1–25. Academic, New York.

Abiko, Y., Ashida, S., and Shimuzu, M. (1972). Purification and properties of D-pantothenate kinase from rat liver. *Biochim. Biophys. Acta* **268**, 364–372.

Alberts, A. W., and Vagelos, P. R. (1966). Acyl carrier protein. VII. Studies of acyl carrier protein and coenzyme A in *Escherichia coli* pantothenate or β-alanine auxotrophs. *J. Biol. Chem.* **241**, 5201–5204.

Angielski, S., and Rogulski, J. (1962). Effect of maleic acid upon the kidney. I. Oxidation of Krebs cycle intermediates by various tissues of maleate-treated rats. *Acta Biochim. Pol.* **9**, 357–365.

Angielski, S., and Rogulski, J. (1975). Metabolic studies in experimental renal dysfunction resulting from maleate administration. *In* "Biochemical Aspects of Renal Function" (S. Angielski and U. C. Dubach, eds.), pp. 86–105. Huber, Bern.

Arias, R. K. (1978). Kinetic study on the reaction mechanism of pantothenase: Existence of an acyl–enzyme intermediate and role of general acid catalysis. *Biochemistry* **17**, 4932–4938.

Axelrod, A. E. (1981). Role of the B vitamins in the immune response. *Adv. Exp. Med. Biol.* **135**, 93–106.

Baker, H., Frank, O., Ziffer, H., Goldfarb, S., Leevy, C. M., and Sobotka, H. (1964). Effect of hepatic disease on liver β-complex vitamin titres. *Am. J. Clin. Nutr.* **14**, 1–6.

Baker, H., Frank, O., Thomson, A. D., and Feingold, S. (1969). Vitamin distribution in red blood cells, plasma and other body fluids. *Am. J. Clin. Nutr.* **22**, 1469–1475.

Barbarat, B., and Podevin, A. (1986). Pantothenate-sodium cotransport in renal brush border membranes. *J. Biol. Chem.* **261**, 14455–14460.

Basu, T. K. (1981). The significance of vitamins in prenatal life. *Int. J. Environ. Stud.* **12**, 31–35.

Basu, A., Subramanian, S., Hiremath, S. S., and Sivaraman, C. (1983). S-Acylated residues of the acyl-carrier protein subunit of *Klebsiella aerogenes* citrate lyase. *Biochem. Biophys. Res. Commun.* **114**, 310–317.

Bean, W. B., and Hodges, R. E. (1954). Pantothenic acid deficiency induced in human subjects. *Proc. Soc. Exp. Biol. Med.* **86**, 693–698.

Beggs, M., and Randle, P. J. (1988). Activity of branched-chain 2-oxo acid dehydrogenase complex in rat liver mitochondria and in rat liver. *Biochem. J.* **256**, 929–934.

Beinlich, C. J., Robishaw, J. D., and Neely, J. R. (1989). Metabolism of pantothenic acid in hearts of diabetic animals. *J. Mol. Cell. Cardiol.* **21**, 641–650.

Beinlich, C. J., Naumovitz, R. D., Song, W. O., and Neely, J. R. (1990). Myocardial metabolism of pantothenic acid in chronically diabetic rats. *J. Mol. Cell. Cardiol.* **22**, 323–332.

Berliner, R. W., Kennedy, T. J., and Hilton, J. G. (1950). Effect of maleic acid on renal function. *Proc. Soc. Exp. Biol. Med.* **75**, 791–799.

Bischoff, E., Tran-Thi, T. A., and Decker, K. F. (1975). Nucleotide pyrophosphatase of rat liver. A comparative study on the enzymes solubilized and purified from plasma membrane and endoplasmic reticulum. *Eur. J. Biochem.* **51**, 353–61.

Bode, C., Kono, H., and Bode, J. C. (1978). Effect of chronic ethanol administration on hepatic content of coenzyme A, carnitine and their acyl esters in rats fed a standard diet or a diet with low protein content. *Hoppe-Seyler's Z. Physiol. Chem.* **359**, 1401–1406.

Bonjour, J.-P. (1980) Vitamins and alcoholism. V. Riboflavin, VI. Niacin, VII. Pantothenic acid, and VII. Biotin. *Int. J. Vitam. Nutr. Res.* **50**, 425–440.

Borutaite, V., Mildaziene, V., Ivanoviene, L., Kholodenko, B., Toleikis, A., and Praskevicius, A. (1989). The role of long-chain acyl-CoA in the damage of oxidative phosphorylation in heart mitochondria. *FEBS Lett.* **243**, 264–266.

Brambl, R., and Plesofsky-Vig, N. (1986). Pantothenate is required in *Neurospora crassa* for assembly of subunit peptides of cytochrome c oxidase and ATPase/ATP synthetase. *Proc. Natl. Acad. Sci. U.S.A.* **83**, 3644–3648.

Brass, E. P., Tahiliani, A. G., Allen, R. H., and Stabler, S. P. (1990). Coenzyme A metabolism in the vitamin B deficient rat. *J. Nutr.* **120**, 290–297.

Bremer, J., Wotjczak, A., and Skrede, S. (1972). The leakage and destruction of CoA in isolated mitochondria. *Eur. J. Biochem.* **25**, 190–197.

Brenner-Holzach, O., and Raaflaub, J. (1954). Effects of swelling on liver mitochondria. *Helv. Physiol. Pharmacol. Acta* **12**, 242–248.

Brown, G. (1959). The metabolism of pantothenic acid. *J. Biol. Chem.* **234**, 370–378.

Brown, G. M., and Williamson, J. M. (1982). Biosynthesis of riboflavin, folic acid, thiamine and pantothenic acid. *Adv. Enzymol.* **53**, 345–381.

Bucovaz, E. T., Tarnowski, S. J., Morrison, W. C., Macleod, R. M., Morrison, J. C., Sobhy, C. M., Rhoades, J. L., and Fryer, J. E. (1980). Coenzyme A-synthesizing protein complex of *Sacchromyces cerevisiae*. *Mol. Cell. Biochem.* **30**, 7–26.

Bull, N. L., and Buss, D. H. (1982). Biotin, pantothenic acid and vitamin E in the British household food supply. *Hum. Nutr.: Appl. Nutr.* **36A**, 190–196.

Carlson, C. A., and Kim, K. H. (1973). Regulation of hepatic acetyl coenzyme A carboxylase by phosphorylation and dephosphorylation. *J. Biol. Chem.* **248**, 378–380.

Cavallini, D., DeMarco, C., Scandurra, R., Dupre, S., and Graziani, M. (1966). The enzymatic conversion of cysteamine to hypotaurine. Purification and properties of the enzyme. *J. Biol. Chem.* **241**, 3189–3196.

Chase, J. F. A. (1967). The substrate specificity of carnitine acetyltransferase. *Biochem. J.* **104**, 510–518.

Ciman, M., and Siliprandi, N. (1968). On the oxidation of alpha-oxobutyrate by isolated mammalian mitochondria. *Biochim. Biophys. Acta* **162**, 164–169.

Cohenour, S. H., and Calloway, D. H. (1972). Blood, urine and dietary pantothenic acid levels of pregnant teenagers. *Am. J. Clin. Nutr.* **25**, 512–517.

Cooper, T. G., and Benedict, C. R. (1968). Regulation of pyruvate carboxylase by coenzyme A and acyl coenzyme A thioesters. *Biochemistry* **7**, 3032–3036.

Corkey, B. E., Brandt, M., Williams, R. J., and Williamson, J. R. (1981). Assay of short chain acyl coenzyme A in tissue extracts by high pressure liquid chromatography. *Anal. Biochem.* **118**, 30–41.

Corkey, B. E., Hale, D. E., Glennon, C., Kelley, R. I., Coates, P. M., and Kilpatrick, L. (1988). Relationship between unusual hepatic acyl coenzyme A profiles and the pathogenesis of Reye syndrome. *J. Clin. Invest.* **82**, 782–788.

Craig, M. C., Dugan, P. E., and Meusing, R. A. (1972). Comparative effects of dietary regimens on the levels of coenzymes regulating the synthesis of fatty acids and cholesterol in rat liver. *Arch. Biochem. Biophys.* **151**, 129–136.

Cronan, J. E., Littel, K. J., and Jackowski, S. (1982). Genetic and biochemical analyses of pantothenate biosynthesis in *Escherichia coli* and *Salmonella typhirium*. *J. Bacteriol.* **149**, 916–922.

Cupo, M. A., and Donaldson, W. E. (1986). Effect of pantothenic acid deficiency on lipogenesis in the chick. *Nutr. Rep. Int.* **33**, 147–155.

Demerec, M., Lahr, E. L., Balbinder, E., Miyake, T., Mack, C., Mackay, D., and Ishidu, J. (1959). Bacterial genetics. *Carnegie Inst. Wash. Yearb.* **58**, 433–439.

Dimroth, P., Dittmar, W., Walther, G., and Eggerer, H. (1973). The acyl carrier protein of citrate lyase. *Eur. J. Biochem.* **37**, 305–315.

Dupre, S. M., Graziani, M., Rosei, M., Fabi, A., and Grosso, E. (1970). The enzymatic breakdown of pantotheine to pantothenic acid and cysteamine. *Eur. J. Biochem.* **16**, 571–578.

Eissenstat, B. R., Wyse, B. W., and Hansen, R. G. (1986). Pantothenic acid status of adolescents. *Am. J. Clin. Nutr.* **44**, 931–937.

Elovson, J., and Vagelos, P. R. (1968). Acyl carrier protein synthatase. X. Acyl carrier protein synthetase. *J. Biol. Chem.* **243**, 3603–3611.

Fenselau, A., and Wallis, K. (1974). Substrate specificity and mechanism of action of acetoacetate coenzyme A transferase from rat heart. *Biochem. J.* **12**, 3884–3888.

Fenstermacher, D. K., and Rose, R. C. (1986). Absorption of pantothenic acid in rat and chick intestine. *Am. J. Physiol.* **250**, G155–160.

Finlayson, H. J., and Seeley, R. C. (1983). The synthesis and absorption of pantothenic acid in the gastrointestinal tract of the adult sheep. *J. Sci. Food Agric.* **34**, 427–432.

Fisher, M. N., and Neely, J. R. (1985). Regulation of pantothenate kinase from various tissues of the rat. *FEBS Lett.* **190**, 293–296.

Fisher, M. N., Robishaw, J. D., and Neely, J. R. (1985). The properties and regulation of pantothenate kinase from rat heart. *J. Biol. Chem.* **260**, 15745–15751.

Food and Nutrition Board (1980). "Recommended Dietary Allowances," 9th Ed. Nat. Acad. Sci., Washington, D.C.

Fox, H. M., and Linkswiler, H. (1961). Pantothenic acid excretion on three levels of intake. *J. Nutr.* **75**, 451–461.

Franklin, J. E., and Trams, E. G. (1971). Metabolism of coenzyme A and related compounds by liver plasma membranes. *Biochim. Biophys. Acta* **230**, 105–116.

Fry, P. C., Fox, H. M., and Tao, H. G. (1976). Metabolic response to a pantothenic acid deficient diet in humans. *J. Nutr. Sci. Vitaminol.* **22**, 339–346.

Funk, G. (1912). The etiology of the deficiency disease. *J. State Med.* **20**, 341–368.

Garland, P. B., and Randle, P. J. (1964). Regulation of glucose uptake by muscle. 10. Effect of alloxan-diabetes. *Biochem. J.* **93**, 678–687.

Garland, P. B., Sheperd, D., and Yates, D. W. (1965). Steady-state concentrations of coenzyme A, acetyl coenzyme A and long chain fatty acyl-coenzyme A in rat liver mitochondria oxidizing palmitate. *Biochem. J.* **97**, 587–594.

Germinario, R. J., and Waller, J. R. (1977). Transport of pantothenic acid in Lactobacillus plantarium. *Can. J. Microbiol.* **23**, 922–930.

Goodhue, C. T., and Snell, E. E. (1966). The bacterial degradation of pantothenic acid. III. Enzymatic formation of aldopantoic acid. *Biochemistry* **5**, 403–408.

Halvorsen, O., and Skrede, S. (1980). Separation of coenzyme A and its precursors by reversed-phase high-performance liquid chromatography. *Anal. Biochem.* **107**, 103–108.

Halvorsen, O., and Skrede, S. (1982). Regulation of the biosynthesis of CoA at the level of pantothenate kinase. *Eur. J. Biochem.* **124**, 211–215.

Harrison, H. E., and Harrison, H. E. (1954). Experimental production of renal glycosuria, phosphaturia and aminoaciduria by injection of maleic acid. *Science* **120**, 606–608.

Hatano, M., Hodges, R. E., Evans, T. C., Hagfemann, R. F., Leeper, D. B., Bean, W. B., and Krehl, W. A. (1967). Urinary excretion of pantothenic acid by diabetic patients and by alloxan-diabetic rats. *Am. J. Clin. Nutr.* **20**, 960–967.

Ho, C. H., and Pande, S. V. (1974). On the specificity of inhibition of adenine nucleotide translocase by long chain acyl-coenzyme A esters. *Biochim. Biophys. Acta* **369**, 86–94.

Hoaglund, M., and Novelli, G. (1954). Biosynthesis of coenzyme A from phosphopantetheine and of pantetheine from pantothenate. *J. Biol. Chem.* **207**, 767–773.

Hodges, R. E., Ohlson, M. A., and Bean, W. B. (1958). Pantothenic acid deficiency in man. *J. Clin. Invest.* **37**, 1642–1657.

Holak, T. A., Nilges, M., Prestegard, J. H., Gronenborn, A. M., and Clore, G. M. (1988). Three-dimensional structure of acyl carrier protein in solution determined by nuclear magnetic resonance and the combined use of dynamical simulated annealing and distance geometry. *Eur. J. Biochem.* **175**, 9–15.

Huang, M. T., and Kies, C. (1981). Vitamin B_6 nutritional status of several strains of mice and rats as affected by pantothenic acid deficiency. *Nutr. Rep. Int.* **23**, 9–17.

Huang, W., Stoops, J. K., and Wakil, S. J. (1989). Complete amino acid sequence of chicken liver acyl carrier protein derived from the fatty acid synthase. *Arch. Biochem. Biophys.* **270**, 92–98.

Hurley, L. S. (1967). Studies on nutritional factors in mammalian development. *J. Nutr.* **91**, 27–38.

Hurley, L. S., and Volkert, N. E. (1965). Pantothenic acid and coenzyme A in the developing guinea pig liver. *Biochim. Biophys. Acta* **104**, 372–376.

Iannucci, J., Milner, R., Arbizo, M. V., and Smith, C. M. (1982). The effect of ethanol and acetaldehyde on [^{14}C]pantothenate incorporation into CoA in cultured rat liver parenchymal cells. *Arch. Biochem. Biophys.* **217**, 15–29.

Idell-Wenger, J. A., Grotyohann, L. W., and Neely, J. R. (1978). Coenzyme A and carnitine distribution in normal and ischemic hearts. *J. Biol. Chem.* **253**, 4310–4318.

Ikeda, M. T., Hosotani, T., Veda, T., Kotaka, Y., and Sakakibara, B. (1979). Effect of vitamin B_6 deficiency on the levels of several water soluble vitamins in germ-free and conventional rats. *J. Nutr. Sci. Vitaminol.* **25**, 141–149.

Israel, B. C., and Smith, C. M. (1987). Effects of acute and chronic ethanol ingestion on pantothenate and CoA status of rats. *J. Nutr.* **117**, 443–451.

Itoh, S., and Kuroshima, A. (1970). Adaptation to cold (1). *Hokkaido Igaku Zasshi* **45**, 1–11.

Jackowski, S., and Rock, C. O. (1981). Regulation of coenzyme A biosynthesis. *J. Bacteriol.* **148**, 926–932.

Jackowski, S., and Rock, C. O. (1983). Ratio of active to inactive forms of acyl carrier protein in *Escherichia coli*. *J. Biol. Chem.* **258**, 15186–15191.

Jackowski, S., and Rock, C. O. (1984). Turnover of the 4'-phosphopantetheine prosthetic group of acyl carrier protein. *J. Biol. Chem.* **259**, 1891–1895.

Johnston, L., Vaughan, L., and Fox, H. M. (1981). Pantothenic acid content of human milk. *Am. J. Clin. Nutr.* **34**, 2205–2209.

Jukes, T. (1939). Pantothenic acid and the filtrate (chick anti-dermatitis) factor. *J. Am. Chem. Soc.* **61**, 975–976.

Jukes, T. H. (1941). The distribution of pantothenic acid in certain products of natural origin. *J. Nutr.* **21**, 193–200.

Kakar, S. S., Huang, W., and Askari, A. (1987). Control of cardiac sodium pump by long-chain acyl coenzymes A. *J. Biol. Chem.* **262**, 42–45.

Kang, E. S., Capaci, M. T., Korones, D. N., and Tekade, N. (1982). Liver coenzyme A ester content: comparison between Reye's syndrome and control subjects. *Clin. Sci.* **63**, 455–460.

Karasawa, T., Yoshida, K., Furukawa, K., and Hosoki, K. (1972). Feedback inhibition of pantothenate kinase by coenzyme A and possible role of the enzyme for the regulation of cellular coenzyme A level. *J. Biochem. (Tokyo)* **71**, 1065–1067.

Karnitz, L. M., Gross, C. J., and Henderson, L. M. (1984). Transport and metabolism of pantothenic acid by rat kidney. *Biochim. Biophys. Acta* **769**, 486–492.

Kathman, J. V., and Kies, C. (1984). Pantothenic acid status of free living adolescents and young adults. *Nutr. Res.* **4**, 245–250.

Kawaguchi, A. K., and Bloch, K. (1976). Inhibition of glutamate dehydrogenase and malate dehydrogenase by palmitoyl coenzyme A. *J. Biol. Chem.* **251**, 1406–1412.

Kerbey, A. L., Radcliffe, P. M., Randle, P. J., and Slugden, P. H. (1979). Regulation of kinase reactions in the pig heart pyruvate dehydrogenase complex. *Biochem. J.* **181**, 427–433.

Kerrey, E., Crispin, S., Fox, H. M., and Kies, C. (1968). Nutritional status of preschool children. I. Dietary and biochemical findings. *Am. J. Clin. Nutr.* **21**, 1274–1279.

Knights, K. M., and Drew, R. (1988). A radioisotopic assay of picomolar concentrations of coenzyme A in liver tissue. *Anal. Biochem.* **168**, 94–99.

Kondrup, J., and Grunnet, N. (1973). The effect of acute and prolonged ethanol treatment on the contents of coenzyme A, carnitine and their derivatives in rat liver. *Biochem. J.* **132**, 373–379.

Koyanagi, T., Hareyama, S., Kikuchi, R., and Kimura, T. (1966). Effect of diet on pantothenic acid content in serum and on the incidence of hypertension among villagers. *Tohoku J. Exp. Med.* **88**, 93–97.

Kumar, S., and Porter, J. W. (1972). The effect of reduced nicotinamide adenine diphosphate, its structural analogues and coenzyme A and its derivatives on the rate of dissociation, conformation and enzyme activity of the pigeon liver fatty acid synthetase complex. *J. Biol. Chem.* **246**, 7780–7789.

Kumar, S., Dorsey, J. A., Meusing, R. A., and Porter, J. W. (1970). Comparative studies of the pigeon liver fatty acid synthetase complex and its subunits. Kinetics of partial reactions and the number of binding sites for acetyl and malonyl groups. *J. Biol. Chem.* **245**, 4732–4744.

Kuwagata, M. (1971). Incorporation of ^{14}C-pantothenic acid into an intermediate of coenzyme A biosynthesis in rat liver. *Vitamins* **43**, 78–86.

Lakin-Thomas, P. L., and Brody, S. (1985). A pantothenate derivative is covalently bound to mitochondrial proteins in *Neurospora crassa*. *Eur. J. Biochem.* **146**, 141–147.

LaNoue, K. F., Bryla, J., and Williamson, J. R. (1972). Feedback interactions in the control of citric acid cycle activity in rat heart mitochondria. *J. Biol. Chem.* **247**, 667–679.

Larrabee, A. R., McDaniel, E. G., Bakerman, H. A., and Vagelos, P. R. (1965). Acyl carrier protein. V. Identification of 4'phosphopantetheine bound to a mammalian fatty acid synthetase preparation. *Proc. Natl. Acad. Sci. U.S.A.* **54**, 267–273.

Leevy, C. M., and Baker, H. (1963). Metabolic and nutritional effects of alcoholism. *Arch. Environ. Health* **7**, 453–459.

Leevy, C. M., George, W. S., Ziffer, H., and Baker, H. (1960). Pantothenic acid, fatty liver and alcoholism. *J. Clin. Invest.* **39**, 1005–1011.

Leevy, C. M., Baker, H., TenHove, W., Frank, O., and Cherrick, G. R. (1965). B-complex vitamins in liver disease of the alcoholic. *J. Clin. Nutr.* **16**, 339–346.

Lewis, C. M., and King, J. C. (1980). Effect of oral contraceptive agents on thiamin, riboflavin and pantothenic acid status in young women. *Am. J. Clin. Nutr.* **33**, 832–838.

Lopaschuk, G. D. (1988). Insulin effects on pantothenic acid uptake in isolated perfused working hearts from diabetic rats. *Diabetes* **37**, 1335–1339.

Lopaschuk, G. D., and Neely, J. R. (1987a). Stimulation of myocardial coenzyme A degradation by fatty acids. *Am. J. Physiol.* **253**, H41–H46.

Lopaschuk, G. D., and Neely, J. R. (1987b). Coenzyme A degradation in the heart: Effects of diabetes and insulin. *J. Mol. Cell. Cardiol.* **19**, 281–287.

Lopaschuk, G. D., Michalak, M., and Tsang, H. (1987). Regulation of pantothenic acid transport in the heart. *J. Biol. Chem.* **262**, 3615–3619.

Lornitzo, F. A., Qureshi, A. A., and Porter, J. W. (1974). Separation of the half-molecular weight nonidentical subunits of pigeon liver fatty acid synthetase by affinity chromatography. *J. Biol. Chem.* **249**, 1654–1656.

Maas, W. K. (1952). Pantothenate studies. III. Description of the extracted pantothenate-synthesizing enzyme of *E. coli*. *J. Biol. Chem.* **198**, 23–32.

Magee, P. T., and Snell, E. E. (1966). The bacterial degradation of pantothenic acid. IV. Enzymatic conversion of aldopantoate to α-ketoisovalerate. *Biochemistry* **5**, 409–416.

Majerus, P. W., Alberts, A. W., and Vagelos, P. R. (1965a). Acyl carrier proteins. III. An enoyl hydrase specific for acyl carrier protein thioesters. *J. Biol. Chem.* **240**, 618–621.

Majerus, P. W., Alberts, A. W., and Vagelos, P. R. (1965b). Acyl carrier protein. VII. The primary structure of the substrate binding. *J. Biol. Chem.* **240**, 4723–4726.

Mantsala, P., (1973). Some characteristics and control of transport in *Escherichia coli* u-5/41. *Acta Chem. Scand.* **27**, 445–452.

Mayo, K. H., and Prestegard, J. H. (1985). Acyl carrier protein from *Escherichia coli*. Structural characterization of short-chain acyl carrier proteins by NMR. *Biochemistry* **24**, 7834–7838.

McAllister, R. A., Campbell, E. H. G., and Calman, K. C. (1982). Metabolic changes in liver of tumor-bearing mice. *J. Surg. Res.* **33**, 500–509.

McAllister, R. A., Fixter, L. M., and Campbell, E. H. G. (1988). The effect of tumor growth on liver pantothenate, CoA, and fatty acid synthetase activity in the mouse. *Br. J. Cancer* **57**, 83–86.

McCall, K. B., Waisman, H. A., and Elvehjem, C. A. (1946). A study of pyridoxine and pantothenic acid deficiency in the monkey (*M. mulatta*). *J. Nutr.* **31**, 685–696.

McCarthy, A. D., Aitken, A., and Hardie, D. G. (1983). The multifunctional polypeptide chain of rabbit mammary fatty acid synthetase contains a domain homologous with the acyl carrier protein of *Escherichia coli*. *Eur. J. Biochem.* **136**, 501–508.

Nakamura, H., and Tamura, Z. 91973). Pantothenate uptake in *E. coli* K-12. *J. Nutr. Sci. Vitaminol.* **19**, 389–400.

Nakamura, T., Nomoto, N., Yagi, R., and Oya, N. (1970). Metabolic vitamin B complex deficiency due to the administration of glucocorticoid. *J. Vitaminol.* **16**, 89–98.

Nakamura, T., Kusonoki, T., Soyama, K., and Kuwagata, M. (1972). Studies on the distribution of pantothenic acid, coenzyme A and their intermediates in rat liver. III. The isolation of pantothenic acid, 4'-phosphopantetheine and coenzyme A by column and paper chromatography. *J. Vitaminol.* **18**, 34–40.

Nakano, K., Sugawara, Y., Ohashi, M., and Harigaya, S. (1986). Glucoside formation as a novel metabolic pathway of pantothenic acid in the dog. *Biochem. Pharmacol.* **35**, 3745–3752.

Neely, J. R., Robishaw, J. D., and Vary, T. C. (1982). Control of myocardial levels of CoA and carnitine. *J. Mol. Cell. Cardiol.* **14**, Suppl. 3, 37–42.

Nelson, R. A. (1968). Intestinal transport, CoA and colitis in pantothenic acid deficiency. *Am. J. Clin. Nutr.* **21**, 495–506.

Nurmikko, V., Salo, E., Hakola, H., Makinen, K., and Snell, E. (1966). The bacterial degradation of pantothenic acid. II. Pantothenate hydrolase. *Biochemistry* **5**, 399–402.

Olson, M. S., Dennis, S. C., DeBuysere, M. S., and Padma, A. (1978). The regulation of pyruvate dehydrogenase in the isolated perfused rat heart. *J. Biol. Chem.* **253**, 7369–7375.

Ono, S., Kameda, K., and Abiko, Y. (1974). Metabolism of pantetheine in the rat. *J. Nutr. Sci. Vitamnol.* **20**, 203–213.

Opie, L. H. (1979). Role of carnitine in fatty acid metabolism of normal and ischemic myocardium. *Am. Heart J.* **97**, 375–388.

Oram, J. R., Bennetch, S. L., and Neely, J. R. (1973). Regulation of fatty acid utilization in isolated perfused rat hearts. *J. Biol. Chem.* **248**, 5299–5309.

Oram, J. F., Idell-Wenger, J., and Neely, J. R. (1975). Regulation of long-chain fatty acid activation in heart muscle. *J. Biol. Chem.* **250**, 73–78.

Orr, M. L. (1969). Pantothenic acid, vitamin B_6 and vitamin B_{12} in foods. *U.S. Dep. Agric. Home Econ. Res. Rep.* No. 36.

Ortega, M. V., Cardenas, A., and Ubiera, D. (1975). panD, a new chromosomal locus of *Salmonella typhirium* for the biosynthesis of beta-alanine. *Mol. Gen. Genet.* **140**, 159–164.

Pacanis, A., and Rogulski, J. (1981). Studies on chemical and enzymatic synthesis of maleyl-CoA. *J. Biol. Chem.* **256**, 13030–13034.

Pacanis, A., Strzelecki, T., and Rogulski, J. (1981). Effects of maleate on the content of CoA and its derivatives in rat kidney mitochondria. *J. Biol. Chem.* **256**, 13035–13038.

Pande, S. V., and Blanchaer, M. C. (1971). Reversible inhibition of adenine diphosphate phosphorylation by long chain acyl coenzyme A esters. *J. Biol. Chem.* **246**, 406–411.

Partin, J. C., Schubert, W. K., and Partin, J. S. (1971). Mitochondrial ultrastructure in Reye's syndrome (encephalopathy and fatty degeneration of the viscere). *N. Engl. J. Med.* **255**, 1339–1343.

Perkins, D. D., Glassey, M., and Bloom, B. A. (1962). New data on markers and rearrangements in *Neurospora*. *Am. J. Genet. Cytol.* **4**, 187–205.

Plesofsky-Vig, N., and Brambl, R. (1984). Three subunit proteins of membrane enzymes in mitochondria of *Neurospora crassa* contain a pantothenate derivative. *J. Biol. Chem.* **259**, 10660–10663.

Polacco, M. L., and Cronan, J. E. (1981). A mutant of *Escherichia coli* conditionally defective in the synthesis of holo-[acyl carrier protein]. *J. Biol. Chem.* **256**, 5750–5754.

Powell, G. L., Elovson, J., and Vagelos, P. R. (1969). Acyl carrier protein. XII. Synthesis and turnover of the prosthetic group of acyl carrier protein *in vivo*. *J. Biol. Chem.* **244**, 5616–5624.

Puri, R., and Porter, J. W. (1981). Isolation of thioesterase and acyl carrier protein activities liberated by elastase digestion of pigeon fatty acid synthetase. *Biochem. Biophys. Res. Commun.* **100**, 1010–1016.

Puri, R. N., and Porter, J. W. (1982). Isolation and characterization of an acyl carrier protein from pigeon liver fatty acid synthetase by controlled proteolysis with elastase. *Biochim. Biophys. Acta* **712**, 576–589.

Rabier, D., Briand, P., Petit, F., Kamoun, P., and Cathelineau, L. (1983). Radioisotopic assay of picomolar amounts of coenzyme A. *Anal. Biochem.* **134**, 325–329.

Rajalakshmi, R., and Nakhasi, H. L. (1975). Effects of neonatal panothenic acid deficiency on brain lipid composition in rats. *J. Neurochem.* **24**, 979–981.

Ramakrishnan, C. V., and Subramaniam, A. (1978). Effects of prenatal and neonatal pantothenic acid deficiency on rat intestinal phosphatases. *Specialia* **15**, 435–437.

Randle, P. J., Garland, P. B., Hales, C. N., Newsholme, E. A., Denton, R. M., and Pogon, G. I. (1966). Interactions of metabolism and the physiological role of insulin. *Recent Prog. Horm. Res.* **22**, 1–48.

Rapp, G. W. (1973). Some systemic effects of malignant tumors. *Cancer (Philadelphia)* **31**, 357–360.

Reibel, D. K., Wyse, B. W., Berkich, D. A., and Neely, J. R. (1981a). Regulation of Coenzyme A synthesis in heart muscle: Effects of fasting and diabetes. *Am. J. Physiol.* **240**, H606–H611.

Reibel, D. K., Wyse, B. W., Berkich, D. A., Palko, W. M., and Neely, J. R. (1981b). Effects of diabetes and fasting on pantothenic acid metabolism in rats. *Am. J. Physiol.* **240**, E597–E601.

Reibel, D. K., Wyse, B. W., Berkich, D. A., and Neely, J. R. (1982). Coenzyme A metabolism in pantothenic acid-deficient rats. *J. Nutr.* **112**, 1144–1150.

Reichelt, K. L. (1971). Isolation of two pantetheine-containing acidic proteins from monkey brain. *J. Neurochem.* **18**, 1317–1328.

Robishaw, J. D., and Neely, J. R. (1984). Pantothenate kinase and control of CoA synthesis in heart. *Am. J. Physiol.* **246**, H532–H541.

Robishaw, J. D., Berkich, D., and Neely, J. R. (1982). Rate-limiting step and control of coenzyme A synthesis in cardiac muscle. *J. Biol. Chem.* **257**, 10967–10972.

Rogulski, J., Pacanis, A., Adamowicz, W., and Angielski, S. (1974). On the mechanism of maleate action in rat kidney mitochondria. Effect of oxidative metabolism. *Acta Biochim. Pol.* **21**, 403–413.

Rogulski, J., Strzelecki, T., Pacanis, A., Kaminska, E., and Angielski, S. (1975). Effects of maleate on renal carbohydrate metabolism *in vivo* and *in vitro*. *In* "Biochemical Aspects of Renal Function" (S. Angielski and U. C. Dubach, eds.), pp. 106–120. Huber, Bern.

Roncari, D. A. K. (1974). Mammalian fatty acid synthetase. I. Purification and properties of human liver complex. *Can. J. Biochem.* **52**, 221–230.

Roy, A. K., and Axelrod, A. E. (1971). Protein synthesis in liver of pancreatic acid-deficient rats. *Proc. Soc. Exp. Biol. Med.* **138**, 804–807.

Said, H. M., and Redha, R. (1987). A carrier-mediated system for transport of biotin in rat intestine *in vitro*. *Am. J. Physiol.* **252**, G52–G55.

Sauberlich, H. E. (1985). Bioavailability of vitamins. *Prog. Food Sci.* **9**, 1–33.

Sauer, F., Pugh, E. L., and Wakil, S. J. (1964). 2-Mercaptoethylamine and beta-alanine as components of acyl carrier protein. *Proc. Natl. Acad. Sci. U.S.A.* **52**, 1360–1366.

Scandurra, R., Barboni, E., Granata, F., Pensa, B., and Costa, M. (1974). Pantothenoylcysteine-4'-phosphate decarboxylase from horse liver. *Eur. J. Biochem.* **49**, 1–9.

Schroeder, H. A. (1971). Losses of vitamins and trace minerals resulting from processing and preservation of foods. *Am. J. Clin. Nutr.* **24**, 562–573.

Schwabedal, P. E., Pietrzik, K., and Wittkowski, W. (1985). Pantothenic acid deficiency as a factor contributing to the development of hypertension. *Cardiology* **72**, Suppl. 1, 187–189.

Scrutton, M. C., and Utter, M. F. (1967). Pyruvate carboxylase. IX. Some properties of the activation by certain acyl derivatives of coenzyme A. *J. Biol. Chem.* **242**, 1723–1735.

Shibata, K., Gross, C. J., and Henderson, L. M. (1983). Hydrolysis and absorption of pantothenate and its coenzymes in the rat small intestine. *J. Nutr.* **113**, 2207–2215.

Shimuzu, S., Kataoka, M., Chung, M. C. M., and Yamada, H. (1988). Ketopantoic acid reductase of *Psuedomonas maltophila* 845. *J. Biol. Chem.* **263**, 12077–12084.

Shug, A. L., and Shrago, E. (1973). Inhibition of phosphoenolpyruvate transport via the tricarboxylate and adenine nucleotide carrier systems of rat liver mitochondria. *Biochem. Biophys. Res. Commun.* **53**, 659–665.

Singh, M., Dempsey, W. B., and Srere, P. A. (1975). Incorporation of pantothenate into citrate lyase by a pantothenateless mutant of *Klebsiella pneumoniae. J. Bacteriol.* **124**, 686–692.

Skeggs, H. R., and Wright, L. D. (1944). The use of *lactobacillus arabinosus* in the microbiological determination of pantothenic acid. *J. Biol. Chem.* **156**, 21–26.

Skrede, S. (1973). The degradation of CoA: subcellular localization and kinetic properties of CoA and dephospho CoA pyrophosphatase. *Eur. J. Biochem.* **38**, 401–407.

Skrede, S., and Halvorsen, O. (1979). Mitochondrial biosynthesis of coenzyme A. *Biochem. Biophys. Res. Commun.* **91**, 1526–1542.

Skrede, S., and Halvorsen, O. (1983). Mitochondrial pantotheinephosphate adenyltransferase and dephospho-CoA kinase. *Eur. J. Biochem.* **131**, 57–63.

Smith, C. M. (1978). The effect of metabolic state on incorporation of [^{14}C]pantothenate into CoA in rat liver and heart. *J. Nutr.* **108**, 863–873.

Smith, C. M., and Savage, C. R. (1980). Regulation of coenzyme A biosynthesis by glucagon and glucocorticoid in adult rat liver parenchymal cells. *Biochem. J.* **186**, 175–184.

Smith, C. M., and Milner, R. E. (1985). The mechanisms of pantothenate transport by rat liver parenchymal cells in primary culture. *J. Biol. Chem.* **260**, 4823–4831.

Smith, C. M., Cano, M. L., and Potyraj, J. (1978). The relationship between metabolic state and total CoA content of rat liver and heart. *J. Nutr.* **108**, 854–862.

Smith, C. M., Israel, B. C., Iannucci, J., and Marino, K. A. (1987). Possible role of acetyl CoA in the inhibition of CoA biosynthesis by ethanol in rats. *J. Nutr.* **117**, 452–459.

Smith, S., and Libertini, L. J. (1979). Specificity and site of action of a mammary gland thioesterase which releases acyl moieties from thioester linkage to the fatty acid synthetase. *Arch. Biochem. Biophys.* **196**, 88–92.

Sobhy, C. (1979). Regulation of fatty acid synthetase activity. The 4'phosphopantetheine hydrolase of rat liver. *J. Biol. Chem.* **254**, 8561–8566.

Solberg, O., and Hegna, I. K. (1979). Microbiological assay of pantothenic acid. *Methods Enzymol.* **62**, 201–204.

Song, W. O., Chan, G. M., Wyse, B. W., and Hansen, R. G. (1984). Effect of pantothenic acid status on the content of the vitamin in human milk. *Am. J. Clin. Nutr.* **40**, 317–324.

Song, W. O., Wyse, B. W., and Hansen, R. G. (1985). Pantothenic acid status of pregnant and lactating women. *J. Am. Diet. Assoc.* **85**, 192–198.

Spector, R. (1986). Development and characterization of pantothenic acid transport in brain. *J. Neurochem.* **47**, 563–568.

Spector, R., and Boose, B. (1984). Accumulation of pantothenic acid by the isolated choroid plexus and brain slices *in vitro. J. Neurochem.* **43**, 472–478.

Srere, P. A., Bottger, B., and Brooks, G. C. (1972). Citrate lyase: A pantothenate-containing enzyme. *Proc. Natl. Acad. Sci. U.S.A.* **69**, 1201–1202.

Srinivasan, V., and Belavady, B. (1976). Alterations in gluconeogenesis in experimental pantothenic aid deficiency. *Ind. J. Biochem. Biophys.* **13**, 387–389.

Srinivasan, V., Christensen, N., Wyse, B. W., and Hansen, R. G. (1981). Pantothenic acid nutritional status in the elderly-institutionalized and non-institutionalized. *Am. J. Clin. Nutr.* **34**, 1736–1742.

Sugarman, B., and Munro, H. N. (1980). ^{14}C-Pantothenate accumulation by isolated adipocytes from adult rats of different ages. *J. Nutr.* **110**, 2297–2301.

Suzuki, T., Abiko, Y., and Shimuzu, M. (1967). Investigations on pantothenic acid and its related compounds. XII. Biochemical studies (7). Dephospho-CoA pyrophosphorylase and dephospho-CoA kinase as a possible bifunctional enzyme complex. *J. Biochem. (Tokyo)* **62**, 642–649.

Swartzentruber, M. S., and Harris, R. A. (1987). Inhibition of metabolic processes by coenzyme A-sequestering aromatic acids. Prevention by *para*-choloro- and *para*-nitrobenzoic-acids. *Biochem. Pharmacol.* **36**, 3147–3153.

Tabachanick, I. I. A., and Bonnycastle, D. D. (1954). The effect of thyroxine on the coenzyme A content of some tissues. *J. Biol. Chem.* **207**, 757–760.

Tahiliani, A. G. (1989). Dependence of mitochondrial coenzyme A transport on the membrane electrical gradient. *J. Biol. Chem.* **264**, 18426–18432.

Tahiliani, A. G., and Neely, J. R. (1987a). A transport system for coenzyme A into isolated rat heart mitochondria. *J. Biol. Chem.* **262**, 11607–11610.

Tahiliani, A. G., and Neely, J. R. (1987b). Mitochondrial synthesis of coenzyme A is on the external surface. *J. Mol. Cell. Cardiol.* **19**, 1161–1168.

Tao, H. G., and Fox, H. M. (1976). Measurements of urinary pantothenic acid excretions of alcoholic patients. *J. Nutr. Sci. Vitaminol.* **22**, 333–337.

Tarr, J. B., Tamura, T., and Stokstad, E. L. R. (1981). Availability of vitamin B$_6$ pantothenate in an average American diet in man. *Am. J. Clin. Nutr.* **34**, 1328–1337.

Taylor, T., Hawkins, D. R., Hathway, D. E., and Partington, H. (1972). A new urinary metabolite of pantothenate in dogs. *Br. Vet. J.* **128**, 500–505.

Taylor, T., Cameron, B. D., Hathway, D. E., and Partington, H. (1974). The disposition of pantothenate in dogs. *Res. Vet. Sci.* **16**, 271–275.

Teller, J. H., Powers, S. G., and Snell, E. E. (1976). Ketopantoate hydroxymethyltransferase. I. Purification and role in pantothenate biosynthesis. *J. Biol. Chem.* **251**, 3780–3785.

Therisod, H., and Kennedy, E. P. (1987). The function of acyl carrier protein in the synthesis of membrane-derived oligosaccharides does not require its phosphopantetheine prosthetic group. *Proc. Natl. Acad. Sci. U.S.A.* **84**, 8235–8238.

Therisod, H., Weissborn, A. C., and Kennedy, E. P. (1986). An essential function for acyl carrier protein in the biosynthesis of membrane derived oligosaccharides of *Escherichia coli. Proc. Natl. Acad. Sci. U.S.A.* **83**, 7236–7240.

Tildon, J. T., and Sevdalian, D. A. (1972). CoA transferase in the brain and other mammalian tissues. *Arch. Biochem. Biophys.* **148**, 382–390.

Trams, E. G., Fales, H. A., and Gal, A. E. (1968). *S*-Palmityl pantetheine as an intermediate in the metabolism of palmityl coenzyme A by rat liver plasma membrane preparations. *Biochem. Biophys. Res. Commun.* **31**, 973–976.

Tsuji, K. (1966). Liquid nitrogen preservation of *Saccharomyces carlsbergensis* and its use in a rapid biological assay of pantothenic acid. *Appl. Microbiol.* **14**, 462–465.

Tsujikawa, M., and Kimura, S. (1981). Effect of exposure to cold on pantothenic acid metabolism in rat liver. *Tohoku J. Exp. Med.* **133**, 457–460.

Tubbs, P. K., and Garland, P. B. (1964). Variations in tissue contents of coenzyme A thioesters and possible metabolic implications. *Biochem. J.* **93**, 550–557.

Turner, J. B., and Hughes, C. D. E. (1962). The absorption of bound forms of B-group vitamins by rat intestine. *Q. J. Exp. Physiol.* **47**, 124–133.

Tweto, J., Liberati, M., and Larrabee, A. R. (1971). Protein turnover and 4′phosphopantetheine exchange in rat liver fatty acid synthetase. *J. Biol. Chem.* **246**, 2468–2471.

Vagelos, P. R., and Larrabee, A. R. (1967). Acyl carrier protein. IX. Acyl carrier protein hydrolase. *J. Biol. Chem.* **242**, 1776–1781.

Vagelos, P. R., Majerus, P. W., Alberts, A. W., Larrabee, A. R., and Ailhaud, G. P. (1966). Structure and function of the acyl carrier protein. *Fed. Proc.* **25**, 1485–1494.

Vallari, D. S., and Rock, C. O. (1985). Pantothenate transport in *E. coli. J. Bacteriol.* **162**, 1156–1161.

Volpe, J. J., and Vagelos, P. R. (1973). Fatty acid synthetase of mammalian brain, liver and adipose tissue. Regulation by prosthetic group turnover. *Biochim. Biophys. Acta* **326**, 293–304.

Voltti, H., and Hassinen, I. E. (1980). A subcellular study of the clofibrate-induced increase in coenzyme A concentration in rat liver. *Biochem. Pharmacol.* **29**, 989–992.

Voltti, H., Savolainen, M. J., Jauhonen, V. P., and Hassinen, I. E. (1979). Clofibrate-induced increase in coenzyme A concentration in rat tissues. *Biochem. J.* **182**, 95–102.

Waldi, D. (1965). Coating materials for thin layer chromatography. *In* "Thin Layer Chromatography" (E. Stahl, ed.), pp. 20–34. Academic Press, New York.

Walsh, J. H., Wyse, B. W., and Hansen, R. G. (1981a). Pantothenic acid content of a nursing home diet. *Ann. Nutr. Metab.* **25**, 178–181.

Walsh, J. H., Wyse, B. W., and Hansen, R. G. (1981b). Pantothenic acid content of 75 processed and cooked foods. *J. Am. Diet. Assoc.* **78**, 140–143.

Weissborn, A. C., and Kennedy, E. P. (1984). Biosynthesis of membrane derived oligosaccharides. Novel glycosyl-transferase system from *Eschrichia coli* for the elongation of beta 1——2-linked polyglucose chains. *J. Biol. Chem.* **259**, 12644–12651.

White, H., and Jencks, W. P. (1976). Mechanism and specificity of succinyl-CoA:3-ketoacid coenzyme A transferase. *J. Biol. Chem.* **251**, 1688–1699.

Whitmer, J. T., Wenger, J. I., Rovetto, M. J., and Neely, J. R. (1978). Control of fatty acid metabolism in ischemic and hypoxic hearts. *J. Biol. Chem.* **253**, 4305–4309.

Williams, R. J., Lyman, C. M., Goodyear, G. H., Truesdail, J. H., and Holiday, D. (1933). "Pantothenic acid", a growth determinant of universal biological occurrence. *J. Am. Chem. Soc.* **55**, 2912–2927.

Williamson, D. H., Bates, M. W., Page, M. A., and Krebs, H. A. (1971). Activities of enzymes involved in acetoacetate utilization in adult mammalian tissues. *Biochem. J.* **121**, 41–47.

Williamson, I. P., and Wakil, S. J. (1966). Studies on the mechanism of fatty acid synthesis. XVIII. Preparation and general properties of acetyl coenzyme A and malonyl coenzyme A-acyl carrier protein translocases. *J. Biol. Chem.* **241**, 2326–2332.

Williamson, J. R., and Corkey, B. (1979). Assay of citric acid cycle intermediates and related compounds—uptake with tissue metabolite levels and intracellular distribution. *Methods Enzymol.* **55.** 200–222.

Witkowski, A., Naggert, J., Mikkelsen, J., and Smith, S. (1987). Molecular cloning and sequencing of a cDNA encoding the acyl carrier protein and its flanking domains in the mammalian fatty acid synthetase. *Eur. J. Biochem.* **165,** 601–606.

Wittwer, C. T., Wyse, B. W., and Hansen, R. G. (1982). Assay of the enzymatic hydrolysis of pantetheine. *Anal. Biochem.* **122,** 213–222.

Wittwer, C. T., Burkhard, D., Ririe, K., Rasmussen, R., Brown, J., Wyse, B. W., and Hansen, R. G. (1983). Purification and properties of a pantetheine hydrolyzing enzyme from pig kidney. *J. Biol. Chem.* **258,** 9733–9738.

Wood, J. M., Bush, B., Pitts, B. J. R., and Schwartz, A. (1977). Inhibition of bovine heart Na$^+$,K$^+$-ATPase by palmityl carnitine and palmityl CoA. *Biochem. Biophys. Res. Commun.* **74,** 677–684.

Wooley, D., Waisman, H., and Elvehjam, C. (1939). Nature and partial synthesis of the chick antidermatitis factor. *J. Am. Chem. Soc.* **61,** 977–978.

Worrall, D. M., and Tubbs, P. K. (1983). A bifunctional complex in coenzyme A biosynthesis: purification of pantotheine phosphate adenyltransferase and dephospho-CoA kinase. *Biochem. J.* **215,** 153–157.

Worthen, H. G. (1963). Renal toxicity of maleic acid in the rat. Enzymatic and morphologic observations. *Lab. Invest.* **13,** 791–799.

Wyse, B. W., Wittwer, C., and Hansen, R. G. (1979). Radioimmunoassay for pantothenic acid in blood and other tissues. *Clin. Chem.* **25,** 108–110.

Yates, D. W., and Garland, P. B. (1966). The partial latency and intramitochondrial distribution of carnitine-palmitoyltransferase (*E.C. 2.3.1.*-), and the CoASH and carnitine permeable space of rat liver mitochondria. *Biochem. Biophys. Res. Commun.* **23,** 460–465.

Yu, H. L., and Burton, D. N. (1974). Adaptive synthesis of rat liver fatty acid synthetase: evidence for *in vitro* formation of active enzyme from inactive protein precursors and 4'phosphopantetheine. *Biochem. Biophys. Res. Commun.* **61,** 483–488.

Zook, E. G., MacArthur, M. J., and Toepfer, E. W. (1956). Pantothenic acid in foods. *U.S. Dep. Agric. Agric. Handb.* No. 97.

VITAMINS AND HORMONES, VOL. 46

Biochemical and Physiological Functions of Pyrroloquinoline Quinone

MINORU AMEYAMA, KAZUNOBU MATSUSHITA, EMIKO SHINAGAWA, AND OSAO ADACHI

Laboratory of Applied Microbiology
Department of Agricultural Chemistry
Yamaguchi University
Yamaguchi 753, Japan

I. INTRODUCTION

It is only 10 years since the chemical structure of pyrroloquinoline quinone (PQQ), 4,5-dihydro-4,5-dioxo-1H-pyrrolo (2,3-f) quino-
line-2,7,9-tricarboxylic acid (Fig. 1), was established independently by
two groups (Salisbury *et al.*, 1979; Duine *et al.*, 1980). Since then there
have been many reports supporting the metabolic significance of PQQ,
and about 20 species of enzymes carrying a PQQ as the prosthetic
group have been identified in organisms from procaryotes to eu-
caryotes (Table I). Thus, PQQ has been evaluated as the third coenzyme following pyridine nucleotide and flavin in biological oxidoreduction. The coenzyme, PQQ, is bound to the apoenzyme protein
through two different mechanisms, covalently and noncovalently, similar to the mode of binding of flavin. However, a relation analogous to
flavin adenine dinucleotide (FAD) and flavin mononucleotide (FMN),
or to NAD and NADP, has not been found in PQQ. As shown in Fig. 1,
PQQ has an orthoquinone structure which is directly responsible for
oxidoreduction. The midpoint redox potential of $+90$ mV (Duine *et al.*,
1981) is distinctly high when compared with those of pyridine nucleotide (-320 mV) and flavin (-45 mV). The redox potential is closely
related with the properties of proteins carrying PQQ (quinoproteins),
as will be mentioned in Sections V and VI.

From the historical point of view, PQQ research can be divided into
four parts: (1) studies on glucose dehydrogenase (EC 1.1.99.17) of
Acinetobacter calcoaceticus and other oxidative bacteria; (2) methanol

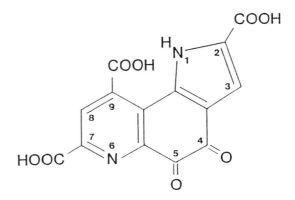

FIG. 1. Pyrroloquinoline quinone.

TABLE I
Enzymes Identified as Quinoprotein

Enzymes	PQQ[a]	Origin	Reference[b]
Methanol dehydrogenase	Free	Methylotrophs	(1)
Methylamine dehydrogenase	Bound	Methylotrophs	(1)
Aliphatic amine dehydrogenase	Bound	*Pseudomonas*	(2)
Aromatic amine dehydrogenase	Bound	*Pseudomonas*	(3)
Glucose dehydrogenase	Free	*Pseudomonas*	(4)
		Acinetobacter	(5)
		Gluconobacter	(4)
		Escherichia	(6)
Alcohol dehydrogenase	Free	*Gluconobacter*	(4,7)
		Acetobacter	(7)
		Pseudomonas	(8,9)
Aromatic alcohol dehydrogenase	Free	*Rhodopseudomonas*	(10)
Polyvinyl alcohol dehydrogenase	Free	*Pseudomonas*	(11)
Polyethylene glycol dehydrogenase	Free	*Flavobacterium*	(12)
Aldehyde dehydrogenase	Free	*Gluconobacter*	(4)
		Acetobacter	(13)
Glycerol dehydrogenase	Free	*Gluconobacter*	(14)
Fructose dehydrogenase	Free	*Gluconobacter*	(15)
Choline dehydrogenase	Bound	Dog kidney	(16)
Methylamine oxidase	Bound	*Fusarium*	(17)
		Arthrobacter	(18)
Amine oxidase	Bound	Fungi	(19)
		Blood plasma	(19)
		Pig kidney	(19)
		Pea seedling	(20)
Lysyl oxidase	Bound	Human placenta	(21)
Nitroalkane oxidase	Bound	*Fusarium*	(22)
Lipoxygenase	Bound	Pea	(23)
Nitrile hydratase	Bound	*Brevibacterium*	(24)
		Pseudomonas	(24)
		Corynebacterium	(25)
Dinitrile hydratase	Bound	*Corynebacterium*	(26)

[a]Free, noncovalently bound; bound, covalently bound.

[b](1)Anthony (1982); (2) Shinagawa *et al.* (1988); (3) Iwaki *et al.* (1983); (4) Ameyama *et al.* (1981a); (5) Duine *et al.* (1979a); (6) Ameyama *et al.* (1986); (7) Ameyama and Adachi (1982); (8) Groen *et al.* (1984, 1986); (9) Gorisch and Rupp (1988); (10) Yamanaka (1988); (11) Shimao *et al.* (1986); (12) Kawai *et al.* (1985); (13) Ameyama *et al.* (1981c); (14) Ameyama *et al.* (1985c); (15) Ameyama (1988b); (16) Ameyama *et al.* (1985f); (17) Adachi and Yamada (1970); (18) van Iersel *et al.*(1986); (19) Ameyama *et al.* (1984a); (20) Glatz *et al.* (21) van der Meer and Duine (1986); (22) Tanizawa *et al.* (1988); (23) van der Meer and Duine (1988); (24) Nagasawa and Yamada (1987); (25) Nagamune *et al.* (1988); (26) Tani *et al.* (1989).

dehydrogenase (Ec 1.1.99.8) and methylamine dehydrogenase which have been developed in the studies on microbial utilization for C_1 compounds; (3) studies on copper-carbonyl-containing amine oxidases (EC 1.4.3.6) and other quinoproteins; and (4) PQQ as the growth factor or growth-stimulating substance for microorganisms. Studies of the former two categories have been completed in terms of discovery and identification of PQQ as the prosthetic group, and now the focus is moving toward elucidation of the reaction mechanism of individual enzymes. The later two categories have been developing rapidly since the discovery of PQQ.

The first report on PQQ appeared in 1959, almost two decades before the identification of the chemical structure of PQQ, when Hauge (1959) described NAD(P)- and flavin-independent glucose dehydrogenase of *Bacterium anitratum* (synonymous *A. calcoaceticus*). Subsequently, Hague isolated a cofactor from the enzyme showing an absorption maximum at 248 nm and a shoulder at 270–280 nm in the oxidized form (Hauge, 1960, 1964). At that time, he concluded that the cofactor was a substituted napthoquinone. Thus began the investigation of PQQ; the development of quinoprotein research thereafter has been reviewed by Anthony (1988).

It is important to compare the function of quinoproteins with pyridine nucleotide- and flavin-dependent enzymes, since they seem to have similar functional properties in the oxidoreductase reaction. In order to adapt to diverse environments, bacteria have developed a variety of respiratory chains to utilize at least two kinds of terminal cytochrome oxidases. Similarly, use of quinoprotein dehydrogenase in addition to NAD enzymes and flavoproteins at the substrate side provides more diverse respiratory chain mechanisms. One might question whether quinoprotein dehydrogenase carries an alternative function in biological oxidation. Some aspects of the functions of quinoprotein dehydrogenase will be described. In addition to PQQ utilization as the prosthetic group of quinoprotein, it functions in microbial growth. It is well known that growth of microorganisms is stimulated markedly by the addition of naturally occurring substances. In the course of investigations on the growth of acetic acid bacteria, it was observed that growth of *Acetobacter* species, which shows no appreciable nutritional requirement, was stimulated markedly by yeast extract in a synthetic medium containing known growth factors such as vitamins, amino acids, and nucleic acids (Ameyama and Kondo, 1966). It has been concluded that the active substance allowing the reduction of lag period in microbial growth was PQQ, or most probably, PQQ adducts.

II. Occurrence and Distribution of PQQ

A. Quinoproteins

It is now known that quinoproteins are distributed widely among procaryotic and eukaryotic organisms. Duine and Jongejan (Vol. 45 in this series) reviewed several aspects of these enzymes, but there are now further questions about several of the quinoproteins to be dealt with critically.

As shown in Table I, most of quinoproteins have been reported from microbial sources and are occupied by oxidoreductases such as methanol, methylamine, glucose, alcohol, aldehyde, glycerol, and fructose dehydrogenases. Novel quinoproteins such as polyvinylalcohol and polyethylene glycol dehydrogenases from symbiotic microbial systems have also been reported. Judging from their metabolic function, one must pose these dehydrogenases to be localized in the periplasmic space or on the periplasmic side of the cytoplasmic membrane of gram-negative bacteria.

The prosthetic group of copper-containing amine oxidases from mammals, plants, and microorganisms have been identified as PQQ bound covalently to the enzyme protein (Table I). There has been controversy over a long period about the entity of the prosthetic group of the enzyme. Adachi and Yamada (1969) isolated two radioactive chromophores from an acid hydrolysate of the enzyme–substrate complex prepared as a Schiff base between the active carbonyl group of the enzyme and [^{14}C]ethylamine with subsequent reduction with borohydride. From spectroscopic properties, the chromophores appeared to be a pyridoxyl peptide, almost identical to PQQ peptide, as now known. Later, Hartmann and Klinman (1987) utilized a reductive trapping of substrate, [^{14}C]-benzylamine, with bovine plasma amine oxidase to provide experimental support for the existence of PQQ at the active site of the enzyme. Like amine oxidase, methylamine oxidase from the gram-positive bacterium *Arthrobacter* has been shown to be a copper-containing quinoprotein (Table I). The same type of enzyme had been purified 15 years before from *Fusarium culmorum*. This enzyme oxidizes methylamine, other short-length aliphatic amines, as well as *N*-methylbenzylamine; the latter yields formaldehyde and benzyl aldehyde. Choline dehydrogenase of mammalian kidney also has proven to be a quinoprotein (Table I); the chromophore isolated is identical with that from copper-containing amine oxidase. Furthermore, nitroalkane oxidase from *Fusarium oxysporum* has been suggested to contain PQQ as the first prosthetic group involved in substrate oxidation prior to the second prosthetic group flavin in the enzyme. (Table I).

Apart from these oxidoreductases, nitrile hydratases from *Brevibacterium* R312 and *Pseudomonas chlororaphis* B23 have been proved to be quinoproteins (Table I). In the latter enzyme reaction, a new function of PQQ in a hydration reaction is apparent. A hydrated form of PQQ, PQQ-H_2O or PQQ-$2H_2O$, probably participates in the activation of H_2O and adds H_2O to the C≡N bond of the nitrile group. Another nitrile hydratase from *Corynebacterium* sp. N-771, activated by photoirradiation, also has proved to be a quinoprotein.

B. NATURALLY OCCURRING SUBSTANCES

Ameyama *et al.* (1985a,c,e) utilized enzymatic, spectroscopic, and bioassay methods to survey for PQQ in naturally occurring substances. Pyrroloquinoline quinone seemed to exist in almost all biological materials. The extracts from naturally occurring biological materials such as yeast extract, meat extract, koji extract, corn steep liquor, potato extract, rumen juice, malt extract, milk, casamino acid and all other extracts prepared commercially or laboratory scale contain PQQ more or less at levels of picograms per milliliter to micrograms per milliliter. Upon gel filtration under defined conditions, PQQ appeared at the same position with assays by either growth stimulation for acetic acid bacteria or glucose dehydrogenase activity. Fermented products, such as beer, wine, sake, vinegar, and soy sauce also contain PQQ, which may derive from the raw materials as well as excretion from microorganisms during fermentation processes. In a culture broth of microorganisms growing in a well-defined synthetic medium, detectable amounts of PQQ are accumulated as the growth reaches the late exponential and stationary phases. Pyrroloquinoline quinone detected in these natural sources probably represents a PQQ adduct formed between the active carbonyl of PQQ and amino groups via Schiff base formation. Since the PQQ–amino acid adduct gives little coenzyme activity when assayed with apo-glucose dehydrogenase, determination of the net content of PQQ in these substances by the enzymatic method is difficult. Pyrroloquinoline quinone accumulation in culture media of methylotrophs grown on methanol or methylamine is discussed in Section IV.

C. BINDING OF PQQ TO SERUM ALBUMIN

Isolation and detection of PQQ chromophore from enzymes containing unknown prosthetic groups requires a reference protein lacking

PQQ. A suitable reference chromophore was obtained from acid hydro-lysates of bovine serum albumin (BSA) (Ameyama *et al.*, 1985a). The chromophore from BSA showed the least coenzyme activity for glucose dehydrogenase but significant growth-stimulating activity for *A. aceti,* lending to BSA apparent properties of a quinoprotein. Addition of excess PQQ to BSA produces spontaneous binding of PQQ to the protein to the extent of 2 mol of PQQ bound per mol of BSA (Adachi *et al.*, 1988a). The resulting PQQ–albumin complex is stable on DEAE chromatography, and is eluted with 0.3 and 1.0 M KCl (BSA appears with 0.1 M KCl). Pyrroloquinoline quinone–albumin exhibits an absorption spectrum with a peak at 336 nm and shows coenzyme activity for glucose dehydrogenase to almost the same level as authentic PQQ. On the other hand, BSA pretreated with pyridoxal 5'-phosphate (PLP) does not bind PQQ. Pyridoxal 5'-phosphate binds to serum albumin via ε-amino groups of lysyl residues to form a Schiff base (Dempsey and Christensen, 1962). The lack of PQQ binding to PLP–albumin suggests that PQQ binds to the same lysyl residues as does PLP.

Although no PQQ has been found free in blood serum, PQQ might exist there as a bound form. Alternatively, a PQQ carrier protein, to which PQQ may bind specifically, and from which it may be discharged, might exist in blood serum. Since BSA is able to bind PQQ *in vitro,* and since isolated BSA itself contains detectable PQQ, serum albumin could be a temporary PQQ carrier protein in mammals.

III. Pyrroloquinoline Quinone as Growth-Stimulating Substance for Microorganisms

Two types of growth-stimulating effects of PQQ for microorganisms are known (Fig. 2). The type I PQQ effect is observed in a symbiotic polyvinyl alcohol (PVA) degradation where one species of *Pseudomo-nas* excretes PQQ, which in turn enables the other species to grow on PVA (Shimao *et al.*, 1984). The latter can produce a carbon source for the former only when PQQ is supplied. Thus, PQQ is regarded as the essential growth factor of the PVA-degrading bacteria when grown on PVA, but not for growth on usual carbon sources.

The Type II growth stimulation by PQQ is characterized by a marked reduction of the lag phase of microbial growth (Ameyama *et al.*, 1984b). In this case, as shown in Fig. 2, the growth rate at the exponential phase and the total cell yield at the stationary phase are not affected by PQQ. Unlike the former type, PQQ is not always an essential growth factor and normal cell growth can be seen even in the

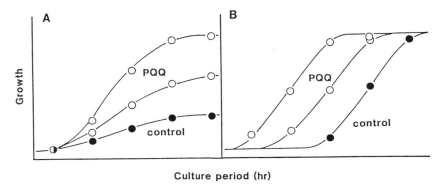

FIG. 2. Schematic drawings of growth stimulation of microorganisms by pyrroloquinoline quinone (PQQ). (A), Type I; (B), Type II.

absence of exogenous PQQ after a relatively prolonged lag time. This
type of PQQ effect was discovered in the course of searching for a
growth-stimulating substance in yeast extract for acetic acid bacteria
(Ameyama and Kondo, 1966). A growth-stimulating effect similar to
that observed with yeast extract is also found with other naturally
occurring substances used as culture ingredients for microorganisms
(Ameyama *et al.*, 1985a). They include peptone, corn steep liquor, malt
extract, koji extract, casamino acid, meat extract, blood powder or
serum, soybean cake, rumen juice, and so forth. Such a growth-stimulating substance has also been isolated from the cultured broths of
various microorganisms (Ameyama *et al.*, 1984c, 1985a; Shimao *et al.*,
1984).

It is also generally accepted that the growth stimulation observed
with such naturally occurring substances is not restricted to only
acetic acid bacteria, but also appears in a variety of microbial genera.
Several lines of evidence indicate that the growth-stimulating substance is quite probably PQQ or PQQ adducts.

A. EVIDENCE FOR THE EXISTENCE OF A GROWTH-STIMULATING
SUBSTANCE FOR ACETIC ACID BACTERIA IN YEAST EXTRACT

The spectra of vitamin requirements have been examined with
acetic acid bacteria (Fig. 3). The upper parts (clear bars) in the figure
for each strain show the effect of a single omission of each vitamin
from the minimal medium containing 10 vitamins. In the lower parts
(solid, dotted, and shaded bars) the effect of the single addition of each
vitamin to the minimal medium is shown. It is clear that

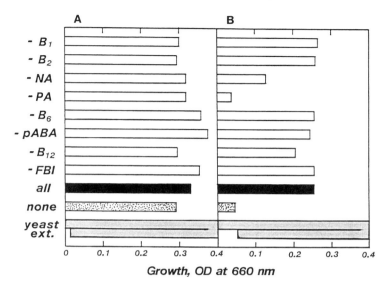

FIG. 3. Vitamin requirements for acetic acid bacteria. (A), *Acetobacter rancens;* (B), *Gluconobacter cerinus.* OD, Optical density; NA, nicotinic acid; PA, pantothenate; pABA, *p*-aminobenzoate; FBI, folic acid/biotion/inositol.

Gluconobacter cerinus requires nicotinic acid and pantothenic acid for growth, whereas no appreciable vitamin requirement is observed for *Acetobacter rancens.* These results are consistent with the vitamin requirements of acetic acid bacteria determined previously (Ameyama and Kondo, 1966), i.e., the genus *Gluconobacter* generally requires pantothenic acid, except for *G. sphaericus,* and some strains require, moreover, thiamine, nicotinic acid, and *p*-aminobenzoic acid to some extent. This is the reason why the four vitamins, pantothenic acid, nicotinic acid, thiamine and *p*-aminobenzoic acid, were included in the basal medium for assaying the growth-stimulating effect. Addition of yeast extract to the medium markedly facilitates the increase in growth of both stains, *Acetobacter* and *Gluconobacter,* of acetic acid bacteria. No appreciable requirement for nucleic acids is observed for either strains. As can be seen, yeast extract contains a growth-stimulating substance for acetic acid bacteria.

B. Fractionation of Naturally Occurring Substances

The growth response of several microbes to yeast extract has been confirmed to be Type II growth stimulation. In order to determine whether such a growth-stimulating effect of yeast extract is specific or universal, a concentrated solution of yeast extract was fractionated by gel filtration. The substance stimulating the growth of *Acetobacter aceti* is found in specific fractions; other fractions show no appreciable growth stimulation. With other bacterial strains, the growth-stimulating activity is found in the same fractions. Likewise, when many kinds of naturally occurring substances were fractionated by gel filtration, the growth-stimulating activity for most of them was observed at the same elution position, indicating that all such growth-stimulating substances are similar in molecular size.

Interestingly, *Escherichia coli* broth of glucose mineral medium was shown to contain growth-stimulating activity; hence, *E. coli*, as well as other microorganisms elaborate the growth-stimulating substance into the culture medium (Ameyama *et al.*, 1984c). Preparations purified from *E. coli* broth, yeast extract, casamino acid, rumen juice, and others (Ameyama *et al.*, 1985a) all show characteristic optical properties almost identical to PQQ. They all can serve as the prosthetic group for apo-glucose dehydrogenase, although the isolated compounds show lower activity than expected from their PQQ contents estimated on the basis of optical density. The PQQ chromophore isolated from quinoproteins by acid hydrolysis usually gives far less coenzyme activity for glucose dehydrogenase than expected (Ameyama *et al.*, 1984a, 1985b; Kawai *et al.*, 1985; Nagasawa and Yamada, 1987; Shinagawa *et al.*, 1988). On the other hand, considerable growth-stimulating activity for *A. aceti* is observed with such PQQ chromophores. We assume that small amounts of PQQ treated with high concentrations of amino compounds in acid hydrolysis, extraction, concentration, etc. are converted to PQQ adducts. We discuss in Section III,B–D the evidence that PQQ becomes less active as the coenzyme for the quinoprotein but retains its growth-stimulating activity conversely, as it forms Schiff base adducts.

C. Effect of PQQ–Amino Acid Adducts on Quinoprotein Glucose Dehydrogenase Activity

Pyrroloquinoline quinone was mixed with L-amino acids and then tested as coenzyme in the assay for glucose dehydrogenase. Almost all L-amino acids examined reduced the coenzyme activity (Ameyama, 1988a; Adachi *et al.*, 1988b). A marked effect was observed with glycine, serine, threonine, tyrosine, arginine, and lysine, which decreased activity to less than 10% of authentic PQQ. Therefore, certain amino acids may selectively bind to the active carbonyl, probably the

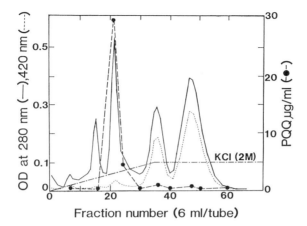

FIG. 4. Chromatographic separation of pyrroloquinoline quinone (PQQ)–serine. OD, Optical density.

5′-carbonyl of PQQ, to form a Schiff base (Lobenstein-Verbeek *et al.*, 1984; Itoh *et al.*, 1984; van der Meer *et al.*, 1986). Schiff base complexes of PQQ with amino compounds such as D-amino acids, amines, amino sugars, carbonyl reagents, and proteins give a yellow band with an absorption spectrum around 420 nm.

D. ISOLATION OF PQQ–SERINE AS A MODEL COMPOUND OF PQQ ADDUCT

As shown in Fig. 4, PQQ adduct formed with serine has been isolated by a DEAE-Sephadex A-25 chromatography (Adachi *et al.*, 1988b). Unreacted serine is excluded by washing the column before gradient elution, and free PQQ, unreacted or dissociated from the adduct, is eluted at about 0.8 M–1.0 M KCl. Thereafter, two peaks of PQQ adduct are eluted from the column somewhat later than free PQQ, since PQQ adducts formed are expected to contain one more carboxylic group than authentic PQQ and thus be eluted from the column at higher salt concentrations. As expected, a marked coenzyme activity for glucose dehydrogenase is found at the positions where free PQQ is eluted, while both peaks of PQQ–serine exhibit a poor coenzyme activity for the enzyme, which is estimated to be over 100 times less active compared with an equimolar amount of authentic PQQ. Conversely, when the growth-stimulating activity was assayed with the PQQ adducts which are administered at a concentration of picomolar to nanomolar level, the two fractions of PQQ–serine equally stimulated the growth of *A. aceti* in the manner of a typical Type II growth stimulation (Ameyama, 1988a). The extent of growth stimulation by these PQQ adducts is roughly 10 times higher than authentic PQQ. Thus, binding of serine to an active carbonyl group of PQQ allows it to be almost inert as coenzyme, whereas the PQQ adduct stimulates the initial stage of proliferation of microorganisms.

The appearance of two Schiff bases each having an absorption maximum at 420 nm could be explained as follows. Since PQQ has an orthoquinone structure as 4,5-dioxo- (Salisbury *et al.*, 1979; Duine *et al.*, 1980, 1987), it is presumed that both carbonyl groups can be enrolled in Schiff base formation to give different species of PQQ–serine. Several amino acids have been reported to form an oxazole compound with PQQ (van Kleef *et al.*, 1988). Similar results have been obtained with other PQQ adducts prepared with other amino compounds. It is interesting to recall that two peaks of PQQ chromophore have been generated from the chromatograms of hydrolysate of quinoproteins such as amine oxidases (Ameyama *et al.*, 1984a), methylamine dehydrogenase (Ishii *et al.*, 1983), choline dehydrogenase (Ameyama *et al.*, 1985f), and aliphatic amine dehydrogenase (Shinagawa *et al.*, 1988).

E. Spectral Properties of Isolated PQQ–Serine

Although such a PQQ–serine adduct exhibits an absorption peak at 420 nm, characteristic for Schiff base formation, the absorption spectrum observed in the ultraviolet region is somewhat different from those obtained with 2,4-dinitrophenylhydrazine (Lobenstein-Verbeek *et al.*, 1984; van der Meer and Duine, 1986; van der Meer *et al.*, 1986) and rather similar to PQQ–oxazole (van Kleef *et al.*, 1988). A characteristic feature is also observed in its fluorescence spectra. A broad peak around 360 nm in excitation spectrum and 460 nm in emission spectrum (Ameyama *et al.*, 1984a) suggests that the compound came from PQQ. Moreover, a sharp fluorescence peak around 420 nm, reflecting the existence of a Schiff base, is characteristic of all.

It is quite probable that the PQQ adduct is formed readily during extraction and isolation from the naturally occurring materials or PQQ chromophore from quinoproteins. Such an adduct must give low PQQ estimates as determined by the enzymatic method. In other words, a small amount of PQQ *in vivo* tends to react with amino compounds to form PQQ adducts in handling, and becomes less active as the prosthetic group. Therefore, though PQQ may exist free or associated with quinoprotein or a PQQ carrier protein *in vivo*, one can not readily obtain PQQ in free form from natural sources. Thus, the growth-stimulating substance purified from naturally occurring materials, which had been concluded to be PQQ (Ameyama *et al.*, 1984c, 1985a), is probably a PQQ adduct. One exception is for PQQ production by methylotrophs where PQQ is excreted into the culture medium as free PQQ and is produced far in excess of amino compounds (Ameyama *et al.*, 1984a, 1988).

F. MEASUREMENT OF GROWTH STIMULATION BY PQQ OR PQQ ADDUCT

As noted in the previous section, PQQ content of biological materials cannot be estimated exactly with the enzymatic assay, but growth-stimulating activity can be measured with the adduct as well as free PQQ. Therefore, PQQ activity must be determined by both coenzyme activity for the quinoprotein and growth-stimulating activity for microorganisms.

The measurement of growth-stimulating activity with PQQ or PQQ adduct can be determined by a conventional microbial assay. In preparing the inoculum, the cell suspension must not be contaminated with free PQQ. Since a fair amount of readily removable PQQ is adsorbed onto the bacterial cell surface, it is necessary for the growth assay to eliminate the readily removable PQQ from the inoculum cell suspension. For this purpose, inoculum cell suspension should be washed several times with water—PQQ disappears after twenty washings. Acidic buffer washing requires only five repeats before PQQ becomes undetectable (Ameyama *et al.*, 1985b). Pyrroloquinoline quinone seems to be easily released from the cell surface by acidic buffers in which PQQ, a kind of tricarboxylic acid, is protonated. Repeated rinsing with water gives an actual pH of around 5–6 wherein PQQ is still in the dissociated form and thus likely bound to the cell surface via ionic bonds. This assumption has been supported by determining the PQQ content of rinsed cells after treating more than 10 times with water or acidic buffer. However, the extensive rinsing with acidic buffer is not recommended because such washing may cause critical removal of the bound form of PQQ from the inoculum and hence interrupt metabolic activity of the organism which requires PQQ as the prosthetic group for several enzyme functions. Therefore, it is recommended that inoculum cells should be thoroughly rinsed with water more than ten times until no PQQ is detected in the supernatant.

The cell suspension with an optical density of 0.1 at 660 nm, prepared as previously described, can be inoculated under sterile conditions. Then, the bacterial growth can be recorded automatically by use of a biophotometer which gives a plot of turbidity at 660 nm periodically with continuous shaking. Thus, reduction in the length of the lag phase is clearly observed in several bacterial growths with exogenous PQQ (Ameyama *et al.*, 1984b). Even with other species, the use of a water-rinsed inoculum is recommended to get clear-cut results with exogenous PQQ.

IV. PRODUCTION OF PQQ

Determination of the chemical structure of PQQ led to a rush of chemical syntheses by several groups, yielding several synthetic routes. The method published by Corey and Tramontano (1981) includes 10 steps with a 20% yield. Other, similar or modified methods have been used for preparation of commercial products. Most of them, however, require several steps and give low yields.

Pyrroloquinoline quinone fermentation was established by Ameyama *et al.* (1984a) with a methylotroph using C_1 compounds as the sole carbon source. In most methylotrophic bacteria, a quinoprotein methanol dehydrogenase is highly developed as the first enzyme for methanol assimilation. Accumulation of PQQ in the culture medium begins at the end of the exponential phase to early stationary phase when methanol in the medium is almost exhausted. Maximal PQQ accumulation is observed at the late stationary phase. When facultative methylotrophs such as *Methylobacterium* AM1 or *Pseudomonas riboflavina* are grown in nutrient broth containing no methanol, neither accumulation of PQQ nor formation of the quinoprotein is observed. Yamanaka and Matsumoto (1977) have reported that methanol dehydrogenase constitutes over 13% of the total extractable protein of a methylotrophic peudomonad. In an obligate methylotroph, *Hyphomicrobium methylovorum*, methanol dehydrogenase exceeds 7% of the total protein in the cell-free extract (Miyazaki *et al.*, 1987). Duine *et al.* (1978) purified methanol dehydrogenase from *Hyphomicrobium* X and reported that one atom each of iron and manganese are involved per mole of enzyme. Adachi *et al.* (1989) purified methanol dehydrogenase from *Methylobacillus glycogenes* and confirmed the presence of one atom of calcium per mole of the enzyme, but found neither iron nor manganese. Calcium ion is bound tightly and cannot be removed without denaturing the enzyme protein. A partial dissociation calcium is achieved by dialyzing the enzyme against high concentrations of urea containing ethylene glycol-bis(β-aminoethyl ether)-N,N,N',N'-tetraacetic acid (EGTA) and 2-mercaptoethanol. The en-

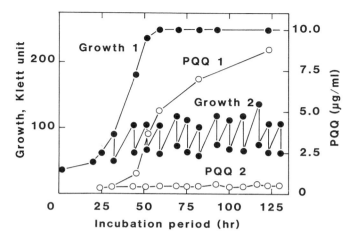

FIG. 5. Effect of culture conditions on pyrroloquinoline quinone (PQQ) formation.

zyme activity of EGTA-dialyzed methanol dehydrogenase is decreased to 10–20% of that of the native enzyme. Addition of calcium restores the original enzyme activity. During denaturation, no release of PQQ from the enzyme is observed. Thus, calcium may be involved in binding up to two enzyme subunits (60 kDa) to form an active enzyme (120 kDa). Holding methylotroph growth to the level of early exponential phase by diluting the culture with fresh medium reduces PQQ concentrations to basal levels as shown in Fig. 5. In exponential growth, methanol dehydrogenase is required for methanol assimilation and the active enzyme must exist without releasing PQQ. In the late stationary phase, where available methanol is almost exhausted and methanol and aldehyde dehydrogenases are no longer necessary for the organism, a rapid turnover of such enzyme proteins should occur. Indeed, methanol dehydrogenase is readily inactivated in the absence of methanol (Yamanaka and Matsumoto, 1977). Thus, it is quite probable that the dissociation of PQQ from the enzymes causes PQQ accumulation in the culture medium; this suggests that the active site of these enzymes must be located on the outer surface of the cytoplasmic membranes. The extent of PQQ accumulation by methylotrophs is variable with strain and culture conditions. A methylotrophic isolate, identified as *M. glycogenes,* by enrichment technique yields 100 μg PQQ/ml after 150 hours incubation (Adachi *et al.,* 1985). In addition to methanol, methylamine can be used as a suitable carbon and nitrogen source for PQQ fermentation, and similar levels of PQQ accumulation are achieved (Urakami, 1986). It has been reported that much-enhanced concentrations, 600 μg PQQ/ml, can be accumulated into the culture medium by controlling and regulating the inorganic ingredients of the culture medium (Urakami, 1987; Urakami *et al.*, 1988). Marine methylotrophs such as *Methylophaga marina* or *M. thalassia*, are also good sources for PQQ production (Urakami, 1987). The isolation and further purification of PQQ obtained by fermentation are easy compared to organic synthesis. Pyrroloquinoline quinone in the culture broth can be adsorbed to anionic ion exchangers with facile isolation from other contaminants. A radioactive PQQ uniformly labeled with ^{14}C also can be readily prepared by adding [^{14}C]methanol to the culture medium (Adachi *et al.*, 1985).

V. Structure and Enzymatic Properties of Quinoprotein Dehydrogenase

Pyrroloquinoline quinone is found mainly as a prosthetic group for primary dehydrogenases of the bacterial respiratory chain. Now, these quinoproteins are recognized as the third group of dehydrogenases, along with NAD(P)-linked dehydrogenases and flavoprotein dehydrogenases. NAD(P)-dependent dehydrogenases are all soluble and linked to a respiratory chain via NADH dehydrogenase which is a membrane-bound flavoprotein. Unlike the NAD(P) enzyme, almost all flavoprotein dehydrogenases are membrane-bound and coupled directly to a respiratory chain. With respect to coupling with a respiratory chain, quinoprotein dehydrogenase more closely relates to flavoprotein but not NAD(P) enzymes, because it transfers reducing equivalents directly to a respiratory chain and binds the prosthetic group tightly in the protein during reaction. Quinoprotein dehydrogenase may differ from flavoprotein in some respects. Although quinoprotein dehydrogenase has been purified as either a soluble or detergent-solubilized (membrane-bound) enzyme, it seems all to be located in the periplasmic space or the periplasmic side of the cytoplasmic membrane of gram-negative bacteria. Quinoprotein dehydrogenase has not so far been found in gram-positive bacteria. Flavoprotein dehydrogenase is mainly located at the inner surface of the cytoplasmic membrane. Further, as expected from its high redox potential, quinoprotein dehydrogenase may couple to a site closer to the terminal end of a respiratory chain than does flavoprotein.

Several quinoprotein dehydrogenases are summarized with reference to structure and enzymatic properties in Table II. Additional in-

TABLE II

STRUCTURE AND PROSTHETIC GROUPS IN QUINOPROTEIN DEHYDROGENASES

Dehydrogenases	Soluble or membrane-bound	Substructure		Prosthetic groups
		Conformation	MW (kDa)	
Glucose dehydrogenase	Soluble	α_2	50	PQQ
	Membrane-bound	α	87	PQQ or PQQ (apo)
Methanol dehydrogenase	Soluble	$\alpha_2\beta_2$	60/12	PQQ (α?)
Methylamine dehydrogenase	Soluble	$\alpha_2\beta_2$	47/15	Pro-PQQ (β)
Alcohol dehydrogenase	Soluble	α_2	60	PQQ
	Soluble	α	67	PQQ (apo)/heme c
	Membrane-bound	$\alpha\beta\gamma$	80/48/12	PQQ/heme c (α)/heme c (β)
Aldehyde dehydrogenase	Membrane-bound	$\alpha\beta$ (γ)	86/55	PQQ (α)/heme c (β)
Aliphatic amine dehydrogenase	Soluble	$\alpha\beta$	60/39	PQQ (α)/heme c (β)

formation may be obtained from reviews by Anthony (1982, 1988), Duine *et al.* (1986, 1987) and Duine and Jongejan (1989).

A. GLUCOSE DEHYDROGENASE

Glucose dehydrogenase is a quinoprotein that catalyzes the direct oxidation of D-glucose to D-gluconate at the outer surface of the cytoplasmic membrane, and serves as an alternative pathway to the phosphotransferase system of bacteria to catalyze D-glucose assimilation (Midgley and Dawes, 1973). The enzyme is found in a variety of bacteria including *Escherichia* or *Klebsiella,* besides oxidative bacteria such as pseudomonads or acetic acid bacteria.

As described previously, glucose dehydrogenase is known to be a classic enzyme for PQQ research; it was initially purified and described by Hauge (1960, 1961, 1964) and subsequently investigated by Duine *et al.* (1979a), who demonstrated glucose dehydrogenase as a quinoprotein. Recently, the same enzyme has been purified and investigated again by two groups (Dokter *et al.,* 1986; Geiger and Gorisch, 1986). The enzymes used by these researchers were those purified from the soluble fraction of *A. calcoaceticus.* This bacterium contains a soluble form of glucose dehydrogenase in addition to the membrane-bound form, the two having been considered for a long time to be the same enzyme or interconvertible forms (Hauge and Hallberg, 1964; Dokter *et al.,* 1987). However, it has been shown that this soluble enzyme is not a typical glucose dehydrogenase, and has been confused with a typical membrane-bound glucose dehydrogenase. The membranes of several strains, *E. coli, Klesbiella aerogenes, Pseudomonas aeruginosa, Glucobacter suboxydans, A. aceti,* and *A. calcoaceticus* all contain antigens cross-reactive with an antibody to glucose dehydrogenase purified from *Pseudomonas fluorescens* (Matsushita *et al.,* 1986). Glucose dehydrogenase from the soluble fraction of *A. calcoaceticus* does not cross-react with the antibody (Matsushita *et al.,* 1988). Subsequently, soluble and membrane-bound glucose dehydrogenases have been purified separately from *A. calcoaceticus* and shown to be distinctive in all aspects, i.e., optimum pH, kinetics, substrate specificity, ubiquinone reactivity, molecular size, and immunoreactivity (Matsushita *et al.,* 1989b). The immunochemical evidence also obviates the possibility that soluble glucose dehydrogenase is a degradation product or a precursor of the membrane-bound enzyme. The notion that soluble and membrane-bound glucose dehydrogenases are independent molecular species is consistent with the genetic evidence obtained by Cleton-Jansen *et al.* (1988a,b) who showed that *A. calcoaceticus* contains two different *gdh* genes with no sequence homology. Furthermore, there are no antigens cross-reacting with the antibody specific for soluble dehydrogenase in either soluble or membrane fractions of any strains tested so far (Matsushita *et al.*, unpublished observations). Thus, *A. calcoaceticus* is exceptional in containing both soluble and membrane-bound glucose dehydrogenases.

Soluble glucose dehydrogenase of *A. calcoaceticus* is a dimer consisting of identical subunits of 48–55 kDa and each subunit contains one molecule of PQQ (Dokter *et al.*, 1986; Geiger and Gorisch, 1986). A gene (*gdh*B) for the enzyme has been cloned and sequenced; the gene product is estimated to be a polypeptide of 52.8 kDa (Cleton-Jansen *et al.*, 1988b). The polypeptide contains a 24-amino acid signal sequence in the N-terminus, and thus is expected to become the mature protein of 50.2 kDa, which does not contain a hydrophobic region. Thus, soluble glucose dehydrogenase seems to be translocated through the cytoplasmic membrane into the periplasmic space. However, the mutant strain containing only *gdh*B gene but not *gdh*A gene (encoding membrane-bound glucose dehydrogenase) does not show any *in vivo* activity for glucose oxidation (Cleton-Jansen *et al.*, 1988a,b). Soluble glucose dehydrogenase characteristically catalyzes the oxidation of disaccharides, lactose, or maltose, as well as D-glucose. The enzyme donates electrons to several artificial dyes; phenazine methosulfate (PMS), dichlorophenol indophenol (DCIP), or Wurster's Blue (WB), as well as the short-chain ubiquinone homologue, Q_1 or Q_2, but does not react with long-chain ubiquinone. Q_6 or Q_9 (Dokter *et al.*, 1986; Geiger and Gorisch, 1986; Matsushita *et al.*, 1989b).

The membrane-bound glucose dehydrogenase, on the other hand, has been solubilized and purified with detergent from membranes of *P. fluorescens*, *G. suboxydans*, and *E. coli*, and also of *A. calcoaceticus* (Matsushita *et al.*, 1980, 1982, 1989a,b; Ameyama *et al.*, 1981b, 1986). The purified enzyme is a single polypeptide of 83–87 kDa (at least in the presence of detergent); probably it exists as a monomer in detergent micelles or in phospholipid membranes. The gene (*gdh*A) for membrane-bound glucose dehydrogenase of *A. calcoaceticus* has been cloned and sequenced; the *gdh*A gene encodes for a protein of 87 kDa and has a very hydrophobic region in the N-terminus (Cleton-Jansen *et al.*, 1988b). The membrane-bound enzymes of all bacterial strains seem closely related structurally since all seven strains tested cross-reacted immunologically (Matsushita *et al.*, 1986). Membrane-bound glucose dehydrogenase exhibits a relatively broad substrate specificity for monosaccharides, including D-glucose, D-fructose, D-galactose, or D-xylose, but the enzyme is incapable of oxidizing lactose as does soluble glucose dehydrogenase. The enzyme can reduce several artificial electron acceptors such as PMS, DCIP, WB, and Q_1 as well as soluble glucose dehydrogenase. Unlike the soluble enzyme, membrane-bound glucose dehydrogenase reduces long-chain ubiquinone, Q_6 or Q_9 (Matsushita *et al.*, 1982, 1989a,b).

The mode of binding of PQQ to apoglucose dehydrogenase seems similar to the enzymes of any origin; the enzyme binds PQQ noncovalently via divalent cation, magnesium, or calcium. The strength of binding, however, is somewhat different from enzyme to enzyme. Pyrroloquinoline quinone can be removed readily by dialysis with EDTA in the enzymes of *P. fluorescens, P. aeruginosa,* or *E. coli,* and can be reconstituted with magnesium or calcium ion (Imanaga *et al.*, 1979; Duine *et al.*, 1983; Ameyama *et al.*, 1985d). On the other hand, PQQ is so tightly bound to the enzymes of *A. calcoaceticus* or *G. suboxydans* that it can not be removed by EDTA dialysis (Duine *et al.*, 1979a; Ameyama *et al.*, 1981b). Instead, PQQ must be removed from the enzyme in *A. calcoaceticus* with heat and reactivated with PQQ in the presence of calcium (Geiger and Gorisch, 1989). In *E. coli* or *K. aerogenes,* almost all of glucose dehydrogenase exists as an apo-form in the membranes; the activity can be reconstituted by the addition of PQQ with magnesium (Homes *et al.*, 1984; Ameyama *et al.*, 1985d). This makes apoglucose dehydrogenase of *E. coli* useful for enzymatic assay of PQQ (Ameyama *et al.*, 1985e; Geiger and Gorisch, 1987). Further, the apoenzyme can be used to study structural requirements for interaction with enzymes. Such studies show tricarboxyl group of PQQ is essential for binding to apoenzyme (Shinagawa *et al.*, 1986).

B. METHANOL AND METHYLAMINE DEHYDROGENASES

Methanol and methylamine dehydrogenases are quinoproteins that catalyze oxidation of methanol or methylamine, to formaldehyde. These quinoproteins are found at high concentrations in the periplasmic space of methylotrophic bacteria growing on these substrates. Detailed descriptions for each enzyme are given in the extensive review of Anthony (1982). Here, the structures and properties of the enzymes are simply summarized with information on recent progress.

Methanol dehydrogenase catalyzes oxidation of diverse primary alcohols, but shows the highest affinity for methanol, unlike alcohol dehydrogenase, described in Section V,C. The activity is assayed with an artificial electron acceptor such as PMS at very high pH with ammonia as activator, the latter probably not physiological.

Methanol dehydrogenase was believed for a long time to be a dimer consisting of identical subunits of 60 kDa (Anthony, 1982, 1988). Genetic studies in *Methylobacterium* AM1, however, show that a possible methanol oxidation operon of this bacterium consists of four sequential genes, *moxFJGI,* which encodes four polypeptides of 60, 30, 20, and 12 kDa, respectively (Anderson and Lidstrom, 1988). There are two additional proteins (30 and 12 kDa), coded by *moxJ* and *moxI* genes, besides the proteins for methanol dehydrogenase (60 kDa) and its physiological electron acceptor, cytochrome c_L (20 kDa). Although the polypeptide encoded by the *moxJ* gene has not been identified, the smallest peptide encoded by the *moxI* gene is a methanol dehydrogenase-associated protein (Anderson and Lidstrom, 1988). Furthermore, methanol dehydrogenase purified from *Methylobacterium* AM1 was shown to contain the second subunit of 8.5 kDa besides the first subunit of 60 kDa at a molar ratio of about 1 : 1 (Nunn *et al.,* 1989). Thus, methanol dehydrogenases can now generally be considered to exist in $\alpha_2\beta_2$ conformation.

Methylamine dehydrogenase oxidizes a variety of primary, but not secondary or tertiary amines. The enzyme activity is measured with an artificial electron acceptor such as PMS, but the enzyme exhibits the activity at normal pH without any activator, which is contrary to that of methanol dehydrogenase.

Methylamine dehydrogenase consists of two large subunits (40–47 kDa) and two small subunits (13–15 kDa) in $\alpha_2\beta_2$ conformation like methanol dehydrogenase. The mode of PQQ binding, however, is different from methanol dehydrogenase in that it bears the prosthetic group noncovalently; PQQ is covalently bound to two amino acid residues of the small subunit of methylamine dehydrogenase (Ishii *et al.,* 1983). Observations suggest that the covalently bound prosthetic group of the enzyme is not PQQ itself, but pro-PQQ (Duine, 1989).

C. ALCOHOL DEHYDROGENASE

Several different types of PQQ-dependent alcohol dehydrogenases have been found in oxidative bacteria such as pseudomonads or acetic acid bacteria. The enzymes catalyze the oxidation of diverse alcohols, but oxidize methanol at low rates or not at all. These alcohol dehydrogenases could be divided into three subgroups according to structure; (1) quinoprotein alcohol dehydrogenase; (2) quinohemoprotein alcohol dehydrogenase; and (3) quinohemoprotein–cytochrome *c* alcohol dehydrogenase (Table II).

Quinoprotein alcohol dehydrogenase has been purified from *P.*

aeruginosa and *Pseudomonas putida*. The enzyme is a dimer of identical subunits of 60 kDa (Gorisch and Rupp, 1988) or a monomer of 100 kDa (Groen *et al.*, 1984), and contains two PQQ moieties per mole. With respect to catalytic properties, these alcohol dehydrogenases are very similar to methanol dehydrogenase; they have a high optimum pH (9.0–9.5) and exhibit enzyme activity with artificial electron acceptors such as PMS or WB in the presence of ammonia or amine. This enzyme, however, is capable of oxidizing a great number of primary (C_1–C_{11}) and secondary (C_3–C_{10}) alcohols and aldehydes (C_2–C_{10}). Though the enzyme is able to oxidize methanol, the K_m for this is 1000 times higher than for ethanol (13–18 μM).

Quinohemoprotein alcohol dehydrogenase has been purified as a monomer of a single polypeptide of 67 kDa from *Pseudomonas testosteroni* (Groen *et al.*, 1986). This enzyme is quite different from quinoprotein alcohol dehydrogenases described previously. It shows a neutral optimum pH (7.7), does not require any activator, and can use ferricyanide as well as PMS or WB as the electron acceptor. It does not catalyze methanol oxidation, but like quinoprotein alcohol dehydrogenase, is active with a variety of primary alcohols (C_2–C_{10}), secondary alcohols, and aldehydes (C_1–C_4). Furthermore, the enzyme characteristically contains one molecule of heme c/mol but not PQQ. The full enzyme activity is reconstituted with one molecule of PQQ/mol of protein with calcium ion. Thus, this enzyme is termed as "quinohemoprotein alcohol dehydrogenase."

Alcohol dehydrogenase of acetic acid bacteria, together with aldehyde dehydrogenase, functions in vinegar fermentation to oxidize ethanol to acetic acid. This alcohol dehydrogenase is totally different from quinoprotein alcohol dehydrogenase, but is similar to quinohemoprotein alcohol dehydrogenase in some respects. This alcohol dehydrogenase is tightly bound to the cytoplasmic membranes, totally unlike other alcohol dehydrogenases existing in soluble form. Alcohol dehydrogenase of acetic acid bacteria has been solubilized and purified in detergent from the membranes of *G. suboxydans* and *A. aceti* (Adachi *et al.*, 1978a,b). Subsequently, the enzyme purified from *G. suboxydans* has been crystallized as large red crystals; it is the first example of crystallization of a membrane-bound dehydrogenase (Adachi *et al.*, 1982). The purified enzyme is composed of three subunits; dehydrogenase peptide of 72–80 kDa, cytochrome c_{553} of 48–53 kDa, and an unknown peptide of 14–17 kDa. The enzyme complex (about 140 kDa) contains one molecule of PQQ and three molecules of heme c as the prosthetic group (Ameyama and Adachi, 1982; K. Matsushita *et al.*, unpublished observations). Heme *c* is bound to both the first and second subunits of the enzyme, and PQQ is probably bound to the first dehydrogenase subunit. Therefore, the dehydrogenase subunit is considered as quinohemoprotein, and alcohol dehydrogenase of acetic acid bacteria should thus be called a quinohemoprotein–cytochrome *c* complex. A gene for the dehydrogenase subunit of alcohol dehydrogenase of *A. aceti* has been cloned and sequenced (Inoue *et al.*, 1989). The gene encodes a polypeptide of 78 kDa and the preceding signal sequence consisting of 35 amino acid residues, which is consistent with the notion that alcohol dehydrogenase of acetic acid bacteria is located on the periplasmic side of the cytoplasmic membrane. Furthermore, of the total amino acid sequence of the 78-kDa dehydrogenase subunit, about 600 amino acid residues of the N-terminal portion exhibits close similarity to the amino acid sequence of quinoprotein methanol dehydrogenase, and the following residues of the C-terminal region contain a heme *c*-binding sequence (Cys-X-X-Cys-His). Thus, the quinohemoprotein dehydrogenase subunit of alcohol dehydrogenase of acetic acid bacteria is considered as a conjugated product of quinoprotein and cytochrome *c* regions.

The quinohemoprotein–cytochrome *c* alcohol dehydrogenase does not require any activator for assay and reacts with ferricyanide as well as PMS, DCIP, or WB, all properties similar to quinohemoprotein alcohol dehydrogenase. The enzyme, however, shows a lower optimum pH (4–6) and relatively restricted substrate specificity compared to quinoprotein or quinohemoprotein alcohol dehydrogenase. It oxidizes only primary alcohols (C_2–C_6) and not methanol, secondary, or tertiary alcohols, or aldehydes (though *Acetobacter* enzyme shows some activity for formaldehyde). Furthermore, the enzyme activity of quinohemoprotein–cytochrome *c* alcohol dehydrogenase is about 10 times higher than that of quinohemoprotein alcohol dehydrogenase. Since a dissociation of cytochrome *c* from the quinohemoprotein–cytochrome *c* complex is known to decrease activity (K. Matsushita *et al.*, unpublished observations), the complex between quinohemoprotein dehydrogenase and cytochrome *c* with or without the third small subunit, may confer particular properties, membrane-binding, increased enzyme activity, and reduced pH optimum to the enzyme.

D. OTHER QUINOPROTEIN DEHYDROGENASES

As shown in Table 1, several enzymes related to alcohol dehydrogenase described in the previous section have been found as quinoproteins, which include aromatic alcohol (Yamanaka and Tsuyuki, 1983; Yamanaka, 1988), polyethylene glycol (Kawai *et al.*, 1980, 1985), and polyvinyl alcohol (Shimao *et al.*, 1986) dehydrogenases. These dehydrogenases are totally inert towards methanol, but exhibit varying specificities for diverse alcohols. Aromatic alcohol dehydrogenase oxidizes well aromatic alcohols such as vannillyl, benzyl, or cinnamyl alcohol, in addition to primary alcohols (C_2–C_{10}), secondary alcohols, and aldehydes. The enzyme is a soluble single protein of 72 kDa, contains heme c, and is thus similar to quinohemoprotein alcohol dehydrogenase. Polyethylene glycol dehydrogenase characteristically catalyzes oxidation of long-chain primary alcohols (C_2–C_{18}) in addition to polyethylene glycol. The enzyme is membrane-bound and has been purified with detergent. The purified enzyme is a tetramer of identical 60-kDa subunits in detergent solution, and appears to be similar to quinoprotein alcohol dehydrogenase since it lacks heme c. Characteristically, polyvinyl alcohol dehydrogenase catalyzes oxidation of secondary alcohols (C_5–C_7) in addition to polyvinyl alcohol, but not primary alcohols. The enzyme is membrane-bound and reduces cytochrome c in the membrane (Shimao *et al.*, 1989). It has not been purified, nor has its structure been determined.

There are other types of quinoprotein dehydrogenases whose structures are known. They are quinoprotein–cytochrome c complexes of which aldehyde dehydrogenases of acetic acid bacteria and aliphatic amine dehydrogenase of *Pseudomonas* are known so far. Aldehyde dehydrogenases are tightly bound to the membranes of acetic acid bacteria, and have been purified with detergent from the membranes of *G. suboxydans* (Adachi *et al.*, 1980) and *A. aceti* (Ameyama *et al.*, 1981c). The purified enzymes are complexes of two to three subunits; the first subunit of 78–86 kDa is a quinoprotein containing non-covalently bound PQQ (Ameyama *et al.*, 1981a), and the second subunit of 45–55 kDa is a cytochrome c_{551}. The enzymes oxidize aliphatic aldehydes, except for formaldehyde, using an electron acceptor such as ferricyanide, PMS, or DCIP at low pH (4–5). Aliphatic amine dehydrogenase has been purified and crystallized from *Pseudomonas* sp. (Shinagawa *et al.*, 1988). The enzyme is a heterodimer (100 kDa) consisting of two subunits; the larger, of 60 kDa, is a quinoprotein containing covalently bound PQQ, and the small subunit, of 39 kDa, is a cytochrome c_{550}. The enzyme catalyzes oxidation of a range of amines, including aliphatic monoamines, aliphatic diamines, aromatic amines, and polyamines, by using PMS, DCIP, or ferricyanide as an electron acceptor.

VI. Coupling of Quinoprotein Dehydrogenase to the Respiratory Chain

Since quinoprotein dehydrogenase composes a part of the respiratory chain and functionally couples with the remaining part of the respiratory chain, it is very important to know how it links to the respiratory chain. The question of the natural electron acceptor for quinoprotein dehydrogenase and how it couples to the respiratory chain is still controversial. This is partly due to the short history, about 10 years, of quinoprotein dehydrogenase research, and partly due to incomplete understanding of the bacterial respiratory chain. Progress in this area, including that summarized by Anthony (1988) is reviewed in Section VI,A–D.

A. Glucose Dehydrogenase

The identity of the natural electron acceptor for glucose dehydrogenase has been a long-standing controversy which now seems to be resolved. Initially, Hauge (1960, 1964) reported that cytochrome b is an electron acceptor of glucose dehydrogenase from *A. calcoaceticus*. On the other hand, Beardmore-Gray and Anthony (1986) suggested that glucose dehydrogenase is linked to the respiratory chain via ubiquinone in *A. calcoaceticus*. Dokter *et al.* (1988) concluded that soluble glucose dehydrogenase of *A. calcoaceticus* donates electrons to the respiratory chain via a cytochrome b_{562} that is reduced at a slow rate. However, such a slow reduction of cytochrome may not necessarily mean an involvement of the cytochrome for the physiological electron transfer, but only its physicochemical redox equilibrium. More importantly, as previously described, *A. calcoaceticus* contains both soluble and membrane-bound glucose dehydrogenase that have been confused with one another, giving rise to controversy on the natural electron acceptor for the enzyme(s) of *A. calcoaceticus*.

On the other hand, membrane-bound glucose dehydrogenases purified from *P. fluorescens* and *G. suboxydans* have been shown to react with the longer chain ubiquinone homologue, Q_6, as well as short-chain homologues Q_1 or Q_2 (Matsushita *et al.*, 1982, 1989a). The reduction rate of Q_6 with membrane-bound glucose dehydrogenase is relatively low. Indeed, work with such a hydrophobic electron acceptor is difficult in aqueous solution, thus suggesting that ubiquinone is the

natural electron acceptor for membrane-bound glucose dehydrogenase. This notion was reinforced by reconstitution of glucose dehydrogenase into a phospholipid bilayer containing ubiquinone. Terminal
oxidase to allow oxidation of resultant ubiquinol had to be reconstituted simultaneously. Thus, glucose dehydrogenases purified from
the membranes of *E. coli* and *G. suboxydans* have been reconstituted
into proteoliposomes together with the respective ubiquinone, Q_8 for
E. coli and Q_{10} for *G. suboxydans,* and cytochrome *o* terminal oxidase
purified from *E. coli* and *G. suboxydans* (Matsushita *et al.,* 1987a,
1989a). The proteoliposomes thus reconstituted are able to catalyze the
oxidation of glucose at a reasonable rate producing an electron transfer reaction which also generates an electrochemical proton gradient
(Table III). The apparent turnover of glucose oxidase with respect to
glucose dehydrogenase in the proteoliposomes is comparable to that of
the native membrane. Since cytochrome *o* has been shown to oxidize
ubiquinol, such an occurrence of glucose oxidase activity indicates that
glucose dehydrogenase is able to reduce Q_8 or Q_{10} to produce Q_8H_2 or
$Q_{10}H_2$, which is in turn oxidized rapidly by the cytochrome *o* in the
proteoliposomes. These reconstitution experiments show that membrane-bound glucose dehydrogenase can donate electrons directly to
ubiquinone in the respiratory chain.

   From *A. calcoaceticus,* both soluble and membrane-bound glucose
dehydrogenases have been purified, separated, and reactivity with
ubiquinone examined (Matsushita *et al.,* 1989b). Although both enzymes are able to react with short-chain ubiquinone homologues, long-
chain homologue, Q_6 or Q_9, is reduced only by membrane-bound enzyme. Furthermore, membrane-bound glucose dehydrogenase has
been reconstituted into proteoliposomes together with Q_9 and *A. calcoaceticus* cytochrome *o* (K. Matsushita *et al.,* unpublished observations). The proteoliposomes are capable of oxidizing glucose as well as
generating a membrane potential (Table III), whereas soluble glucose
dehydrogenase exhibits no glucose oxidase activity in spite of binding
to proteoliposomes. Thus, even in *A. calcoaceticus* as well as *E. coli* or
G. suboxydans, ubiquinone is the likely natural electron acceptor for
membrane-bound glucose dehydrogenase. The natural electron acceptor for the soluble glucose dehydrogenase of *A. calcoaceticus* remains
unclear and has been further questioned (Cleton-Jansen *et al.,*
1988a,b).

   Thus, it is reasonable to conclude that membrane-bound glucose
dehydrogenase, present in a wide variety of bacteria, is coupled to the
respiratory chain via ubiquinone.

TABLE III
RECONSTITUTION OF GLUCOSE OXIDASE RESPIRATORY CHAIN

Strains	Systems	GDH (units/mg)	Glucose oxidase (units/mg)	Turnover number[a] (e/s/mol)	Membrane potential (mV)	Terminal oxidase functioning
E. coli GR 1 9N[b]	Native membranes	0.24	0.16	573	–	Cytochrome o
	Proteoliposomes	10.0	5.89	517	-124	Cytochrome o
G. suboxydans[c]	Native membranes	2.86	1.08	676	–	Cytochrome o
	Proteoliposomes	40.0	9.00	435	-112	Cytochrome o
A. calcoaceticus	Native membranes	4.00	0.75	228	–	Cytochrome o/d
LMD 79.41[d]	Proteoliposomes	90.8	10.7	122	-130	Cytochrome o

[a]The values are expressed per mole of GDH.
[b]Proteoliposomes for E. coli system are prepared from glucose dehydrogenase (GDH) and cytochrome o, both purified from the organism, Q_8, and E. coli phospholipids (Matsushita et al., 1987a).
[c]Proteoliposomes for G. suboxydans system from GDH and cytochrome o both purified from the organism, Q_{10}, and G. suboxydans phospholipids (Matsushita et al., 1989a).
[d]Proteoliposomes for A. calcoaceticus from membrane-bound GDH and cytochrome o of the organism, Q_9, and E. coli phospholipids (K. Matsushita et al., unpublished observations).

B. METHANOL DEHYDROGENASE

The problem of coupling of methanol dehydrogenase to the respiratory chain is still unresolved. Although there is general agreement that cytochrome c_L is the natural electron acceptor for methanol dehydrogenase, the reduction rate of the cytochrome c with methanol dehydrogenase *in vitro* is extraordinarily low (Anthony, 1982, 1988). There are two controversial notions to explain this apparent slow reaction rate with cytochrome c_L.

An autoreduction phenomenon is found in purified cytochrome c_L that becomes reduced as an intramolecular electron transfer reaction at high pH without reductant. The autoreduction is proposed to be involved in the mechanism of electron transfer between methanol dehydrogenase and cytochrome c_L (O'Keeffe and Anthony, 1980; Elliott and Anthony, 1988). The autoreduction occurs at abnormally high pH but the addition of methanol dehydrogenase decreases the pH to the physiological range. This suggests that the reaction may be physiological. Furthermore, the autoreduction rate of cytochrome c_L with methanol dehydrogenase is sufficient to account for the respiration rate *in vivo*, which is 60 times faster than the reduction rate of methanol-dependent cytochrome c catalyzed *in vitro* by methanol dehydrogenase (Elliott and Anthony, 1988). It is nevertheless unclear whether the autoreduction phenomenon occurs *in vivo* during electron transfer from methanol to oxygen, and to what extent such electron transfer is constituted by autoreduction.

Another possible explanation is that a mediator between dehydrogenase and cytochrome or one of the components is inactivated during preparation of the cell-free extract. This idea has been developed by Duine and colleagues, who showed that the electron transfer from methanol to cytochrome c_L occurs when cell-free extract of *Hyphomicrobium* X is prepared anaerobically but not aerobically (Duine *et al.*, 1979b). They also suggested that the reduction step of methanol dehydrogenase with methanol is rate limiting and requires some activator, while the reduction step of cytochrome c_L with reduced methanol dehydrogenase is not rate limiting (Dijkstra *et al.*, 1988a, 1989). Moreover, the activator capable of stimulating cytochrome c_L reduction can be isolated from anaerobically prepared cell-free extracts and is an oxygen-sensitive low molecular weight component (Dijkstra *et al.*, 1988b). Unfortunately, however, the factor does not activate the electron transfer to physiological rates and the component has not been identified chemically.

Thus, neither of the two notions just above provides a definitive answer as to how methanol dehydrogenase is linked to the respiratory chain to form the methanol oxidase system. Before proving the reaction *in vivo*, one must reproduce it *in vitro*. In this respect, Froud and Anthony (1984) have tried to reconstitute methanol oxidase respiratory chain from methanol dehydrogenase, cytochrome c_L and cytochrome *co* terminal oxidase purified from *Methylophilus methylotrophus*. The reconstituted system shows significant methanol oxidase activity which is sensitive to EDTA or azide, like an intact system. For the reconstitution, all three components are indispensable and cytochrome c_L is not replaced by cytochrome c_H, which stimulates the electron transfer from cytochrome c_L to cytochrome *co*, suggesting that the methanol oxidase respiratory chain of *M. methylotrophus* is composed of methanol dehydrogenase, cytochrome c_L, cytochrome c_H, and cytochrome *co* in sequence. However, the reconstituted activity is very low compared to that of whole cells. This may reflect the fact that cytochrome c_L reduction is slow and that the system has been reconstituted under "unnatural" conditions with simple mixing of purified enzymes at low concentrations, thus not favoring association of components. Hence, there remain many unsolved problems of the methanol oxidase respiratory chain. Is there an oxygen-sensitive factor involved in electron transfer from methanol to cytochrome c_L? Is structural interaction among components required for full electron transfer? What is the function of the newly found small subunit of methanol dehydrogenase in electron transfer? What is the function in electron transfer of the *moxJ* gene, identified genetically (Anderson and Lidstrom, 1988) between the *moxF* gene (methanol dehydrogenase large subunit) and the *moxG* gene (cytochrome c_L) encoding a polypeptide of 30 kDa?

C. METHYLAMINE DEHYDROGENASE

The coupling of methylamine dehydrogenase, in contrast to methanol dehydrogenase to the respiratory chain is much more clear. There is, however, still some controversy as to the natural electron acceptor for methylamine dehydrogenase and mechanisms of structural interaction between the dehydrogenase and a blue copper protein, amicyanin.

Although there is a general agreement that amicyanin is the physiological electron acceptor for methylamine dehydrogenase, it is not necessarily detected in all methylotrophs grown on methylamine. Some authors, moreover, imply that methylamine dehydrogenase reacts with a cytochrome *c* (Anthony, 1982, 1988). In order to elucidate whole process of electron transfer in methylamine oxidase respiratory chain, the methylamine oxidase system of two methylotrophs has been reconstituted by the same procedure as used for reconstitution of the methanol oxidase system, unlike that for the glucose oxidase system, which is performed by simply mixing the purified components. Initially, significant methylamine oxidase activity was obtained by mixing methylamine dehydrogenase with cytochrome c_H and cytochrome aa_3 terminal oxidase purified from *Methylobacterium* AM1 (Fukumori and Yamanaka, 1987). In this system, amicyanin was not required for oxygen consumption coupled to the oxidation of methylamine, but the activity obtained (21 electron/sec/mol of cytochrome aa_3) was small. The same oxidase system has been reconstituted using the dehydrogenase, amicyanin, cytochrome c_H, or azurin, and cytochrome *co* terminal oxidase purified from the obligate methylotroph 4025 (Auton and Anthony, 1989). Here, amicyanin is indispensable, not replaced by cytochrome c_L or c_H, and electron transfer between amicyanin and cytochrome *co* can be mediated by cytochrome c_H or a second blue copper protein, azurin. The maximum electron transfer rate from methylamine to oxygen is 115 electron/sec/mol of cytochrome *co*, which is about 20% of that in the whole cells. However, this requires a 1000-fold excess of amicyanin or azurin relative to cytochrome *co*. Hence, the turnover value obtained with respect to cytochrome *co* does not necessarily imply a rapid electron transfer from methylamine dehydrogenase to azurin via amicyanin. Although some ambiguity remains about details, it is reasonable to conclude that the methylamine oxidase respiratory chain of at least organism 4025 consists of methylamine dehydrogenase, amicyanin, cytochrome c_H or azurin, and cytochrome *co* in sequence.

The structural interactions among respiratory components of the methylamine oxidase respiratory chain, as well as the methanol oxidase respiratory chain, have not been studied extensively. In methylamine oxidase systems of organism 4025 (Lawton and Anthony, 1985) and *Thiobacillus versutus* (Wielink *et al.*, 1988), it has been speculated from results on *in vitro* rate constants and assumed high concentrations of components in the periplasm, that freely soluble and collisional interaction between methylamine dehydrogenase and amicyanin can explain the respiration rate of whole cells. On the other hand, in *Paracoccus denitrificans,* methylamine dehydrogenase reportedly forms a 1:2 complex with amicyanin under low ionic strength (Gray *et al.*, 1988). This complex produces a decrease in a redox potential of amicyanin, thereby enabling amicyanin to transfer electrons to the next electron acceptor, cytochrome c_{551}. Thus, it remains unknown whether the respiratory system of methylamine oxidase functions with freely soluble or tightly associated components.

In any event, since terminal oxidase is embedded in the phospholipid membrane *in vivo*, cytochrome *c* mediating electron transfer between amicyanin and the terminal oxidase must have some structural interaction with the terminal oxidase. If the whole methylamine oxidase respiratory chain can be reconstituted maintaining such a structural relationship, physiological rates of methylamine oxidase activity might be attained *in vitro*.

D. Alcohol Dehydrogenase

There is little information on coupling of alcohol dehydrogenase to the respiratory chain. Since quinoprotein alcohol dehydrogenase of *P. aeruginosa* and *P. putida* are analogous to methanol dehydrogenase in terms of structure and kinetics, the natural electron acceptor for the alcohol dehydrogenase would be expected to be a soluble cytochrome *c*. There is, however, no report of such a cytochrome *c*, and coupling of quinoprotein alcohol dehydrogenase to the respiratory chain is unknown. The natural electron acceptor for quinohemoprotein alcohol dehydrogenase of *P. testosteroni* is also unknown. Since the enzyme is different from quinoprotein alcohol dehydrogenase in several respects, quinohemoprotein alcohol dehydrogenase may be coupled to the respiratory chain by mechanisms distinct from that of quinoprotein alcohol dehydrogenase.

The coupling mechanism of alcohol dehydrogenase of acetic acid bacteria to the respiratory chain has been investigated (Ameyama, 1989). This alcohol dehydrogenase is distinctive in several respects from quinoprotein or quinohemoprotein alcohol dehydrogenase. It forms a complex with cytochrome *c* and is tightly bound to the membrane. Furthermore, acetic acid bacteria, including both *Acetobacter* and *Gluconobacter* genera, display highly active respiratory chains terminated by cytochrome *o* or cytochrome a_1, now known to be a ubiquinol oxidase (Matsushita *et al.*, 1987b, and unpublished observations). Thus, the ethanol oxidase respiratory chain has been reconstituted in the manner similar to the glucose oxidase system. Alcohol dehydrogenase purified from *G. suboxydans* or *A. aceti* was reconstituted together with ubiquinone, Q_{10} or Q_9, and terminal oxidase, cytochrome *o* or a_1. Unlike glucose dehydrogenase, alcohol dehydrogenase could be incorporated successfully into preformed proteoliposomes. This is explained by hydrophobicity differences between the two dehydrogenases. The proteoliposomes thus prepared exhibit ethanol oxidase activity with 10 times higher specific activity than is found in the intact membrane. This represents about 50% of the *in vivo* turnover number for alcohol dehydrogenase. Thus, alcohol dehydrogenase of acetic acid bacteria seems to be linked to the respiratory chain via ubiquinone, which is just like glucose dehydrogenase. However, this alcohol dehydrogenase consists of three subunits, quinohemoprotein, cytochrome *c,* and an unknown protein. Neither the intramolecular electron transfer mechanisms among these subunits nor the components donating electrons to ubiquinone are known.

E. Conclusions on the Role of Quinoproteins in the Respiratory Chain

As shown in Fig. 6, methanol and methylamine dehydrogenases are coupled with cytochrome c_L and amicyanin, respectively, which may or may not form a relatively weak complex, and may be freely soluble in the periplasmic space or loosely bound to the periplasmic side of the cytoplasmic membrane. Such a putative complex donates electrons to a terminal oxidase embedded in the membrane via cytochrome *c,* which seems to be loosely bound to the periplasmic side of the cytoplasmic membrane by analogy with the mitochondrion. The terminal oxidase involved in methanol or methylamine oxidase system must, therefore, be a cytochrome *c* oxidase, of which only cytochrome aa_3 and cytochrome *co* are known.

On the other hand, glucose dehydrogenase, as well as the alcohol dehydrogenase complex of quinohemoprotein and cytochrome *c,* are bound relatively tightly to the periplasmic side of the cytoplasmic membrane, and donate electrons to ubiquinone embedded in membrane phospholipids. The resulting ubiquinol is subsequently oxidized by a terminal oxidase in the membrane. Thus, the terminal oxidase involved in glucose or alcohol oxidase system must be a ubiquinol oxidase, the activity of which has been found in cytochrome *o,* cytochrome *d* and cytochrome a_1.

The methylotrophic acetic acid bacteria *Acetobacter methanolicus* is interesting in that it contains both methanol and alcohol oxidase systems in the respiratory chain (Loffhagen and Babel, 1984). If both oxidase systems bear completely different respiratory chains and terminal oxidases as described, there must be in this organism two independent respiratory chains containing the respective terminal oxidase. Further research on the respiratory chain of *A. methanolicus* should provide a clear answer on the difference between methanol and alcohol respiratory chains.

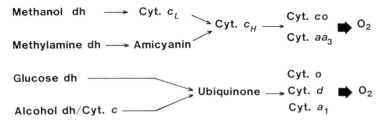

FIG. 6. Schematic respiratory chains in which quinoprotein hydrogenases are involved. Cyt, Cytochrome; dh, dehydrogenase.

Generally, respiratory chain systems involving quinoprotein as primary dehydrogenases are simple and only the terminal oxidase generates an electrochemical proton gradient. Such a truncated respiratory chain may be favorable for rapid oxidation of large amounts of substrate. This notion also is suggested by the periplasmic location of quinoprotein dehydrogenase, since there is no requirement for energy-consuming transport of the substrates into the cells.

VII. Physiological Role of PQQ in Mammals

One of the most interesting questions is whether PQQ represents a newly discovered vitamin. As noted, several mammalian enzymes contain quinoproteins, and PQQ itself has been detected in some naturally occurring mammalian preparations. Pyrroloquinoline quinone has also been found in human serum, urine, cerebrospinal fluid (Paz *et al.*, 1988), and adrenal tissue (Killgore *et al.*, 1989). Thus, there is an increasing body of evidence to show that PQQ and quinoproteins function in mammalian tissues.

A. Function of PQQ in Connective Tissue Formation

The discovery that lysyl oxidase contains PQQ as the prosthetic group (van der Meer and Duine, 1986; Williamson *et al.*, 1986) generated a great deal of interest in the function of PQQ in connective tissue. Lysyl oxidase is involved in the formation of covalently cross-linked collagen bridges through catalysis of semialdehyde formation produced by the enzyme reaction, and thus PQQ is predicted to be critical for connective tissue formation. More recently, Killgore *et al.* (1989) reported that PQQ deprivation in the diet causes decreased levels of lysyl oxidase in mice, leading to lathyrism, poor growth, and impaired reproduction. Indeed, skin friability was the most striking feature in mice fed PQQ-deficient diets. This was chemically confirmed by finding abnormally increased collagen extractability from skin.

In addition to its role in lysyl oxidase function, PQQ and its structurally related compounds, 3,4-dihydroxyphenylacetate and 3,4-dihydroxymandelate, both generating from dopamine and noradrenaline, respectively (Hanauske-Abel *et al.*, 1987; Gunzler *et al.*, 1988), inhibit prolyl hydroxylase. Prolyl hydroxylase intracellularly catalyzes the formation of peptidyl hydroxyproline which makes stable triple-helical collagen. The hydroxylated collagen helix is then secreted to the extracellular compartment and is converted to stable matrix collagen by the action of lysyl oxidase. Thus, the catabolic products of amines may act as catalytic inhibitors of prolyl hydroxylase and as biosynthetic inhibitors of lysyl oxidase.

Although it is not easy to understand why PQQ is an inhibitor for prolyl hydroxylase yet in spite of being the prosthetic group of lysyl oxidase, it is reasonable to conclude that PQQ has an indispensable role for the formation of stable collagen matrix and thus connective tissue.

B. FUNCTION OF PQQ IN THE CRYSTALLINE LENS

Pyrroloquinoline quinone has been found to have a repressive effect on formation of lens cataracts. Hydrocortisone-induced cataract in chicken embryos was clearly repressed by administration of PQQ (Nishigori *et al.*, 1989; Katsumata *et al.*, 1988). It is postulated that these cataracts are induced by the accumulation of quinoid or polyol substances, such as dopaquinone or sorbitol, produced by tyrosinase or aldose reductase, respectively. Both of these enzymes are inhibitable by PQQ, with K_i values of 0.7 mM (for tyrosinase) and for aldose reductase, 0.3–5 μM (Katsumata *et al.*, 1988).

Thus, it is obvious that PQQ may have an important role on metabolism in the crystalline lens although investigations in this area are still evolving.

C. PQQ AS A RADICAL SCAVENGER

There are at least two reports on PQQ as a radical scavenger in mammals. Matsumoto *et al.* (1988) have reported that exogenous administration of PQQ markedly reduced mortality rate and improved hematological parameters during endotoxin shock induced with an *E.*

coli toxin in rats. Since endotoxin is known to generate superoxide anion by causing membrane damage and disseminated intravenous coagulopathy, they have speculated that PQQ acts as a radical scavenger to reduce the mortality rate of rats. More directly, Hamagishi *et al.* (1989) have shown that PQQ is able to repress the generation of superoxide anion intraperitoneally induced by the administration of carrageenan in mice, or by the enzyme reaction with xanthine oxidase.

Thus, it is possible that PQQ functions as a radical scavenger to remove the harmful superoxide anion in mammalian tissues.

D. Other Possible Functions of PQQ in Mammalian Systems

As noted, information is accumulating to suggest that PQQ is a vitamin in mammalian as well as bacterial systems. Although direct evidence is not available, other important functions for PQQ in systems could be posed: (1) Since PQQ is a prosthetic group of some enzymes for metabolism of amines (Duine and Jongejan, 1989, and Vol. 45 in this series) and is found in cerebrospinal fluid (Paz *et al.*, 1988), it has significance in neurological disorders; and (2) Since PQQ is detected in egg yolk and milk at relatively high levels (Paz *et al.*, 1988; Killgore *et al.*, 1989), it may be a vital nutrient for developing embryos and for newborn mammals. Thus, studies on PQQ in mammals may be leading to the establishment of PQQ as a vitamin, as well as to better understanding of PQQ in physiology and pathophysiology.

REFERENCES

Adachi, O., and Yamada, H. (1969). Amine oxidase of microorganisms (Part VII). An improved purification procedure and further properties of amine oxidase of *Aspergillus niger*. *Agric. Biol. Chem.* **33,** 1707–1716.

Adachi, O., and Yamada, H. (1970). Amine oxidase of microorganisms (Part VIII). Purification and properties of amine oxidase of *Fusarium culmorum*. *Mem. Res. Inst. Food Sci. Kyoto Univ.* **31,** 10–18.

Adachi, O., Tayama, K., Shinagawa, E., Matsushita, K., and Ameyama, M. (1978a). Purification and characterization of particulate alcohol dehydrogenase from *Gluconobacter suboxydans*. *Agric. Biol. Chem.* **42,** 2045–2056.

Adachi, O., Miyagawa, E., Shinagawa, E., Matsushita, K., and Ameyama, M. (1978b). Purification and properties of particulate alcohol dehydrogenase from *Acetobacter aceti*. *Agric. Biol. Chem.* **42,** 2332–2340.

Adachi, O., Tayama, K., Shinagawa, E., Matsushita, K., and Ameyama, M. (1980). Purification and characterization of membrane-bound aldehyde dehydrogenase from *Gluconobacter suboxydans*. *Agric. Biol. Chem.* **44,** 503–515.

Adachi, O., Shinagawa, E., Matsushita, K., and Ameyama, M. (1982). Crystallization of membrane-bound alcohol dehydrogenase of acetic acid bacteria. *Agric. Biol. Chem.* **46,** 2859–2863.

Adachi, O., Hayashi, M., Shinagawa, E., Matsushita, K., Takimoto, K., and Ameyama, M. (1985). Fermentative production of a novel prosthetic group, pyrroloquinoline quinone (Part III). *Proc. Annu. Meet. Agric. Chem. Soc.* p. 463. (In Jpn.)

Adachi, O., Shinagawa, E., Matsushita, K., Nakashima, K., Takimoto, K., and Ameyama, M. (1988a). Binding of pyrroloquinoline quinone to serum albumin. *In* "PQQ and Quinoproteins" (J. A. Jongejan and J. A. Duine, eds.), pp. 145–147. Kluwer, The Hague.

Adachi, O., Okamoto, K., Shinagawa, E., Matsushita, K., and Ameyama, M. (1988b). Adduct formation of pyrroloquinoline quinone and amino acid. *BioFactors* **1**, 251–254.

Adachi, O., Matsushita, K., Shinagawa, E., and Ameyama, M. (1990). Purification and properties of methanol dehydrogenase and aldehyde dehydrogenase from *Metylobacillus glycogenes*. *Agric. Biol. Chem.* **54**, 3123–3129.

Ameyama, M. (1988a). Growth stimulating effect of pyrroloquinoline quinone for microorganisms. *In* "PQQ and Quinoproteins" (J. A. Jongejan and J. A. Duine, eds.), pp. 149–157. Kluwer, The Hague.

Ameyama, M. (1988b). Biochemistry of acetic acid bacteria. *Nippon Nogeikagaku Kaishi* **62**, 1185–1193. (In Jpn.)

Ameyama, M. (1989). Quinoproteins and oxidative fermentation in acetic acid bacteria. *FEBS Meet., 19th, Abstr. Book* MO 61 L.

Ameyama, M., and Adachi, O. (1982). Alcohol dehydrogenase from acetic acid bacteria, membrane-bound. *Methods Enzymol.* **89**, 450–457.

Ameyama, M., and Kondo, K. (1966). Carbohydrate metabolism by the acetic acid bacteria. Part V. On the vitamin requirement for the growth. *Agric. Biol. Chem.* **30**, 203–211.

Ameyama, M., Matsushita, K., Ohno, Y., Shinagawa, E., and Adachi, O. (1981a). Existence of a novel prosthetic group. PQQ, in membrane-bound electron transport chain-linked, primary dehydrogenases of oxidative bacteria. *FEBS Lett.* **130**, 179–183.

Ameyama, M., Shinagawa, E., Matsushita, K., and Adachi, O. (1981b). D-Glucose dehydrogenase of *Gluconobacter suboxydans*. Purification and characterization. *Agric. Biol. Chem.* **45**, 851–861.

Ameyama, M., Osada, K., Shinagawa, E., Matsushita, K., and Adachi, O. (1981c). Purification and characterization of aldehyde dehydrogenase of *Acetobacter aceti*. *Agric. Biol. Chem.* **45**, 1889–1890.

Ameyama, M., Hayashi, M., Matsushita, K., Shinagawa, E., and Adachi, O. (1984a). Microbial production of pyrroloquinoline quinone. *Agric. Biol. Chem.* **48**, 561–565.

Ameyama, M., Shinagawa, E., Matsushita, K., and Adachi, O. (1984b). Growth stimulation of microorganisms by pyrroloquinoline quinone. *Agric. Biol. Chem.* **48**, 2909–2911.

Ameyama, M., Shinagawa, E., Matsushita, K., and Adachi, O. (1984c). Growth stimulating substance for microorganisms produced by *Escherichia coli* causing the reduction of the lag phase in microbial growth and identity of the substance with pyrroloquinoline quinone. *Agric. Biol. Chem.* **48**, 3099–3107.

Ameyama, M., Shinagawa, E., Matsushita, K., and Adachi, O. (1985a). Growth stimulating activity for microorganisms in naturally occurring substances and partial characterization of the substance for the activity as pyrroloquinoline quinone. *Agric. Biol. Chem.* **49**, 699–709.

Ameyama, M., Shinagawa, E., Matsushita, K., and Adachi, O. (1985b). How many times should the inoculum be rinsed before inoculation in the assay for growth stimulating activity of pyrroloquinoline quinone? *Agric. Biol. Chem.* **49**, 853–854.

Ameyama, M., Shinagawa, E., Matsushita, K., and Adachi, O. (1985c). Solubilization, purification and properties of membrane-bound glycerol dehydrogenase from *Gluconobacter industrious. Agric. Biol. Chem.* **49**, 1001–1010.

Ameyama, M., Nonobe, M., Hayashi, M., Shinagawa, E., Matsushita, K., and Adachi, O. (1985d). Mode of binding of pyrroloquinoline quinone to apo-glucose dehydrogenase. *Agric. Biol. Chem.* **49**, 1227–1231.

Ameyama, M., Nonobe, M., Shinagawa, E., Matsushita, K., and Adachi, O. (1985e). Methods of enzymatic determination of pyrroloquinoline quinone. *Anal. Biochem.* **151**, 263–267.

Ameyama, M., Shinagawa, E., Matsushita, K., Takimoto, K., Nakashima, K., and Adachi, O. (1985f). Mammalian choline dehydrogenase is a quinoprotein. *Agric. Biol. Chem.* **49**, 3623–3626.

Ameyama, M., Nonobe, M., Shinagawa, E., Matsushita, K., Takimoto, K., and Adachi, O. (1986). Purification and characterization of the quinoprotein D-glucose dehydrogenase apoenzyme from *Escherichia coli. Agric. Biol. Chem.* **50**, 49–57.

Ameyama, M., Matsushita, K., Shinagawa, E., and Adachi, O. (1988). Pyrroloquinoline quinone: excretion by methylotrophs and growth stimulation for microorganisms. *BioFactors* **1**, 51–53.

Anderson, D. J., and Lidstrom, M. E. (1988). The *mox*FG region encodes four polypeptides in the methanol-oxidizing bacterium *Methylobacterium* sp. strain AM1. *J. Bacteriol.* **170**, 2254–2262.

Anthony, C. (1982). "The Biochemistry of Methylotrophs," pp. 167–218. Academic Press, New York.

Anthony, C. (1988). Quinoproteins and energy transduction. *In* "Bacterial Energy Transduction" (C. Anthony, ed.), pp. 293–316. Academic Press, San Diego, California.

Auton, K. A., and Anthony, C. (1989). The 'methylamine oxidase' system of an obligate methylotroph. *Biochem. J.* **260**, 75–79.

Beardmore-Gray, M., and Anthony, C. (1986). The oxidation of glucose by *Acinetobacter calcoaceticus:* Interaction of the quinoprotein glucose dehydrogenase with the electron transport chain. *J. Gen. Microbiol.* **132**, 1257–1268.

Cleton-Jansen, A.-M., Goosen, N., Wenzel, T. J., and van de Putte, P. (1988a). Cloning of the gene encoding quinoprotein glucose dehydrogenase from *Acinetobacter calcoaceticus:* Evidence for the presence of a second enzyme. *J. Bacteriol* **170**, 2121–2125.

Cleton-Jansen, A.-M., Goosen, N., Vink, K., and van de Putte, P. (1988b). Cloning of the genes encoding the two different glucose dehydrogenases from *Acinetobacter calcoaceticus. In* "PQQ and Quinoproteins" (J. A. Jongejan and J. A. Duine, eds.), pp. 79–85. Kluwer, The Hague.

Corey, E. J., and Tramontano, A. (1981). Total synthesis of the quinonoid alcohol dehydrogenase coenzyme of methylotrophic bacteria. *J. Am. Chem. Soc.* **103**, 5599–5600.

Dempsey, W. B., and Christensen, H. N. (1962). The specific binding of pyridoxal 5'-phosphate to bovine serum albumin. *J. Biol. Chem.* **237**, 1113–1120.

Dijkstra, M., Frank, J., van Wielink, J. E., and Duine, J. A. (1988a). The soluble cytochrome *c* of methanol-grown *Hyphomicrobium* X. *Biochem. J.* **251**, 467–474.

Dijkstra, M., Frank, J., and Duine, J. A. (1988b). Methanol oxidation under physiological conditions using methanol dehydrogenase and a factor isolated from *Hyphomicrobium* X. *FEBS Lett.* **227**, 198–202.

Dijkstra, M., Frank, J., and Duine, J. A. (1989). Studies on electron transfer from methanol dehydrogenase to cytochrome c_L, both purified from *Hyphomicrobium* X. *Biochem. J.* **257**, 87–94.

Dokter, P., Frank, J., and Duine, J. A. (1986). Purification and characterization of quinoprotein glucose dehydrogenase from *Acinetobacter calcoaceticus* L.M.D. 79.41. *Biochem. J.* **239**, 163–167.

Dokter, P., Pronk, J. T., van Schie, B. J., van Dijken, J. P., and Duine, J. A. (1987). The *in vivo* and *in vitro* substrate specificity of quinoprotein glucose dehydrogenase of *Acinetobacter calcoaceticus* LMD 79.41. *FEMS Microbiol. Lett.* **43**, 195–200.

Dokter, P., van Wielink, J. E., van Kleef, M. A. G., and Duine, J. A. (1988). Cytochrome *b*-562 from *Acinetobacter calcoaceticus* L.M.D. 79.41. *Biochem. J.* **254**, 131–138.

Duine, J. A. (1989). Quinoproteins, a novel class of enzymes. *FEBS Meet., 19th, Abstr. Book* MO 56 L.

Duine, J. A., and Jongejan, J. A. (1989). Quinoproteins, enzymes with pyrroloquinoline quinone as cofactor. *Annu. Rev. Biochem.* **58**, 403–426.

Duine, J. A., Frank, J., and Westerling, J. (1978). Purification and properties of methanol dehydrogenase from *Hyphomicrobium* X. *Biochim. Biophys. Acta* **524**, 277–287.

Duine, J. A., Frank, J., and van Zeeland, J. K. (1979a). Glucose dehydrogenase from *Acinetobacter calcoaceticus*. A "quinoprotein." *FEBS Lett.* **108**, 443–446.

Duine, J. A., Frank, J., and de Ruiter, L. G. (1979b). Isolation of a methanol dehydrogenase with a functional coupling to cytochrome *c*. *J. Gen. Microbiol.* **115**, 523–526.

Duine, J. A., Frank, J., and Verwiel, P. E. J. (1980). Structure and activity of the prosthetic group of methanol dehydrogenase. *Eur. J. Biochem.* **108**, 187–192.

Duine, J. A., Frank, J., and Verwiel, P. E. J. (1981). Characterization of the second prosthetic group in methanol dehydrogenase from *Hyphomicrobium* X. *Eur. J. Biochem.* **118**, 395–399.

Duine, J. A., Frank, J., and Jongejan, J. A. (1983). Detection and determination of pyrroloquinoline quinone, the coenzyme of quinoproteins. *Anal. Biochem.* **133**, 239–243.

Duine, J. A., Frank, J., and Jongejan, J. A. (1986). Pyrroloquinoline quinone and quinoprotein enzymes in microbial oxidations. *FEMS Microbiol. Rev.* **32**, 165–178.

Duine, J. A., Frank, J., and Jongejan, J. A. (1987). Enzymology of quinoproteins. *Adv. Enzymol.* **59**, 169–212.

Elliott, E. J., and Anthony, C. (1988). The interaction between methanol dehydrogenase and cytochrome *c* in the acidophilic methylotroph *Acetobacter methanolicus. J. Gen. Microbiol.* **134**, 369–377.

Froud, S. J., and Anthony, C. (1984). The purification and characterization of the *o*-type cytochrome oxidase from *Methylophilus methylotrophus*, and its reconstitution into a 'methanol oxidase' electron transport chain. *J. Gen. Microbiol.* **130**, 2201–2212.

Fukumori, Y., and Yamanaka, T. (1987). The methylamine oxidizing system of *Pseudomonas* AM1 reconstituted from purified components. *J. Biochem. (Tokyo)* **101**, 441–445.

Geiger, O., and Gorisch, H. (1986). Crystalline quinoprotein glucose dehydrogenase from *Acinetobacter calcoaceticus*. *Biochemistry* **25**, 6043–6048.

Geiger, O., and Gorisch, H. (1987). Enzymatic determination of pyrroloquinoline quinone using crude membranes from *Escherichia coli*. *Anal. Biochem.* **164**, 418–423.

Geiger, O., and Gorisch, H. (1989). Reversible thermal inactivation of the quinoprotein glucose dehydrogenase from *Acinetobacter calcoaceticus*. *Biochem. J.* **261**, 415–421.

Glatz, Z., Kovar, J., Macholan, L., and Pec, P. (1987). Pea (Pisumsativum) diamine oxidase contains pyrroloquinoline quinone as a cofactor. *Biochem. J.* **242**, 603–606.

Gorisch, H., and Rupp, M. (1988). Quinoprotein ethanol dehydrogenase from *Pseudomonas*. In "PQQ and Quinoproteins" (J. A. Jongejan and J. A. Duine, eds.), pp. 23–33. Kluwer, The Hague.

Gray, K. A., Davidson, V. L., and Knaff, D. B. (1988). Complex formation between methylamine dehydrogenase and amicyanin from *Paracoccus denitrificans*. *J. Biol. Chem.* **263**, 13987–13990.

Groen, B. W., Frank, J., and Duine, J. A. (1984). Quinoprotein alcohol dehydrogenase from ethanol-grown *Pseudomonas aeruginosa*. *Biochem. J.* **223**, 921–924.

Groen, B. W., van Kleef, D. A. M., and Duine, J. A. (1986). Quinoprotein alcohol dehydrogenase apoenzyme from *Pseudomonas testosteroni*. *Biochem. J.* **234**, 611–615.

Gunzler, V., Hanauske-Abel, H. M., Duine, J. A., Kivirikko, K. I., and Corey, E. J. (1988). Inhibition of collagen hydroxylases by PQQ reveals its domain structure. In "PQQ and Quinoproteins" (J. A. Jongejan and J. A. Duine, eds.), pp. 227–232. Kluwer, The Hague.

Hamagishi, Y., Murata, S., Kamei, H., Oki, T., and Ameyama, M. (1989). Novel pharmacological activity of a novel cofactor PQQ. Radical scavenger-like activity. *Abstr. Annu. Meet. Jpn. Pharmacol. Soc., 109th* p. 42.

Hanauske-Abel, H. M., Tschank, G., Gunzler, V., Baader, E., and Gallop, P. (1987). Pyrroloquinole quinone and molecules mimicking its functional domains. Modulators of connective tissue formation? *FEBS Lett.* **214**, 236–243.

Hartmann, C., and Klinman, J. P. (1987). Reductive trapping of substrate to bovine amine oxidase. *J. Biol. Chem.* **262**, 962–965.

Hauge, J. G. (1959). Purification and properties of a bacterial glucose dehydrogenase. *Acta Chem. Scand.* **13**, 2125.

Hauge, J. G. (1960). Purification and properties of glucose dehydrogenase and cytochrome *b* from *Bacterium anitratum*. *Biochim. Biophys. Acta* **45**, 250–262.

Hauge, J. G. (1961). Mode of action of glucose dehydrogenase from *Bacterium anitratum*. *Arch. Biochem. Biophys.* **94**, 308–318.

Hauge, J. G. (1964). Glucose dehydrogenase of *Bacterium anitratum*: an enzyme with a novel prosthetic group. *J. Biol. Chem.* **239**, 3630–3639.

Hauge, J. G., and Hallberg, P. A. (1964). Solubilization and properties of the structurally-bound glucose dehydrogenase of *Bacterium anitratum*. *Biochim. Biophys. Acta* **81**, 251–256.

Homes, R. J. W., Postma, P. W., Neijssel, O. M., Tempest, D. W., Dokter, P., and Duine, J. A. (1984). Evidence of a quinoprotein glucose dehydrogenase apoenzyme in several strains of *Escherichia coli*. *FEMS Microbiol. Lett.* **24**, 329–333.

Imanaga, Y., Hirano-Sawatake, Y., Arita-Hashimoto, Y., Itou-Shibouta, Y., and Katoh-Semba, R. (1979). On the cofactor of glucose dehydrogenase of *Pseudomonas fluorescens*. *Proc. Jpn. Acad.* **55**, 264–269.

Inoue, T., Sunagawa, M., Mori, A., Imai, C., Fukuda, M., Takagi, M., and Yano, K. (1989). Cloning and sequencing of the gene encoding the 72-kilodalton dehydrogenase subunit of alcohol dehydrogenase from *Acetobacter aceti*. *J. Bacteriol.* **171**, 3115–3122.

Ishii, Y., Hase, T., Fukumori, Y., Matsubara, H., and Tobari, J. (1983). Amino acid sequence studies of the light subunit of methylamine dehydrogenase from *Pseudomonas* AM1: existence of two residues binding the prosthetic group. *J. Biochem. (Tokyo)* **93**, 107–119.

Itoh, S., Kato, N., Ohshiro, Y., and Agawa, T. (1984). Oxidative decarboxylation of α-amino acids with coenzyme PQQ. *Tetrahedron Lett.* **25**, 4753–4756.

Iwaki, M., Yagi, T., Horiike, K., Saeki, Y., Ushijima, T., and Nozaki, M. (1983). Crystallization and properties of aromatic amine dehydrogenase from *Pseudomonas* sp. *Arch. Biochem. Biophys.* **220**, 253–262.

Katsumata, M., Ohsawa, Y., Nakagiri, C., and Nakano, S. (1988). Anti-cataract agent. *Jpn. Pat.* 63-41421.

Kawai, F., Kimura, T., Tani, Y., Yamada, H., and Kurachi, M. (1980). Purification and characterization of polyethylene glycol dehydrogenase involved in the bacterial metabolism of polyethylene glycol. *Appl. Environ. Microbiol.* **40**, 701–705.

Kawai, F., Yamanaka, H., Ameyama, M., Shinagawa, E., Matsushita, K., and Adachi, O. (1985). Identification of the prosthetic group and further characterization of a novel enzyme, polyethylene glycol dehydrogenase. *Agric. Biol. Chem.* **49**, 1071–1076.

Killgore, J., Smidt, C., Duich, L., Romero-Chapman, N., Tinker, D., Reiser, K., Melko, M., Hyde, D., and Rucker, R. B. (1989). Nutritional importance of pyrroloquinoline quinone. *Science* **245**, 850–852.

Lawton, S. A., and Anthony, C. (1985). The role of blue copper proteins in the oxidation of methylamine by an obligate methylotroph. *Biochem. J.* **228**, 719–725.

Lobenstein-Verbeek, C. L., Jongejan, J. A., Frank, J., and Duine, J. A. (1984). Bovine serum amine oxidase: A mammalian enzyme having covalently-bound PQQ as prosthetic group. *FEBS Lett.* **170**, 305–309.

Loffhagen, N., and Babel, W. (1984). Localization of primary alcohol-oxidizing enzymes in the facultative methylotrophic *Acetobacter* sp. MG 70. *A. Allg. Mikrobiol.* **24**, 143–149.

Matsumoto, T., Suzuki, O., Hayakawa, H., Ogiso, S., Hayakawa, N., Nimura, Y., Takahashi, I., and Shionoya, S. (1988). Effects of exogenous PQQ on mortality rate and some biochemical parameters during endotoxin shock in rats. *In* "PQQ and Quinoproteins" (J. A. Jongejan and J. A. Duine, eds.), pp. 162–164. Kluwer, The Hague.

Matsushita, K., Ohno, Y., Shinagawa, E., Adachi, O., and Ameyama, M. (1980). Membrane-bound D-glucose dehydrogenase from *Pseudomonas* sp.: solubilization, purification and characterization. *Agric. Biol. Chem.* **44**, 1505–1512.

Matsushita, K., Ohno, Y., Shinagawa, E., Adachi, O., and Ameyama, M. (1982). Membrane-bound, electron transport-linked, D-glucose dehydrogenase of *Pseudomonas fluorescens*. Interaction of the purified enzyme with ubiquinone or phospholipid. *Agric. Biol. Chem.* **46**, 1007–1011.

Matsushita, K., Shinagawa, E., Inoue, T., Adachi, O., and Ameyama, M. (1986). Immunological evidence for two types of PQQ-dependent D-glucose dehydrogenase in bacterial membranes and the location of the enzyme in *Escherichia coli*. *FEMS Microbiol. Lett.* **37**, 141–144.

Matsushita, K., Nonobe, M., Shinagawa, E., Adachi, O., and Ameyama, M. (1987a). Reconstitution of pyrroloquinoline quinone-dependent D-glucose oxidase respiratory chain of *Escherichia coli* with cytochrome *o* oxidase. *J. Bacteriol.* **169**, 205–209.

Matsushita, K., Shinagawa, E., Adachi, O., and Ameyama, M. (1987b). Purification, characterization and reconstitution of cytochrome *o*-type oxidase from *Gluconobacter suboxydans*. *Biochim. Biophys. Acta* **894**, 304–312.

Matsushita, K., Shinagawa, E., Adachi, O., and Ameyama, M. (1988). Quinoprotein D-glucose dehydrogenase in *Acinetobacter calcoaceticus* LMD 79.41: the membrane-bound enzyme is distinct from the soluble enzyme. *FEMS Microbiol. Lett.* **55**, 53–58.

Matsushita, K., Shinagawa, E., Adachi, O., and Ameyama, M. (1989a). Reactivity with ubiquinone of quinoprotein D-glucose dehydrogenase from *Gluconobacter suboxydans*. *J. Biochem. (Tokyo)* **105**, 633–637.

Matsushita, K., Shinagawa, E., Adachi, O., and Ameyama, M. (1989b). Quinoprotein D-glucose dehydrogenase of the *Acinetobacter calcoaceticus* respiratory chain: membrane-bound and soluble forms are different molecular species. *Biochemistry* **28**, 6276–6280.

Midgley, M., and Dawes, E. A. (1973). The regulation of transport of glucose and methyl α-glucoside in *Pseudomonas aeruginosa*. *Biochem. J.* **132**, 141–154.

Miyazaki, S. S., Yoki, S., Izumi, Y., and Yamada, H. (1987). Purification and characterization of methanol dehydrogenase of a serine-producing methylotroph, *Hyphomicrobium methylovorum*. *J. Ferment. Technol.* **65**, 371–377.

Nagamune, T., Endoh, I., Kurata, H., Hirata, M., Iijima, M., Hirata, A., Smeds, A. L., and Sudoh, M. (1988). Studies on photoactivating enzymes. Purification and properties of nitrile hydratase from *Corynebacterium* sp. N-771. *Proc. Annu. Meet. Agric. Chem. Soc.* **62**, 129.

Nagasawa, T., and Yamada, H. (1987). Nitrile hydratase is a quinoprotein. A possible new function of pyrroloquinole quinone : activation of H₂O in an enzymatic hydration reaction. *Biochem. Biophys. Res. Commun.* **147**, 701–709.

Nishigori, H., Yasunaga, M., and Iwatsuru, M. (1989). Effect of PQQ on corticoid-induced cataract and hepatic metabolism in chicken embryo. *Abstr. Annu. Meet. Jpn. Phamacol. Soc., 109th* p. 5.

Nunn, D. N., Day, D., and Anthony, D. (1989). The second subunit of methanol dehydrogenase of *Methylobacterium extorquens* AM1. *Biochem. J.* **260**, 857–862.

O'Keeffe, D. T., and Anthony, C. (1980). The interaction between methanol dehydrogenase and the autoreducible cytochromes *c* of the facultative methylotroph *Pseudomonas* AM1. *Biochem. J.* **190**, 481–484.

Paz, M. A., Fluckinger, R., Henson, E., and Gallop, P. M. (1988). Direct and amplified redox-cycling measurements of PQQ in quinoproteins and biological fluids: PPQ-peptides in pronase digests of DBH and DAO. *In* "PQQ and Quinoproteins" (J. A. Jongejan and J. A. Duine, eds.), pp. 131–143. Kluwer, The Hague.

Salisbury, S. A., Forrest, H. S., Cruse, W. B. T., and Kennard, O. (1979). A novel coenzyme from bacterial primary alcohol dehydrogenase. *Nature (London)* **280**, 843–844.

Shimao, M., Yamamoto, H., Ninomiya, K., Kato, N., Adachi, O., Ameyama, M., and Sakazawa, C. (1984). Pyrroloquinoline quinone as an essential growth factor for a poly (vinyl alcohol)-degrading symbiont, *Pseudomonas* sp. VM15C. *Agric. Biol. Chem.* **48**, 2873–2873.

Shimao, M., Ninomiya, K., Kuno, O., Kato, N., and Sakazawa, C. (1986). Existence of a novel enzyme, pyrroloquinoline quinone dependent polyvinyl alcohol dehydrogenase, in a bacterial symbiont, *Pseudomonas* sp. strain VM15C. *Appl. Environ. Microbiol.* **51**, 268–275.

Shimao, M., Onishi, S., Kato, N., and Sakazawa, C. (1989). Pyrroloquinoline quinone-dependent cytochrome reduction in polyvinyl alcohol-degrading *Pseudomonas* sp. strain VM15C. *Appl. Environ. Microbiol.* **55**, 275–278.

Shinagawa, E., Matsushita, K., Nonobe, M., Adachi, O., Ameyama, M., Ohshiro, Y., Itoh, S., and Kitamura, Y. (1986). The 9-carboxyl group of pyrroloquinoline quinone, a novel prosthetic group, is essential in the formation of holoenzyme of D-glucose dehydrogenase. *Biochem. Biophys. Res. Commun.* **139**, 1279–1284.

Shinagawa, E., Matsushita, K., Nakashima, K., Adachi, O., and Ameyama, M. (1988). Crystallization and properties of amine dehydrogenase from *Pseudomonas* sp. *Agric. Biol. Chem.* **52**, 2255–2263.

Tani, Y., Kurihara, M., and Nishise, H. (1989). Characterization of nitrile hydratase and amidase, which are responsible for the conversion of dinitriles to monotriles. *Agric. Biol. Chem.* **53**, 3151–3158.

Tanizawa, K., Moriya, T., Kido, T., Tanaka, H., and Soda, K. (1988). Structural studies on the PQQ-like cofactor of nitroalkane oxidase from *Fusarium oxysporum. In* "PQQ and Quinoproteins" (J. A. Jongejan and J. A. Duine, eds.), pp. 43–45. Kluwer, The Hague.

Urakami, T. (1986). Production of pyrroloquinoline quinone. *Jpn. Pat.* 61-247397.

Urakami, T. (1987). Production of pyrroloquinoline quinone. *Jpn. Pat.* 62-19094.

Urakami, T., Yashima, K., Yoshida, A., and Itoh, C. (1988). Fermentative production of pyrroloquinoline quinone by a methylotrophic bacteria. *Proc. Annu. Meet. Agric. Chem. Soc.* **62**, 304.

van der Meer, R. A., and Duine, J. A. (1986). Covalently-bound pyrroloquinoline quinone is the organic prosthetic group in human placental lysyl oxidase. *Biochem. J.* **239**, 789–791.

van der Meer, R. A., and Duine, J. A. (1988). Pyrroloquinoline quinone (PQQ) is the organic cofactor in soybean lipoxygenase-1. *FEBS Lett.* **235**, 194–200.

van der Meer, R. A., Jongejan, J. A., Frank, J., and Duine, J. A. (1986). Hydrazone formation of 2,4-dinitrophenylhydrazine with pyrroloquinoline quinone in porcine kidney diamine oxidase. *FEBS Lett.* **206**, 111–114.

van Iersel, J., van der Meer, R. A., and Duine, J. A. (1986). Methylamine oxidase from *Arthtrobacter* P1: a bacterial copper-quinoprotein amine oxidase. *Eur. J. Biochem.* **161**, 415–419.

van Kleef, M. A. G., Jongejan, J. A., and Duine, J. A. (1988). Factors relevant in the reaction of PQQ with amino acids. Analytical and mechanistic implications. *In* "PQQ and Quinoproteins" (J. A. Jongejan and J. A. Duine, eds.), pp. 217–226. Kluwer, The Hague.

van Wielink, J. E., Frank, J., and Duine, J. A. (1988). Electron transport from methylamine to oxygen in the Gram-negative bacterium *Thiobacillus versutus. In* "PQQ and Quinoproteins" (J. A. Jongejan and J. A. Duine, eds.), pp. 269–278. Kluwer, The Hague.

Williamson, P. R., Moog, R. S., Dooley, D. M., and Kagan, H. R. (1986). Evidence for pyrroloquinoline quinone as the carbonyl cofactor in lysyl oxidase by absorption and resonance raman spectroscopy. *J. Biol. Chem.* **261**, 16302–16305.

Yamanaka, K. (1988). New PQQ-enzyme: aromatic alcohol and aldehyde dehydrogenase in *Rhodopseudomonas acidophila* M402. *In* "PQQ and Quinoproteins" (J. A. Jongejan and J. A. Duine, eds.), pp. 40–42. Kluwer, The Hague.

Yamanaka, K., and Matsumoto, K. (1977). Purification, crystallization and properties of primary alcohol dehydrogenase from methanol-oxidizing *Pseudomonas* sp. No. 2941. *Agric. Biol. Chem.* **41**, 467–475.

Yamanaka, K., and Tsuyuki, Y. (1983). A new dye-linked alcohol dehydrogenase (vanillyl alcohol dehydrogenase) from *Rhodopseudomonas acidophila* M402. Purification, identification of reaction product and substrate specificity. *Agric. Biol. Chem.* **47**, 2173–2183.

Index

A

Absorption, intestinal, pantothenic acid, 174–176

Acetazolamide, effects on bone resorption, 44–47

Acetic acid bacteria
alcohol dehydrogenase
electron acceptor for, 259
functions, 250
aldehyde dehydrogenase, 252
growth stimulating substance (yeast extract), 236–237
vitamin requirements for, 237

Acetobacter
A. aceti, growth stimulating substance in, 238
A. methanolicus, methanol and alcohol oxidase systems, 260
alcohol dehydrogenase coupling to respiratory chain, 259
fractions with growth-stimulating activity, 238
vitamin requirements, 237

Acetyl CoA, regulation of CoA synthesis, 191, 207

Acidification, extracellular hemivacuole by osteoclasts, 48–49

Acinetobacter calcoaceticus
electron acceptor for glucose dehydrogenase, 253–254
gdh genes, 246–247
glucose dehydrogenase, 246–248

ACP (*see* Acyl carrier proteins)

Acyl carrier proteins
alpha helices, 211
from bacteria, birds, mammals, and plants, 210–211
and CoA, precursor—product relationship, 212
4'-phosphopantetheine prosthetic group, 210–211

prosthetic group turnover, nutritional status effects, 214

protein complexes containing, 214–215

Adenine nucleotide translocation, effects of CoA long-chain acyl esters, 209

Adhesion, osteoclasts to bone surfaces, 42–44

Adhesion receptors, on human osteoclasts, 42–43

Adhesion systems, for osteoclast migration, 63

Adipocytes, pantothenic acid transport in, 178

Adrenal glands, CoA concentrations, 195

β-Adrenergic receptor kinase, phosphorylation of G protein-coupled receptors, 15, 18–21

Adrenergic receptors
chimeric α_2—β_2, cytoplasmic loop coupling to G proteins, 15
conserved amino acids, 3
proline residue in transmembrane spanning domain II, 3, 8

α_2-Adrenergic receptors, phosphorylation by protein kinase C, 15

β_2-Adrenergic receptors
Asp-113 in, 3
cAMP response element identification, 29–31
cytoplasmic loops
amino acids after deletion/substitution mutations, 16
regions coupling to G proteins, 15–16
size of, 3
deletion mutants, coupling to G proteins, 16
densensitization, 17–23
disulfide bond formation in, 14
gene expression, posttranscriptional mechanisms affecting, 26–28